DRUGS FOR THE RESPIRATORY SYSTEM

Edited by

Reuben M. Cherniack, M.D.
*Professor of Medicine
Department of Medicine
National Jewish Center for Immunology
   and Respiratory Medicine
University of Colorado
Denver, Colorado*

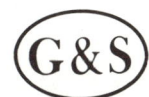

Grune & Stratton, Inc.
Harcourt Brace Jovanovich, Publishers
Orlando   New York   San Diego   Boston   London
San Francisco   Tokyo   Sydney   Toronto

© 1986 by Grune & Stratton, Inc.

All rights reserved. No part of this publication
may be reproduced or transmitted in any form or
by any means, electronic or mechanical, including
photocopy, recording, or any information storage
and retrieval system, without permission in
writing from the publisher.

Grune & Stratton, Inc.
Orlando, Florida 32887

Distributed in the United Kingdom by
Grune & Stratton, Ltd.
24/28 Oval Road, London NW 1

Library of Congress Catalog Number 86-080740
International Standard Book Number 0-8089-1818-4
Printed in the United States of America
86 87 88 89   10 9 8 7 6 5 4 3 2 1

Contents

    Preface   v

    Contributors   vii

1. **β_2 Agonists**
   Enrique Fernandez and Reuben M. Cherniack   1

2. **Theophylline and Methylxanthine Derivatives**   21
   Stanley J. Szefler

3. **Cromolyn Sodium and Other Mast-Cell-Stablizers**
   Lynn M. Marshall   43

4. **Anticholinergic, Antimuscarinic Drugs (Atropine Sulfate, Ipratropium Bromide)**
   Robert A. Bethel and Charles G. Irvin   61

5. **Corticosteroids**
   Shih-Wen Chang and Talmadge E. King   77

6. **Cytotoxic Drugs for Nonneoplastic Disorders of the Respiratory System**
   Leslie C. Watters   139

7. **Drug Therapy in the Management of Cough**
   Gary R. Cott   165

8. **Respiratory Stimulants**
   Richard J. Martin and Robert D. Ballard   191

9. **Pulmonary Vasodilators**
   G.S. Worthen   213

10. **Newer Agents**
    Robert A. Sandhaus   227

    Index   237

Preface

Pulmonary disease and particularly chronic respiratory disease is increasing in prevalence at a rapid rate, but only a few truly new drugs are available for the therapeutic armamentarium. Most new agents are modifications of older drugs, with emphasis on more prolonged action and fewer side effects. In most of the respiratory diseases, the pathogenesis remains cloudy. Many of the drugs are still directed at reducing symptoms and/or preventing progression of disease; none are curative.

The book essentially emanates from the members of the Respiratory Division of the Department of Medicine at the National Jewish Center for Immunology and Respiratory Medicine. We have attempted to discuss the different groups of medications currently utilized in the management of respiratory disorders: beta agonists, theophylline, mast-cell stabilzers, corticosteroids, cytotoxic agents, cough medications, respiratory stimulants, pulmonary vasodilators, and newer agents that are still under investigation. While respiratory infection often plays a major role in acute disability associated with pulmonary disease, antibiotics have been omitted deliberately, as it was felt they would constitute another text.

In each chapter we discuss what is known and what is not known about the mechanisms of action of these agents, critically evaluate clinical results and present the indications for their use, the contraindications, recommended dosage and side effects, as well as their interaction with other drugs. We hope an understanding of the mechanism of action of each of the agents described in this book will lead to an improved understanding of their use and appropriate prescription in order to induce improvement and prevent side effects, as well as obviate the deleterious effects that develop as a result of interaction with other drugs. We have provided a moderately extensive bibliography to allow the reader to access more detailed information if so desired.

I wish to thank Mary Peterson for her extensive efforts in collecting and coordinating the manuscripts and the secretaries of the contributors to this book: Helga Cole, Sue Hirsch, Toni Peterson, Kathy Kloss, Wanda Mohatt, Cindi Houk, Catheryne Booker, Marialyce Austin, and Mary Peterson who accepted our suggested revisions graciously and cooperated with deadlines.

Contributors

Robert D. Ballard, M.D.
Pulmonary Fellow, Departments of Medicine, National Jewish Center for Immunology and Respiratory Disease and University of Colorado, Denver, Colorado.

Robert A. Bethel, M.D.
Assistant Professor of Medicine, Departments of Medicine, National Jewish Center for Immunology and Respiratory Medicine and University of Colorado, Denver, Colorado.

Shih-Wen Chang, M.D.
Senior Pulmonary Fellow, Departments of Medicine, National Jewish Center for Immunology and Respiratory Medicine and University of Colorado, Denver, Colorado.

Reuben M. Cherniack, M.D.
Professor of Medicine, Departments of Medicine, National Jewish Center for Immunology and Respiratory Medicine and University of Colorado, Denver, Colorado.

Gary R. Cott, M.D.
Assistant Professor of Medicine, Departments of Medicine, National Jewish Center for Immunology and Respiratory Medicine and University of Colorado, Denver, Colorado.

Enrique Fernandez, M.D.
Associate Professor of Medicine, Departments of Medicine, National Jewish Center for Immunology and Respiratory Medicine and University of Colorado, Denver, Colorado.

Charles G. Irvin, Ph.D.
Assistant Professor of Medicine, Departments of Medicine, National Jewish Center for Immunology and Respiratory Medicine and University of Colorado, Denver, Colorado.

Talmadge E. King, M.D.
Director, Adult Clinical Services, and Clinic, National Jewish Center for Immunology and Respiratory Medicine and Associate Professor of Medicine, University of Colorado, Denver, Colorado.

Lynn M. Marshall, BSN
Adult/Geriatric Nurse Practitioner, Denver, Colorado

Richard J. Martin, M.D.
Associate Professor of Medicine, Departments of Medicine, National Jewish Center for Immunology and Respiratory Medicine and University of Colorado, Denver, Colorado.

Robert Sandhaus, M.D.
Assistant Professor of Medicine, Departments of Medicine, National Jewish Center for Immunology and Respiratory Medicine and University of Colorado, Denver, Colorado.

Stanley J. Szefler, M.D.
Director of Pediatric Clinical Pharmacology, National Jewish Center for Immunology and Respiratory Medicine and Associate Professor of Pediatrics and Pharmacology, University of Colorado, Denver, Colorado.

Leslie C. Watters, M.D.
Associate Professor of Medicine, Departments of Medicine, National Jewish Center for Immunology and Respiratory Medicine and University of Colorado, Denver, Colorado, Veterans Administration Hospital, Denver, Colorado.

G. Scott Worthen, M.D.
Assistant Professor of Medicine, Departments of Medicine, National Jewish Center for Immunology and Respiratory Medicine and University of Colorado, Denver, Colorado.

Enrique Fernandez
Reuben M. Cherniack

1

β_2 Agonists

Sympathomimetic drugs have been utilized since antiquity, the Chinese having used Ma Huang (derived from the plant Ephedra equisetina), for more than 5,000 years. Tablets of the dessicated adrenal gland were first prescribed for the treatment of asthma in 1900.[1] Takamine[2] isolated a benzoyl derivative compound he called *epinephrine*. Later the purified adrenal extract was named *adrenaline,* and the active constituent, of the dessicated adrenals, ephedrine, was described in 1926.[3]

All of the important sympathomimetic bronchodilators are either catecholamines or related compounds, epinephrine being the prototype drug. Extensive investigations have elucidated the physiologic properties of the naturally occurring catecholamines that act as neurotransmitters in the sympathetic nervous system and to the development of highly efficacious analogues with great therapeutic value. These synthetic compounds may differ from one another in chemical structure, absorption, and metabolism; but their fundamental action is the same. When administered in sufficient quantity by the appropriate route, they relieve smooth muscle constriction, facilitate mucocilliary transport, activate ion pumps within the airways, and down-regulate the release of mast cell constituents. Thus, they are the drugs of choice for treatment of acute episodes of bronchospasm and for the prevention of exercise-induced bronchospasm.

DRUGS FOR THE RESPIRATORY SYSTEM
ISBN 0-8089-1818-4

Copyright © 1986 by Grune & Stratton, Inc.
All rights of reproduction in any form reserved.

PHARMACOLOGY OF BRONCHIAL SMOOTH MUSCLE

There is smooth muscle in the airway from the trachea down to the alveolar ducts, and it is under the control of the autonomic nervous system. Parasympathetic innervation of the bronchi occurs via the vagus nerve as far down as the terminal bronchioles, but evidence for direct innervation by the sympathetic nervous system is incomplete.[4] On the other hand, adrenoceptor agonist drugs are used extensively in the management of bronchoconstriction, while cholinergic antagonists have only a limited role. In addition, despite the lack of evidence of direct sympathetic innervation of human muscle, it is clear that adrenoceptors are present in bronchial smooth muscle. In 1940, Ahlquist[5] suggested division of adrenoceptors into α- and β-receptors, and demonstrated that the order of potency for *alpha* tissue responses was epinephrine, norepinephrine, and isoproterenol, and for β responses, isoproterenol, epinephrine, and norephinephrine. The β-adrenoreceptors have been further subdivided in β_1 and β_2 receptors,[6] a concept supported by the development of specific β_1 and β_2 adrenoceptor antagonists and selective β_2 agonist agents, which have minimal β_1 mediated side effects.[7,8]

The major effects of stimulation of the alpha and beta-receptor groups in the human are summarized in Table 1-1. Adrenoreceptor antagonists affect bronchial challenge with inhaled histamine, exercise, and allergens.[9-11] How the adrenoreceptors are stimulated in the absence of nervous control has not been elucidated.

Table 1-1
Effects of Adrenoreceptor Stimulation in Humans

Alpha:
   Decreased adenyl cyclase activity
   Constriction of smooth muscle of arteries, veins, bronchi
   Constriction of gastrointestinal, urinary bladder, trigone sphincters.
   Enhanced histamine release
   Contraction of pilomotor muscles
   Hepatic glycogenolysis
Beta:
   Increased adenyl cyclase activity
Beta$_1$
   Cardiac stimulation: isotropic and inotropic
   Increased lipolysis in free fatty acids
Beta$_2$
   Vasodilation
   Bronchodilation
   Inhibition of histamine release
   Skeletal muscle tremor
   Lactic acidemia

β₂ Agonists

It is known, however, that various forms of stimulation of the lung cause release of mediators that in turn stimulate irritant receptors in the lung to trigger a vagal reflex with release of acetylcholine, which acts on the muscle cells to produce bronchoconstriction.

As is depicted in Figure 1-1, airway patency normally depends on the balance between relaxant (via beta-adrenergic receptors) and contractile (through α-adrenergic and cholinergic receptors) influences on bronchial smooth muscle cells. Cyclic AMP apparently produces cell relaxation and is counteracted by cyclic GMP, which tends to cause cell contraction. Activation of the β receptors results in stimulation of the enzyme, adenyl cyclase, and this increases the production of cyclic AMP, which appears to produce relaxation by inhibiting protein kinase and stimulating binding of calcium ions to the cytoplasmic reticulum and the cell membrane, thus reducing mycoplasmal calcium concentration in both polarized and depolarized smooth muscle.[12] Conversely, cholinergic and alpha receptor stimulation enhances cyclic GMP production, while α-receptor stimulation also reduces cAMP. Thus β-adrenergic agents are important agents for reversal of bronchoconstriction. In addition to relaxation of respiratory smooth muscle, β-adrenergic agents reduce mast cell degranulation, decrease mucous gland secretion, and increase cilia beat frequency, thus enhancing mucocilliary clearance from the lungs.

The biochemical characteristics of the naturally occurring catecholamine and its synthetic analogues are shown in Figure 1-2. It can be seen that catecholamine bronchodilators such as norepinephrine, epinephrine, isoproterenol, isoetharine, rimeterol, and hexaprenaline have a phenolic ring with hydroxyl groups

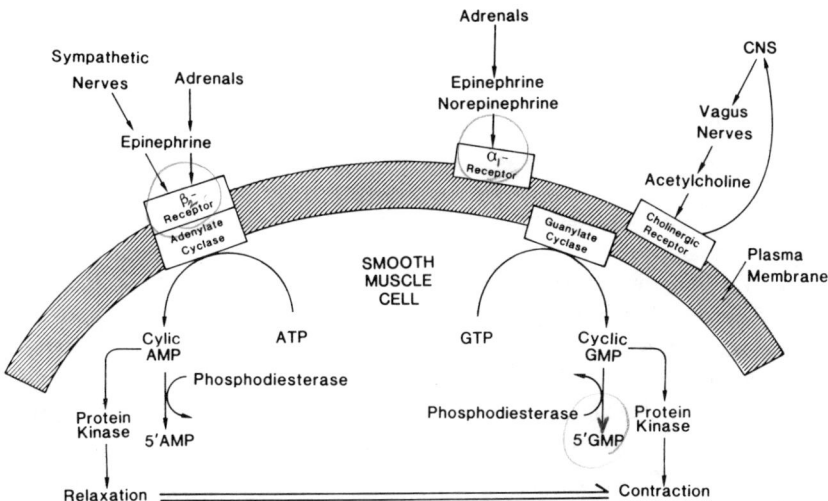

Fig. 1. Mechanism of bronchoconstriction and pharmacologic control of bronchodilation. (Farr RS., by permission.[50])

1. Synthesis Of The Naturally Occuring Catecholamines

2. Catecholamines Bronchodilators

3. Resorcinol Bronchodilators

4. Saligenin Bronchodilators

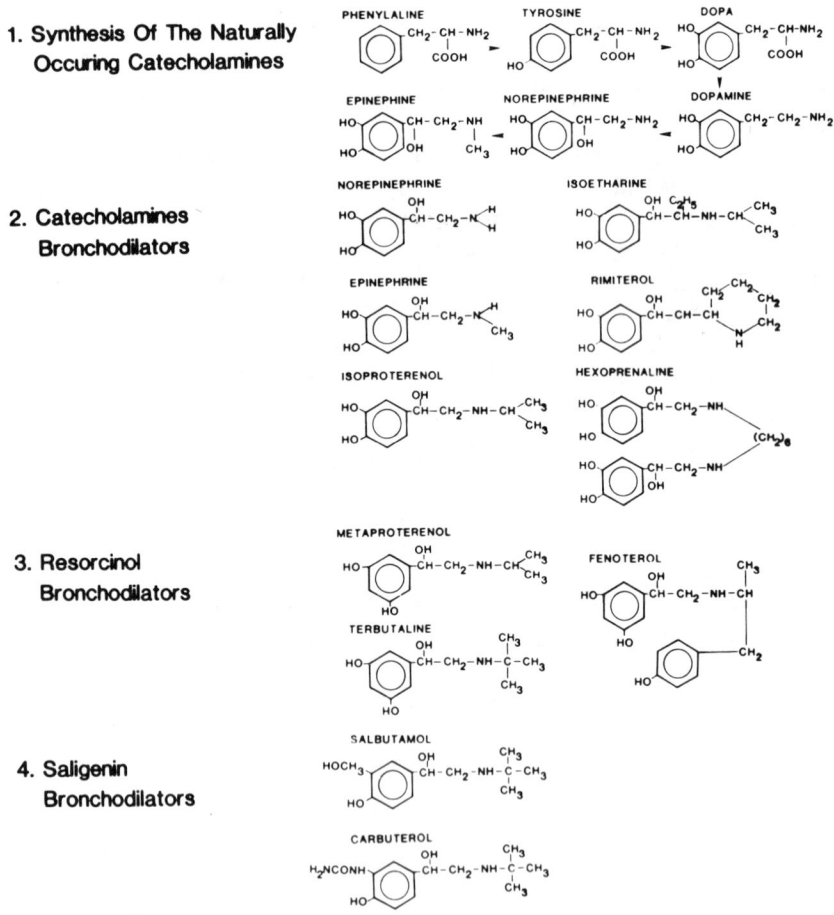

Fig. 2. The biochemical structure of the adrenergic bronchodilators.

at the 3 and 4 positions, an ethyl amino moiety in the number 1 position, and a hydroxyl group in the β carbon. They differ from one another in the size of the N substituent. In addition, isoetharine is distinguished by the addition of an ethyl group in the α carbon of the side chain.

An increase in N substituent increases β activity and decreases α activity. Thus, addition of a methyl group to norepinephrine, which has only α activity, creates epinephrine, which has equal α and β effects. A second methyl group transforms epinephrine to isoproterenol, which has predominantly β activity. The introduction of an α alkyl group in the ethanolamine side chain also increases a drug's activity as a β-receptor stimulant, but this diminishes when the amino moiety exceeds a certain size. β-receptor stimulation is markedly reduced by removal of the phenolic hydroxy group and almost abolished with the loss of the β-hydroxyl group.

The position of the two phenolic hydroxyl groups and the nature and size of the N substituent are important in catecholamine metabolism. Through the monoamine oxidase (MAO) intracellular pathways, epinephrine, and isoproterenol give rise to metanephrine and 3-methoxy isoproterenol, both of which are weak β-blockers. Further, degradation of catechols is accomplished by intestinal sulfokinase and other conjugating enzymes. Because of their rapid metabolism, the catecholamines are short-acting and ineffective by oral administration.

Replacement of the catechol nucleus by a resorcinol or saligenin ring results in the formation of compounds that are far more selective and longer-acting. The resorcinols, such as metaproterenol, terbutaline, and fenoterol, differ from the catecholamines in that the hydroxyl groups are shifted from the 3-4 position on the ring to a 3-5 configuration. The saligenins, such as salbutamol and carbuterol, are derived by substitutions at the 3-hydroxy position, and this increases their specificity. In addition, they no longer serve as substrates for catechol-o-methyltranferase (COMT) and/or MAO enzymes, so that they are effective when given orally and have a longer duration of action.

In vitro and *in vivo* animal studies suggest that all sympathomimetics dilate bronchial smooth muscle, the most potent agent being isoproterenol followed by salbutamol, terbutaline, fenoterol, and metaproterenol. Salbutamol, terbutaline, and fenoterol are much less active in cardiac tissue than are isoproterenol, metaproterenol, and the rest of the catecholamines. Although evaluation of studies of these agents in humans is difficult because of differences in study design, selection of end-point, dose administered and/or route of administration, and the severity of illness, it would appear that isoproterenol, salbutamol, terbutaline, and fenoterol have equal potency as bronchodilators, and that metaproterenol and the rest of the agents are somewhat less effective.[13-18] As is seen in Table 1-2, the duration of action of catecholamines, in general, is about 2-3 hours, while the cardiac effects only last a few minutes. Resorcinols and/or saligenins, on the other hand, last 4-6 hours, and any cardiac effects last longer.

Improvement in lung function can be measured within 20-30 minutes following administration of orally active drugs (resorcinols and saligenins) in both healthy individuals and those with reversible airway obstruction. Following inhalation improvement can be measured within 30 seconds, and in minutes when given subcutaneously.

ADRENORECEPTOR AGONISTS

Ephedrine

Synthetic ephedrine (phenylisopropanol-methylamine), which is the levorotatory isomer 1-ephedrine, differs from epinephrine in that it has no 3- and 4-hydroxyl groups. This structural alteration prevents the action of COMT, and reduces potency, so that ephedrine must be taken in milligram doses. Addition of

Table 1-2
Adrenergic Bronchodilators

Generic Name	Brand Name	Alpha Effect	Beta-1 Effect	Beta-2 Effect	Peak Response Time (Min)	Duration of Effect (Min)
Catecholamines						
Ephedrine	Ephedrine	+	+	+		2–3
Epinephrine 0.25% and 0.5%	Adrenaline Asmolin Asma-Meter* (0.2 mg) Medihaler-EPI* (0.16 mg)	+	+	+	5	1–2
Racemic Epinephrine 2.25%	Vaponefrin Asthmanefrin Micronefrin Solution A	+	+	+	5	1–2
Racemic Epinephrine 2.25% with Atropine 0.5%	Dylephrin Also Anticholinergic	+	+	+	5–10	2–3
Isoproterenol HCl	Isuprel 0.5–1% Vapo-N-ISO 0.5% Isuprel Mistome* Ter (0.125 mg) Norisodrine Aerotrol[a] (0.12 mg)	−	+	+	10–15	2–3
Isoproterenol Sulfate Metered Dose 0.075 mg	Medihaler-ISO LUF-ISO	−	+	+	5–15	2–3
Isoproterenol HCl Phenylephrine Bitartate MDI 0.16 mg ISO 0.24 mg PHENYL.	Medihaler-DUO	−	+	+	5–15	2–4

Drug	Brand	β1	β2	Onset (min)	Duration (min)
Isoproterenol	Aerolone	−	+	5-15	2-3
HCl 0.25% Compound					
Cyclopentamine 0.5%					
Isoetharine HCl 1%	Bronkosol	−	±	5-15	2-3
Phenylephrine HCl 0.25%	Bronkometer				
MDI*					
0.34 ISO with					
0.07 PHENYL.					
Rimeterol					
Hexoprenaline					
Resorcinols					
Metaproterenol	Alupent	−	±	30-45	3-5
MDI* (0.65 mg)	Metaprel				
Tablets 10 and 20 mg					
Fenoterol	Berotec	−	+	120-180	240-480
Tablets 5 and 10 mg					
MDI* (0.2 mg)					
Terbutaline	Brincanyl	−	±	120-180	4-6
Tablets 2.5 and 5 mg	Brethine				
Injectable Solution				15-60	120-240
1.0 mg/ml					
MDI*				30-60	240-300
(0.25 mg)					
Saligenins					
Salbutamol	Ventolin	−	±	120-180	360-480
or Albuterol	Proventil				
Tablets 2 and 4 mg					
MDI* (0.2 mg)				30-60	240-300
Intravenous					
Carbuterol**	Bronsecur	−	±	120-180	360-480
Tablets 2 and 4 mg					

*Metered dose mg/discharge
**Not available in the United States

a methyl group at the carbon ring renders the drug resistant to MAO, so that, unlike epinephrine, it is effective orally. The pharmacologic effect of ephedrine is primarily indirect through the release of norepinephrine from sympathetic nerve endings, although it also has a small direct effect on adrenoreceptors. Since norepinephrine is a relatively weak β_2 agonist, ephedrine is less potent than the newer oral β_2 agonist agents.[18-19] Thus, ephedrine is a poor choice for the management of bronchospasm.

When used alone, the usual dose for adults is 15–20 mg four times a day. The appropriate dose for children aged 2–6 years is 0.3–0.5 mg/kg every four hours up to a maximum of 2 mg/kg per day, and 6.25–12.5 mg every four hours, up to a maximum of 75 mg/day for older children.

Ephedrine is contraindicated in patients suffering from hypertension or cardiac disease, because of its α and β_1-adrenergic effects. In addition, it is not recommended for nervous or agitated patients, or for those who sleep poorly.

Epinephrine

Epinephrine is taken up actively by sympathetic nerve endings and smooth muscle, and is metabolized through the MAO and COMT enzyme pathways. It stimulates both α- and β-adrenoreceptors, but its powerful β-effects render it an important component of the treatment of bronchospasm. For many years, subcutaneous ephinephrine (1:1000 solution) was the treatment of choice in status asthmaticus. It is prescribed at a dose of 0.1–0.5 mg (0.01 mg/kg in small children), which may be repeated at 15–20 minute intervals. The effect of an aqueous suspension of epinephrine (1:200) may persist for as long as 8–10 hours. The intramuscular and intravenous routes of administration are rarely used in the management of bronchospasm. It has also been utilized as an aerosol (1:100 solution), and metered-dose products of epinephrine, such as primetine, can be purchased without prescription. One should not use a solution of epinephrine that has developed a brown color, as the responsible adrenochromes have been reported to cause adverse reactions such as hallucinations. With the advent of more selective β_2 agonist agents, the use of epinephrine in the management of bronchospasm is decreasing.

Epinephrine can be applied topically to arrest surface bleeding, injected to reduce blood flow to help hemostasis, or to limit removal of a primary drug (such as a local anesthetic). It can also be used in the management of acute allergic emergencies, the emergency treatment of hypoglycemia, or by intracardiac injection to resuscitate a patient with cardiac arrest.

Isoproterenol

Isoproterenol is a potent bronchodilator, although it is nonselective and short-acting. An effect of aerosol administration usually persists for 90–120 minutes. Isoproterenol is as efficacious as epinephrine in the emergency therapy of asthma, but because of the proven superiority of the newer β-adrenergic agonists, there is little justification for prescription of isoproterenol.[20] Since it has strong β_1 effects, it is also used in the treatment of cardiovascular diseases, mainly in Stokes-Adams attacks. The drug is rapidly metabolized to 3-methoxyisoproterenol, an agent that can cause weak blockade of the β_2 receptor site by COMT.

Isoproterenol can be administered by aerosol, orally, sublingually, or intravenously. The ratio of bronchodilation to cardiostimulatory effects depends on the route of administration, and differs considerably when it is given by other than the inhalation route. An aerosol can be administered with a powered or hand-held nebulizer, utilizing a 1:200 solution, or by a metered-dose inhaler that delivers from 0.04 to 0.125 mg/puff, depending on the preparation used. Oral and sublingual administration (5–20 mg) are less satisfactory alternatives. Intravenous therapy is used mainly in children in a dosage of 0.8 mcg/kg/minute, while the appropriate dose for adults is 0.03–0.2 mcg/kg/minute. Intravenous delivery should be controlled by a constant infusion pump and the patient carefully monitored in an intensive care setting.

Isoetharine

Isoetharine, the first new agent to demonstrate a greater β_2 agonist effect, has relatively little β_1 activity and negligible α-activity. Although its duration of action is slightly longer than that of isoproterenol (because it is resistant to MAO), its pattern of bronchodilation is very similar. In the United States, isoetharine is available as an aerosol product (Bronkosol and Bronkometer Breon Laboratories Inc, New York, New York 10016), which also contains phenylephrine is thought to decrease side effects and prolong the duration of action. Isoetharine is safe and has few cardiovascular side effects at the usual dose, although the blood pressure may fall slightly, and the heart rate might rise slightly. Its use would appear to be limited to rapid relief of acute attacks of bronchoconstriction.

Rimeterol and Hexoprenaline

These agents are short-acting β-selective agents of moderate potency with pharmacologic actions that are similar to those of isoetharine.

Metaproterenol

The cardiac and bronchial effects of metaproterenol do not differ significantly from those of isoproterenol.[21] Intravenous metaproterenol is as effective as isoproterenol for the treatment of acute asthma and as an aerosol, but it is not superior to other long-acting bronchodilators. By virtue of a shift of the hydroxyl groups to the third and fifth carbons on the benzene ring, metaproterenol is not susceptible to inactivation by COMT and, therefore, can be administered orally. However, because it is still susceptible to MAO, its duration of action is somewhat shorter than that of selective β_2-adrenergic agonists whether administered orally or by inhalation. The recommended oral dose for adults is 20 mg three times a day, but many patients develop tremor and tachycardia, so it is advisable to start with 10 mg three times a day.

Fenoterol

Fenoterol, a derivative of metaproterenol, is also resistant to COMT, so that it can also be given by mouth as well as by aerosol. It has very selective β_2-receptor properties and its potency is comparable to that of terbutaline and salbutamol. The optimal oral dose for adults appears to be 7.5 mg two or three times a day. The corresponding aerosol dose is about 400 mg.

Terbutaline

Terbutaline is a long-acting resorcinol and thus is not affected by COMT or by sulfatization. It is effective by all routes of administration and is available for oral and subcutaneous administration and as a metered-dose aerosol. It is highly β-selective resulting in greater bronchodilation and lasting longer than metaproterenol. The recommended oral dose is 5 mg three or four times a day, although it is usually better to start with the lower dosage (2.5 mg three to four times a day). Terbutaline offers an important alternative for subcutaneous treatment, and is preferable in patients who can not tolerate epinephrine, such as those with hypertension or cardiac disease. The dose for subcutaneous use is 0.25 mg, which can be repeated in 15–30 minutes, but a total dose of 0.5–0.75 mg during a 4 hour period should not be exceeded.

Salbutamol

This saligenin is resistant to COMT and sulfatization. It is a very selective β_2 stimulant, and perhaps the most potent and safest of the sympathomimetic bronchodilators. The oral dose is 4 mg four times a day, although 2 mg is often effective and does not produce side effects. The recommended dose intravenously in adults is 100 mcg, followed by 300 mcg in 15 minutes if the response is inadequate. It can also be given by continuous infusion over one hour (4 mcg/minute, or 0.05–0.2 mcg/kg/minute). A total dose of 0.2 mg given over a period of five minutes may be optimal. Intravenous administration of salbutamol inhibits premature labor. It can cause a fall in serum potassium, probably because of intracellular migration of potassium, because of insulin release, brought about by stimulation of pancreatic β_2 adrenoreceptors. The drug has been reported to be useful in treatment of hyperkalemia associated with attacks of familial periodic paralysis.

Carbuterol

This agent is pharmacologically similar to salbutamol, and is a highly selective β_2 stimulator with a long duration of action.

ROUTES OF ADMINISTRATION

The β_2 agonist agents may be administered by inhalation, orally, subcutaneously or intravenously. Theoretically, aerosol administration has certain advantages, because the drug is applied directly to receptors in the airways. This is shown in Figure 1-3, which indicates that the onset and extent of bronchodilation produced by terbutaline is most rapid following inhalation and that the extent was greater with higher dosage.[22] Conversely, oral, subcutaneous or intravenous administration delivers the drug via the systemic circulation, and the plasma concentration that must be achieved to produce bronchodilation may result in

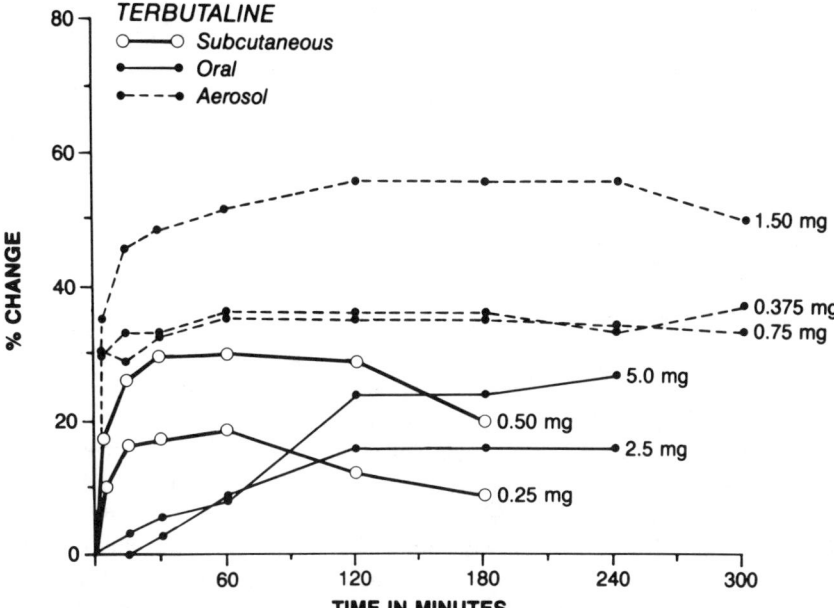

Fig. 3. The change in FEV_1 following three different routes of administration of terbutaline. (Dulfano MJ, Glass P., by permission.[22])

greater side effects.[22,23] The relative dosage utilized and the extent of bronchodilation resulting when administered orally, subcutaneously, and by inhalation is also illustrated in Figure 1-3.[22]

Oral Administration

As indicated earlier, catecholamines are rapidly degraded by COMT and are ineffective when taken orally. Oral administration of medications such as metaproterenol, terbutaline, and salbutamol have a lower potential for abuse and produce a peak effect in two to four hours and the bronchodilation persists for up to six hours. These advantages are counterbalanced, however, by an increased incidence of skeletal muscle tremor and cardiac side effects. In order to minimize side effects, treatment is usually begun with ½ the recommended therapeutic dose and gradually increased toward full dosage, as tolerated. It has been suggested that oral medication has a greater effect on peripheral airways. Consequently, oral aminophylline and/or a β-agonist, in doses which do not cause troublesome side effects, along with inhaled β-adrenergic agonists have been advocated on a regular basis if significant symptoms persist.[24]

Parenteral Administration

Although terbutaline and salbutamol are available for intravenous administration in other countries, they are not available in the U.S.A. On theoretical grounds, terbutaline should be superior to epinephrine when used parenterally, but the incidence of side effects and magnitude or duration of bronchodilation is apparently no different. Epinephrine, ethylnorepinephrine, and terbutaline are available in this country for subcutaneous administration. In any case, several studies have failed to demonstrate an advantage of parenteral adrenergic therapy over inhaled β_2 adrenergic agents in acute severe asthma.[24-26]

Aerosol Administration

As indicated in Figure 1-3, inhaled beta-adrenergic bronchodilator results in more rapid and greater improvement in lung function than oral or subcutaneous administration. In addition, the ratio of bronchodilation to side effects is greatly increased over the other routes of administration. On the other hand, greater patient abuse is possible, and hypoxemia may develop. The inhalation of catecholamines such as isoproterenol and isoetharine result in maximal bronchodilation within a few minutes, but the effect declines progressively and is essentially undetectable after one to two hours. The bronchodilation following inhalation of more selective β_2 agents begins and peaks a little later than isoproterenol, but their action persists longer (two or more hours for metaproterenol and up to six hours for salbutamol). For these reasons salbutamol is preferred for chronic administration, whereas isoproterenol or isoetharine are chosen in the acute situation.

The delivery of inhaled bronchodilator by IPPB provides no advantage over the use of a metered dose freon-propelled nebulizer, a hand-held nebulizer, or a compressor-powered nebulizer.[27,28] Similarly, the response to inhaled adrenergic bronchodilators has been shown to be equal or superior to that of a loading dose of aminophylline followed by continuous infusions in the emergency treatment of severe asthma.[29,30] This suggests that the use of aminophylline in the emergency treatment of asthma has been overemphasized, and may have led to underusage of adrenergic bronchodilators.

Optimal inhalation of an aerosol requires appropriate education of the patient about the correct method of inhalation, and ensurance of deposition of aerosolized particles in the peripheral airways, (i.e. the rate of inspiration, the size of the breath, and the size of the droplets delivered).[31] When a metered dose inhaler (MDI) is used, over 80 percent of the dose is deposited in the oropharynx because of impaction of the high-speed aerosol particles, and only about 10 percent reaches the conducting airway.[32] Extension tubes or aerochambers have helped overcome this problem as well as poor "hand-lung" coordination. Delivery of aerosol into an aerochamber slows the speed of the particles and fosters reduction in particle size through propellant evaporation, thereby enhancing penetration to smaller airways.[33,34] In well-trained subjects, extenders with a volume of less than 300 ml apparently do not provide additional benefit over MDI's alone, while those that are 750 ml or greater augment the response significantly.[35]

At our institution, we prefer to deliver the aerosolized bronchodilator with a hand-held bulb-type nebulizer, utilizing a dilute solution of the β-agonist (50:50 in saline or water). A simple plastic flex-tube between the nebulizer and the mouthpiece fosters delivery of predominantly small droplets and avoids deposition of large drops in the oropharynx, trachea, and major bronchi, where they are readily absorbed. We believe that the mode of inhalation of the aerosol is very important and recommend the following technique. The nebulizer bulb (or in patients who cannot squeeze a bulb, the MDI) is repeatedly squeezed, (or compressed air is continuously activated through the nebulizer) and the aerosol inhaled continuously during a very slow full inspiration from functional residual capacity to total lung capacity. The mouthpiece is removed, the breath is held at full inspiration for about ten seconds, then followed by a very slow exhalation back to FRC through pursed lips. The patient should then breathe normally for about a minute, before determining whether: (1) subjective relief is *felt* in the lower lateral aspects of the chest, (2) the cardiac rate has risen by 10 beats/min., or (3) a mild tremor has developed. In the absence of any of these events, the slow deep inhalation of aerosol, breath held, slow exhalation, and then relaxed breathing for at least a minute, are repeated, over and over again, until either full penetration to the periphery of the lung is felt, or mild side effects develop.

The number of inhalations necessary with each *treatment* and the number of treatments/day depend on the severity of airway obstruction, and thus, will vary considerably from patient to patient and, within a particular patient, from time to time. Our patients are, therefore, advised to inhale the β-agonist daily in this manner before going to bed and on arising, even though feeling *well*. In addition, a full *treatment* should be taken whenever chest tightness, cough, wheezing, or dyspnea develop during the day or night, and before being exposed to agents, or undertaking an activity, known to precipitate symptoms. Clearly then, it is our feeling that there is no particular dose of medication or number of treatments in a day for a given patient. The amount of medication inhaled and the number of times the patient should take full *treatments* will depend on the degree and frequency of bronchoconstriction. On the other hand, it is extremely important that patients understand that an increase in the daily requirement of inhaled beta agonists is indicative of increasing airway obstruction, and the need for more frequent *treatments* should be considered as a warning necessitating contact of the attending physician immediately.

ADVERSE EFFECTS OF ADRENORECEPTOR AGONISTS

The adverse effects of adrenoreceptor agonists are shown in Table 1-3. In the late 1960s there was a significant increase in the mortality of asthmatic patients in Great Britain,[36] and although the evidence for a relationship was not convincing, self-medication with pressurized aerosols of isoproterenol was implicated.[37]

Table 1-3
Side Effects of Sympathomimetic Bronchodilators

Cardiovascular:	Tachycardia, palpitations, arrhythmias, changes in blood pressure, angina, myocardial necrosis, vasoconstriction or vasodilation.
Nervous System:	Agitation, anxiety, tremulousness, insomnia, faintness, dizziness.
Genito Urinary:	Urinary retention (mainly in men with prostatic hypertrophy).
Opthalmic:	Glaucoma.
Metabolic:	Hyperglycemia, hyperthyroidism.
Gastrointestinal:	Dry mouth, gagging, nausea, vomiting.
Respiratory:	Tracheal irritation, bronchial irritation, bronchospasm.
Pregnancy:	Inhibition of premature labor.
Blood Gases:	Decrease in PaO_2.
Interaction with other drugs:	Monoamine oxidase inhibitors, general anesthetics hypotensive agents, pressor agents, thyroid hormone, insulin, oral hypoglycemic agents.
Other:	Tachyphylaxis, paradoxic response (bronchospasm).

Cardio Vascular Effects

In the doses employed clinically, the resorcinols and saligenins do not stimulate the heart directly. However, all share the same dose-limiting side effects–tremor, which is due to stimulation of β_2 receptors in skeletal muscles, tachycardia, and increased cardiac output, which are due to a decrease in peripheral vascular resistance because of stimulation of the smooth muscle in blood vessels supplying skeletal muscles. The tremor is particularly troublesome in individuals with an increased sympathetic drive.

Cardiac Arrythmias

Compounds that produce vasoconstriction and cardiac stimulation are much more arrhythmogenic. While the cardiac effect of β-agonists is likely to be relatively harmless in normal subjects, it may be serious in susceptible individuals. Collins and co-workers[38] demonstrated that small doses of intravenous isoproterenol could result in asystole in animals, if they were hypoxemic. Under these circumstances, the stimulant effect of a small dose of β-agonist can be converted to severe cardiac depression.[39]

The more selective β_2 agents are not devoid of cardiovascular consequences. These can develop from the direct activation of β-receptors, or reflexly in order to maintain cardiac output in the face of a drug-induced fall in peripheral vascular resistance.[40] Although these findings tend to be more frequent and severe following subcutaneous or intraveneous injection, they can also occur following oral administration. Indeed, terbutaline has been reported to increase ventricular ectopy in a patient with preexisting arrhythmias.[41] Because of the relatively slow metabolism of the newer agents, (i.e., resorcinols and saligenins) tachyarrhythmias tend to last longer than those seen with catecholamines.

Effects on Gas Exchange

The arterial oxygen tension (PaO_2) has been reported to fall following administration of atropine, aminophylline, and the adrenoreceptor agents, even though airway function improves. The fall in PaO_2 is most likely due to greater mismatching of ventilation and perfusion, resulting in more of the blood flow being directed through poorly ventilated areas, so that the PaO_2 falls. The fall in PaO_2 is usually short lived, and spontaneous recovery occurs within 30 minutes. However, this phenomenon is important, and if during bronchodilator therapy there is any reason to suspect that oxygenation is inadequate, supplemental O_2 should be administered.

Metabolites

The metabolite of isoproterenol (3-O-methyl-isoproterenol) has been shown to possess weak beta-blocking properties.[42] Because this metabolite can be formed in the lung after the inhalation of isoproterenol, it is possible for its local concentration to be high. No β-blocking metabolite has been demonstrated with other β-agonist agents.

Non-specific Effects

As is shown in Table 1-3, nonspecific side effects can occur with all the sympathomimetic drugs. Dry mouth, gagging, nausea, and occasionally, vomiting may occur. Headache, dizziness, faintness, and sweating may be related to cardiovascular effects. Irritation of the tracheobronchial tree, and even tracheobronchitis may be induced by aerosol therapy. In particular, it may induce bronchospasm after the initial inhalation in patients with very reactive airways, and paradoxic bronchoconstriction following inhaled bronchodilator has also been reported.[43]

Development of Tolerance

Tolerance or subsensitivity, (i.e., diminished responsiveness to bronchodilators), may occur when receptors are repeatedly exposed to high concentrations of β-adrenergic agonists. *In vitro* studies of nonpulmonary tissue from patients said to have adrenergic subsensitivity indicate a markedly decreased number of available β-adrenergic receptors and a diminished generation of cAMP following stimulation of adenyl cyclase. This does not appear to be important clinically, however, as tolerance to a particular dose after one or two weeks is generally minimal, and no further loss of bronchodilator effect occurs with continuing observation for up to 12 months. Nevertheless the response to inhaled β agonists is generally reduced considerably in patients with prolonged bronchospasm. In such cases, corticosteroids have been reported to restore responsiveness to isoproterenol and albuterol.[44,45] Since adrenergic responsiveness can be restored in as little as one hour by corticosteroids, the prompt use of moderate doses of corticosteroids during exacerbations of asthma that are not responsive to the usual adrenergic therapy is highly recommended.

Adverse Effects of Freon Propellants

Freon is far from being biologically inert,[46] since it is a fluorinated hydrocarbon that is closely related to chloroform and halothane. It has been shown that conscious dogs breathing moderate concentrations of flurocarbon may develop severe ventricular arrhythmias following intravenous epinephrine, but not isoproterenol.[47,48] The arterial blood concentration of flurocarbons 11 and 12 required to sensitize the heart were 20 and 35 mcg/ml, respectively. Because the half-life of these fluorocarbons is short, it is reasonable to conclude the flurocarbons in inhalers present little hazard if they are used as recommended. Based on the animal data, a patient would have to take as much as 12–24 consecutive inhalations of fluorocarbon to achieve a myocardial concentration sufficient to sensitize the heart.[49]

REFERENCES

1. Solis-Cohen: The use of adrenal substance in the treatment of asthmas. JAMA 34:1164–1166, 1900
2. Takamine J: Adrenaline: The active principle of the suprarenal gland. Scott Med Surg J 10:131–138, 1902
3. Chen KK, Schmidt GF: The action and clinical use of ephedrine. JAMA 87:836–841, 1926
4. Staub NC: Some aspects of airways structure and function. Postgrad Med J 51:(Suppl 7):21–34, 1975
5. Ahlquist RP: A study of the adrenoreceptors. Am J Physiol 153:586–600, 1948
6. Lands AM, Arnold A, McAuliff JP, et al: Differentiation of receptor system activated by sympathomimetic amines. Nature 214:597–598, 1967
7. Fitzgerald JD: Perspective in adrenergic beta receptor blockade. Clin Pharmacol Ther 10:298–306, 1969
8. Moran NC: Pharmacological characterization of adrenergic receptors. Pharmacol Rev 18:503–512, 1966
9. Seale JP, Andersen SD, Lindsay DA: A trial of an alpha adrenoreceptor blocking drug (indorumin) in exercise-induced bronchoconstriction. Scand J Respir Dis 57:261–266, 1976
10. Gaddie J, Legge JS, Petrie G, et al: The effects of an alpha adrenergic receptor blocking drug on histamine sensitivity in bronchial asthma. Br J Dis Chest 66:141–146, 1972
11. Patel KR, Kerr JW: Effect of alpha receptor blocking drug, thymoxamine, on allergen induced bronchoconstriction in extrinsic asthma. Clin Allergy 5:311–316, 1975
12. Anderson RGG, Nilsson KB: Role of cyclic nucleotides metabolism and mechanical activity in smooth muscle, in Stephens NL, (ed): Biochemistry of smooth muscle. Baltimore, University Park Press, pp 203, 1977
13. Choo-Karg YFJ, Simpson WT, Grant IWB: Controlled comparison of bronchodilating effects of three beta-adrenergic stimulant drugs administered by inhalation to patients with asthma. Br Med J 2:287–289, 1969
14. Turnhein K, Kraupp O: Pulmonary and systemic circulatory effects and beta-adrenergic selectivity of hexoprenaline, salbutamol, oxyfedrine, and isoproterenol. Eur J Pharmacol 15:231–239, 1971
15. Shenfield GM, Patersen JW: Clinical assessment of bronchodilator drugs delivered by aerosol. Thorax 28:124–128, 1973
16. Gurwitz D, Levison H: Dose-response study of oral fenoterol in asthmatic children. Dev Pharmacol Ther 1:265–273, 1980
17. Steen SN, Smith R, Kuo J, et al: Comparison of the bronchodilator effects of aerosol fenoterol and isoproterenol. Chest 72:724–730, 1977

18. Kennedy MCS, Jackson SLO: Oral sympathomimetic amines in treatment of asthma. Br Med J 2:1506, 1963
19. Lal S, Bhalla KK, Davey AJ: Slow release salbutamol and tedral in the treatment of reversible airway obstruction. Postgrad Med J 47 (suppl):89–92, 1971
20. Rossing TH, Fanta CH, Goldstein DGH, et al: Emergency therapy of asthma: Comparison of the acute effects of parenteral and inhaled sympathomimetics and infused aminophylline. Am Rev Respir Dis 122:365–371, 1980
21. McEvoy JDS, Vall-Spinosa A, Paterson JW: Assessment of orciprenaline and isoproterenol infusion in asthmatic patients. Am Rev Respir Dis 108:490–500, 1973
23. Dulfano MJ, Glass P: The bronchodilator effects of terbutaline. Route of administration and patterns of response. Ann Allergy 37:357–366, 1976
24. Thringer G, Svedmyr N: Comparison of infused and inhaled terbutaline in patients with asthma. Scand J Respir Dis 57:17–24, 1976
25. Ben Zvi Z, Lam C, Hoffman J: An evaluation of the initial treatment of acute asthma. Pediatrics 70:348–353, 1982
26. Pancordo S, Fifield G, Davis S: Subcutaneous epinephrine versus nebulized terbutaline in the emergency treatment of asthma. Clin Pharmacol 2:45–48, 1983
27. Lawford G, Jones BJM, Milledge JS: Comparison of intravenous and nebulized salbutamol in initial treatment of severe asthma. Br Med J 1:84, 1978
28. Cherniack RM, Goldberg I: The effect of nebulized bronchodilator delivered with and without IPPB on ventilatory function in chronic obstructive emphysema. Am Rev Respir Dis 91:13–20, 1965
29. Cherniack RM, Svanhill E. Long term use of intermittent positive pressure breathing (IPPB) in chronic obstructive pulmonary disease. Am Rev Respir Dis 113:721–728, 1976
30. Rossing T, Fanta G, Snapfer SR, et al: Emergency therapy of asthma: Comparison of the acute effects of parenteral and inhaled sympathomimetics and infused aminophylline. Am Rev Respir Dis 122:365–371, 1979
31. Appel D, Shim CS, Williams MH Jr: Comparative effect of epinephrine and aminophylline in the treatment of acute asthma. Am Rev Respir Dis 177 (part 2) 91, 1978
32. Dolovich M, Ruffin RE, Roberts R, et al: Optimal delivery of aerosols from metered dose inhalers. Chest 80 (Supp):911–918, 1981
33. Ryan G, Dolovich MB, Olbminski G: Standardization of inhalation provocation tests: Influence of nebulizer output, particle size and method of inhalation. J Allergy Clin Immunol 67:156–161, 1981
34. Newman SP, Moren F, Pavia D, et al: Deposition of pressurized aerosols inhaled through extended devices. Am Rev Respir Dis 124:317–320, 1981
35. Ellul-Micallef R, Moss F, Welterlin K, et al: Use of a special inhaler attachment in asthmatic children. Thorax 35:620–623, 1980
36. Riulin J, Mindorff C, Reilly P, et al: Pulmonary response to a bronchodilator delivered from three inhalation devices. J Pediatr 104(3):470–473, 1984
22. Speizer FE, Doll R, Heaf P: Observations on recent increase in mortality from asthma. Br Med J 1:335–339, 1968
37. Speizer FE, Doll R, Heaf P, Strang LB: Investigation into use of drugs preceding death from asthma. Br Med J 1:339–343, 1968
38. Collins JM, McDevitt DG, Shanks RG, Swanton JG: The cardiotoxicity of isoproterenol during hypoxia. Br J Pharmacol 36:35–45, 1969

39. Lockett MF: Dangerous effects of isoproterenol in myocardial failure. Lancet 2:104-106, 1965
40. Sackner MA, Daugherty R, Watson H, et al: Hemodynamic effects of epinephrine and terbutaline in normal man. Chest 68:616-624, 1975
41. Banner AS, Sunderrajan EV, Agarroal MK, et al: Arrhythmogenic effects of orally administered bronchodilators. Arch Intern Med 139:434-437, 1979
42. Paterson JW, Connolly ME, Davies DS, et al: Isoprenaline resistance and the use of pressurized aerosols in asthma. Lancet 2:426-429, 1968
43. Reisman RE: Asthma induced by adrenergic aerosol. J Allergy 46:162-177, 1970
44. Ellul-Micallef R, Fench FF: Effect of intravenous prednisolone in asthmatics with diminished adrenergic responsiveness. Lancet 2:1269-1270, 1975
45. Holgate ST, Baldwin CJ, Tattersfield AE: Beta-adrenergic agonists resistance in normal human airways. Lancet 2:375-377, 1977
46. Dollery CT: The toxicity of propellant gases in: An evaluation of bronchodilator drugs, in Asthma Research Council Symposium London: Trust for Education and Research and Therapeutics, 183-189, 1974
47. Bass M: Sudden death. JAMA 212:2075-2079, 1970
48. Reinhardt CF, Azar A, Maxfield ME, Smith PE, Mullin LS: Cardiac arrhythmias and aerosol "sniffing." Arch Environ Health 22:265-279, 1971
49. Dollery CT, Williams FM, Draffan GH: Arterial blood levels of flurocarbons in asthmatic patients following use of pressurized aerosol. Clin Pharmacol Ther 15:59-66, 1974
50. Farr RS: Asthma in adults: The ambulatory patient. Hospital Practice 13:113-123, 1978

Stanley J. Szefler

2

Theophylline and Other Methylxanthine Derivatives

Theophylline (1,3-dimethylxanthine) is a bronchodilator that plays a primary role in the treatment of reactive airways disease. Although bronchodilator properties were recognized in the early 1920s, it was not used clinically until the mid 1930s. After a period of uncertainty regarding the risk-benefit considerations of theophylline therapy, the use of theophylline was rejuvenated by several major events. Of significant importance was the development of techniques to measure serum theophylline concentrations (STC). It was soon recognized that theophylline toxicity could be related to STC and there was considerable variability among patients in the rate of theophylline elimination. This ultimately led to the identification of individualized dosage regimens. With the observation that certain patients required frequent dosing to maintain therapeutic STC, this problem was resolved with the application of controlled-release delivery systems to reduce the frequency of dosing to three times a day, then twice daily, and recently even once daily.

Despite the recognized benefits of theophylline therapy, there are certain disadvantages, primarily related to adverse effects. The risk for certain severe effects including seizures, gastrointestinal distress, insomnia, and potential behavior alterations, prompt an ongoing assessment regarding the position of theophylline in the therapeutic armamentarium for reactive airways disease. This issue is particularly relevant when one considers the availability of other effective agents with limited risk for adverse effects, particularly cromolyn, inhaled selective β_2-adrenergic agents, and aerosol corticosteroids. Nevertheless,

DRUGS FOR THE RESPIRATORY SYSTEM   Copyright © 1986 by Grune & Stratton, Inc.
ISBN 0-8089-1818-4   All rights of reproduction in any form reserved.

theophylline occupies a position of superiority in the treatment of reactive airways disease in the United States.

The advantages of theophylline include its rapid onset of action, relatively long duration of action, ease of administration, and the ability to individualize the dose to obtain optimal response. In addition to the previously described undesirable effects, however, there is a relatively narrow margin of safety necessitating therapeutic drug monitoring and careful assessment for the multiple conditions that may alter theophylline diposition. A framework will be developed in the following discussion to provide the clinician sufficient information to evaluate the role of theophylline in individual patients and to use it in a safe and effective manner.

Mechanisms of Action

Originally it was proposed that the cellular mechanism of bronchodilator action was related to the inhibition of the enzyme phosphodiesterase that is responsible for metabolism of cyclic AMP. It is now apparent that STCs commonly generated are insufficient to adequately inhibit phosphodiesterase activity.[1] Several other mechanisms for theophylline were proposed, including activity as a prostagladin antagonist, ability to alter intracellular calcium and the potential to compete for adenosine receptor binding. Also identified as possibilities are the reduction of catecholamine uptake or metabolism.[2]

Of interest is the failure of enprofylline (3-propylxanthine), a recently developed xanthine derivative bronchodilator, to inhibit adenosine receptors, consequently reducing the significance of this mechanism.[3] Further investigations are therefore necessary to identify the primary mechanism of action for theophylline. While it is clearly useful to evaluate the mechanism at the primary site of action, specifically bronchial smooth muscle, it is equally important to investigate mechanisms at extrapulmonary sites. This will assist in the understanding of undesirable effects and perhaps lead to the development of site-specific derivatives to maintain the beneficial response and minimize risks for adverse effects.

Besides a bronchodilator effect, manifested by bronchial smooth muscle relaxation, theophylline has other systemic effects including: central nervous system stimulation, cardiovascular effects (decreased peripheral vascular resistance, potential cardiac stimulation, and increased cerebrovascular resistance), a diuretic effect, and increased gastric secretion. Some of these effects may be used therapeutically, such as the application of central nervous stimulating properties, for the treatment of apnea of the newborn. In addition, the effect of theophylline on increasing diaphragmatic contractility may provide additional benefits in the treatment of obstructive airways disease.[4,5] It is not clear at the present time whether theophylline has the potential to inhibit the late phase pulmonary response following antigen challenge. There is at least one study that

Theophylline and Other Methylxanthine Derivatives

demonstrates that single doses of theophylline significantly attenuate the airway response to histamine and methacholine.[6]

Indications

Theophylline is used in the following situations: (1) treatment of acute respiratory distress secondary to reactive airways disease, (2) for continuous therapy to alleviate symptoms of chronic asthma, and (3) prevention of recurrent apnea in the newborn. In addition, theophylline is frequently prescribed for the treatment of chronic obstructive pulmonary disease, although the benefits are less clear.

ACUTE RESPIRATORY DISTRESS

Sympathomimetic bronchodilators are the drugs of choice for acute asthma since they provide a rapid onset of action with the parenteral or inhaled route of administration. Theophylline is given following ineffective response with β-adrenergic agents. For acute asthma, it is recommended that aminophylline, the ethylenediamine salt of theophylline, be delivered by the intravenous route to assure rapid and total systemic availability.

Before initiating theophylline treatment, it is essential to determine if the patient is receiving chronic theophylline therapy. If the patient has been receiving theophylline, the serum theophylline concentration should be measured. The response to theophylline is maximized by selecting a dose sufficient to provide an STC between 10–20 µg/ml. In the absence of previous theophylline therapy, this is achieved with an intravenous aminophylline dose of 6 mg/kg (1 mg aminophylline=0.79 mg theophylline). This is based on the assumption that 1 mg/kg theophylline will increase the STC by 2 µg/ml, as determined by the following equation:

$$C_p = \frac{DOSE}{Vd}$$

where C_P is the STC desired and Vd the average volume of distribution, 0.5 L/kg. If the patient has been receiving theophylline therapy, a partial loading dose (in mg/kg body weight) can be administered to achieve a desired concentration:

$$Dose = (C_p^{desired} - C_p^{measured})/(0.5 \text{ L/kg})$$

In each case, the dose should be based on the patient's ideal body weight. Since the Vd for individual patients may vary between 0.3 to 0.7 L/kg, a follow-up

STC should be obtained 30 minutes after the infusion to assess the need for additional theophylline.

After the initial infusion, theophylline is continued via the intravenous route until respiratory distress is adequately resolved. The dose of aminophylline varies in relation to the patient's age, smoking status, and the presence of conditions that may impair theophylline elimination, such as liver disease or congestive heart failure. Table 2-1 summarizes a standard theophylline dosing regimen for the initial maintenance dose.[7] This may be administered by a constant intravenous infusion or by dividing the dose into every four or six hour intervals. Since elimination may vary considerably among patients, STC should be measured to assess the adequacy of the dose.

When the episode of respiratory distress is adequately resolved, theophylline therapy may be continued with an oral preparation. The dose is divided into equal parts and administered at intervals consistent with the absorption properties of the formulation chosen.

CHRONIC ASTHMA

Theophylline is frequently used as the first choice and only medication for the treatment of chronic asthma. Certain patients, however, may obtain equivalent therapeutic response with cromolyn and/or β-adrenergic agonists, such as aerosol metaproterenol, terbutaline, or albuterol. Patients who do not receive adequate response from theophylline, may benefit from the addition of inhaled β-adrenergic agonists, cromolyn and inhaled corticosteroids. Patients with respiratory distress refractory to these medications may require a short course of oral corticosteroids.

Response to theophylline is dose related and it is commonly recommended to derive dosage regimens that provide STC between 10–20 μg/ml. However, the

Table 2-1
Recommended Initial Theophylline Dosage Regimens*

	mg/kg†/24 hrs
Children: 6 months to 9 years	20
Children: 9 years to 16 years, and young adult smokers	16
Healthy non-smoking adults	10
Older patients and patients with cor pulmonale	6
Patients with congestive heart failure or liver disease	2.4

*F.D.A. Drug Bulletin 1980; 10:4–6
†Based on estimated lean (ideal) body weight.

goal of therapy should be to produce maximal bronchodilation (i.e., the highest $FEV_{1.0}$). It appears that certain patients can be maintained adequately with STC as low as 5 µg/ml. Although the risk for severe adverse effects increases as STC exceeds 20 µg/ml, some patients will identify undesirable effects with STC below 20 µg/ml. Doses should therefore, be individualized and generally STC should be maintained between 8–15 µg/ml or at the level that is associated with the highest $FEV_{1.0}$ and no side effects.

Initial dosage regimens for chronic therapy are consistent with those listed in Table 2-1. Very frequently, when these doses are initiated, patients will identify discomforting effects such as nausea, abdominal pain, irritability, and restlessness at night. These undesirable symptoms can be minimized by beginning therapy with a lower dose, such as one half the total daily dose, and gradually increasing to the recommended maintenance dose.[8]

Once the full maintenance dose is achieved, an STC should be measured. The guidelines presented in Table 2-1 are designed to provide an average STC of 10 µg/ml; therefore, a proportion of patients will be below and others well within the therapeutic range. Dosage adjustments can then be made to result in a more desirable STC, dependent upon clinical response ($FEV_{1.0}$). For most patients, there is a linear relationship between the dose and the resultant STC. Thus, a 25 percent increase in dose should result in a 25 percent increase in STC. For some patients, however, as the dose is increased, the capacity for theophylline metabolism is eventually attained. In this situation, the resultant STC may greatly exceed that expected from the increase in dose. This phenomenon, referred to as dose-dependent elimination, may occur in certain patients even with STC in the therapeutic range.[9] Dosage increments should not exceed 25 percent, and further dose adjustments should be preceded by an STC measurement.

Adequate maintenance theophylline therapy will reduce symptoms in patients with chronic respiratory distress. Most patients will achieve better symptom control during the day, as well as the night. Patients with exercise-induced asthma may also notice improved exercise tolerance, although additional benefits may be derived from pretreatment with cromolyn or β-adrenergic agents or a combination thereof. The effect of single dose theophylline therapy before exercise is highly individualized among patients.

RECURRENT APNEA

Theophylline and caffeine are routinely used in the treatment of neonatal apnea. Their efficacy is considered secondary to stimulation of the central nervous system. In addition, suggested mechanisms of action include: increased sensitivity to carbon dioxide, increased transmission of neural impulses, and improved skeletal muscle contraction, to name a few.[10] Caffeine has advantages over theophylline since it has a wide therapeutic index with fewer peripheral effects. Unfortunately, a commercial preparation is not readily available, resulting in the dependence on theophylline.

Effective use of theophylline with its narrow margin of safety necessitates careful dose selection and monitoring STC. The theophylline dose should be much lower in premature newborns corresponding to the slow rate of elimination and a lower range of desired STC.[11,12] The recommended initial loading dose is 6 mg/kg theophylline and a maintenance dose of 1 mg/kg theophylline every eight hours.[10] Further dosage adjustments can be derived following measurement of STC. The desired range for effective therapy with minimal risk for adverse effects ranges between 5–15 μg/ml. The efficacy of theophylline may also be related to the conversion and subsequent accumulation of caffeine. The suggested range of plasma caffeine concentration is between 5–20 μg/ml, although no significant toxic effects are observed with concentrations up to 50 μg/ml.[10] Risks for toxicity may be further minimized by monitoring theophylline and caffeine concentrations simultaneously.

In patients with apnea who are unresponsive to theophylline therapy, preliminary information suggests that the addition of doxapram, an analeptic drug, may be beneficial.[12] The primary disadvantage of this agent is the requirement for intravenous administration and relatively short duration of action.

CHRONIC OBSTRUCTIVE PULMONARY DISEASE (COPD)

While the efficacy of theophylline is well established in the treatment of reactive airways disease, specific benefits for patients with COPD associated with chronic bronchitis and emphysema remain to be defined. Due to the nature of the disease, reversibility in $FEV_{1.0}$ is marginal along with subjective feelings of improvement.[13-15] The pathophysiologic mechanisms of COPD, however, differ from reactive airways disease since there is significant mucus gland hypertrophy, excessive mucus production, and airway collapse secondary to emphysema.

Beneficial effects may be related to the limited degree of reversibility present in some patients as well as improvement in respiratory muscle contractility, increase in cardiac output, and an increase in hypoxic ventilatory drive. More information is needed regarding the role of theophylline in the treatment as well as prevention of episodes of acute respiratory distress in these patients.

Contraindications

The only specific contraindication to the use of theophylline is for patients who develop hypersensitivity reactions to theophylline or xanthine derivatives. Severe hypersensitivity reactions are almost exclusively associated with aminophylline (theophylline ethylenediamine). To date there are no reported hypersensitivity reactions to theophylline. The reaction is attributed to the ethylenediamine component, a chemical used as a preservative for industrial purposes, with well known sensitizing capacities.

Although the adverse effects of theophylline include gastrointestinal distress, arrhythmias, and seizures, there are no specific contraindications for the use of theophylline in patients with gastrointestinal disorders (ulcers, colitis), cardiac dysrhythmias, or convulsive disorders. With available alternatives such as cromolyn, inhaled β_2-adrenergic agonists, and aerosol corticosteroids, it would be prudent to consider these agents over theophylline in patients with these conditions. If theophylline is required, a combination of low dose theophylline and an inhaled or low dose oral β_2-adrenergic agonist agents, cromolyn, or inhaled corticosteroids may be sufficient to obtain optimal clinical response and minimal risk for adverse effects.

Dosage and Special Considerations

Theophylline therapy requires special considerations for the choice of the dosage regimen, product formulation and the application of therapeutic drug monitoring. Safe and effective use of theophylline necessitates an understanding of principles related to these subjects.

DOSAGE REGIMEN

As previously described, the Food and Drug Administration has recognized the necessity to provide guidelines to individualize initial theophylline doses in patients and require that this information be included in product literature (Table 2-1). These recommendations consider the effect of age, smoking status, and the presence of certain diseases that may affect theophylline elimination such as cor pulmonale, congestive heart failure, or liver disease.

Since theophylline is eliminated primarily by biotransformation, its elimination may be altered by the numerous conditions that affect metabolic capacities. These include age, disease, and other medications. In general, theophylline elimination is slowest in premature newborns and increases with age.[11,16] On the basis of mg per kg body weight, dosage requirements in young children, ages 1–9 years, are the highest and then decrease in adolescence and gradually approach adult requirements.[17-19] With advancing age, metabolic rate is assumed to decrease; however, this is likely due to the development of diseases directly related to the liver or indirectly affecting hepatic function, such as congestive heart failure. A summary of pharmacokinetic parameters, as related to age, is included in Table 2-2. The term half-life is used to describe the time it takes to eliminate one half of the drug from the body or the time required to reduce the

Table 2-2
Theophylline half-life and clearance values related to age*

	Half-life (hours)	Clearance (ml/kg/hr)
Premature newborn	25	28
Term infants less than 6 months	10	48
6 months to 1 year	4	120
Children: 1 to 4 years	3.4	100
4 to 12 years	not available	100
12 to 17 years	3.7	60
Adults: healthy non-smoking	8	45
Elderly: non-smokers	8.6	35

*modified from data compiled by Hendeles and Weinberger, Pharmacotherapy 1983; 3:2–44

serum theophylline concentration by 50 percent. While this parameter is familiar to most clinicians, the elimination half-life in itself is not useful in estimating dosage requirements. The more reliable dosing estimate is obtained through a determination of theophylline clearance. Clearance indicates the volume of plasma cleared of theophylline per unit time. Additional information in regard to the application of principles of pharmacokinetics to treatment courses can be obtained with the assistance of several excellent reviews prepared for clinicians.[20-22]

In addition to age and disease, there are a number of conditions that may alter theophylline elimination. In general, any condition that affects drug metabolism or may be associated with hepatoxicity is likely to modify theophylline disposition. These factors are listed in Table 2-3, and those identified by an asterisk have been verified by specific clinical studies. The presence of these conditions should be considered in the identification of a maintenance theophylline dose. Removal of medications or resolution of diseases implicated in altered theophylline metabolism may also necessitate adjustments in the theophylline dose.

PRODUCT FORMULATION

One of the advantages of theophylline is the availability of several routes of administration, specifically, parenteral, oral, and rectal. Parenteral administration is limited to the intravenous route since the irritating effect of the solution does not facilitate intramuscular or subcutaneous administration. Theophylline may be administered rectally via suppositories or a specially formulated solution. Since absorption from rectal suppositories is erratic and often incomplete, the rectal solution is preferred if this route is considered necessary and compliance

Table 2-3
Conditions or Medications That Alter Drug Metabolism

Increased Drug Metabolism	Decreased Drug Metabolism
Enzyme Inducers	Disease
barbiturates*	liver disease*
carbamazepine*	pulmonary edema*
phenytoin*	congestive heart failure*
phenylbutazone	Enzyme Inhibitors
rifampin*	allopurinol
Smoking	chloramphenicol
cigarettes*	cimetidine*
marijuana*	phenylbutazone
Diet	Hepatotoxic Agents
high protein*	acetaminophen
low methylxanthine*	anabolic steroids
charcoal broiled foods*	L-asparaginase
brussel sprouts	azathioprine
cabbage	cyclophosphamide
	halothane
	isoniazid
	macrolide antibiotics*
	(erythromycin, troleandomycin)
	mercaptopurine
	methotrexate
	methyldopa
	oral contraceptives*
	phenytoin
	propranolol*
	rifampin
	Viral infections*
	Viral immunizations
	(Influenza trivalent vaccine*)

Presented with modifications from Szefler, S.J., Ped Clin N Amer 1983; 30(5):949
*Demonstrated specifically with theophylline

assured.[23,24] An additional advantage of the rectal solution over the suppository is the opportunity to individualize the dose. Prolonged rectal application may be associated with the development of proctitis.

The oral route is the most frequently used and formulations available include rapidly absorbed solutions and tablets, and sustained-release preparations. Advantages of rapidly absorbed solutions include the ability to individualize the dose to small increments, complete absorption, and immediate availability for pharmacologic effect. Disadvantages include the unpleasant taste and the necessity for frequent administration, especially in rapid theophylline metabolizers, in order to maintain therapeutic serum theophylline concentrations.

Sustained-release delivery systems were developed to take advantage of the ability to reduce the rate of absorption, and therefore, facilitate prolonged time intervals between doses while minimizing fluctuations in serum theophylline concentrations. The popularity of these products is substantiated by the number available, well over 20 different preparations. Initially success was recognized by the ability to dose three times a day. Additional technical modifications provided the opportunity to dose twice daily. The most recent development is the introduction of formulations suitable for once daily dosing. The proposed advantage is that of compliance and patient acceptance. The introduction of the *ultraslow* release products generated considerable controversy in relation to the reliability of theophylline absorption, specifically concerning the extent of absorption and the effect of food on the rate of absorption. These issues will be discussed in more detail.

Performance of sustained-release theophylline (SRT) formulations is described in one of two ways. One method is to present average serum theophylline concentrations from a group of patients over a single dosage interval. This method tends to provide a smooth STC-time profile over time and minimizes the variation in STC within individual patients. For twice-daily preparations a single 12-hour daytime dosage interval is usually examined.

Another method of examining SRT products is to generate absorption data after single doses of the study preparation. Mean absorption rates are derived and used to develop computer simulations of multiple dose treatment regimens. This methodology tends to minimize the influence of intrasubject variability in theophylline absorption and elimination. The variation in theophylline absorption from controlled-release delivery systems may be significant and may have considerable effect on the resultant STC-time profile.[25,26] Furthermore, elimination may be altered by the numerous conditions previously discussed (Tables 2-1 and 2-3).

Recently, Scott et al[27] identified a diurnal pattern in the STC-time profile in a group of pediatric patients. Higher STCs occurred during the daytime dosing interval, while the lowest STC followed the evening dose. Very often the lowest STC occurs at 12 MN. Studies by Rogers et al[28] attributed these variations in STC to inconsistencies in the rate of theophylline absorption from the SRT formulation. This was based on the identification of consistent theophylline clearance over a 24-hour study period with a continuous intravenous aminophylline infusion. Unfortunately, very little information is available on the absorption of theophylline from the available SRT formulations over multiple dosage intervals (24–48 hours). This information is essential to examine the performance of these products under actual clinical conditions.

THERAPEUTIC DRUG MONITORING

The early application of STC measurements identified the significant interpatient differences in the required dose necessary to achieve therapeutic STCs. It is now considered essential to monitor STC to optimize effect, minimize toxicity and avoid medicolegal retribution. Obviously, this should be combined with a measurement of clinical response, such as symptom control and pulmonary function. The application of STC monitoring was facilitated by technical advances that make it feasible to not only measure STC accurately and efficiently in the laboratory, but also in an office practice. It will soon be possible to rapidly analyze STC without an instrument,[29] making is possible to measure STC even in the home. Unfortunately, the responsibility for the interpretation of the resultant measurement has gradually shifted away from those trained in the principles of pharmacokinetics. The obvious consequence is the potential oversight of significant factors essential to the accurate interpretation of the STC measurement.

In order to analyze an STC, the following conditions should be clearly identified:[30]

1. Patient characteristics—age and weight (specifically lean or ideal body weight in the obese patient).
2. Dosage characteristics—amount, dosing interval, and dosage form (liquid, tablet, parenteral, or sustained-release).
3. Sampling conditions—time of last dose and time of blood sample.
4. Other medications—specifically drugs that may effect theophylline elimination and drugs (or metabolites) that may interfere with the theophylline assay.

The most frequent question relates to the appropriate time to measure an STC. This depends primarily on the question to be addressed. If it is related to the relative risk for toxicity, then it is desirable to measure the highest or peak STC. If therapeutic efficacy is questioned, then it is important to identify the lowest or trough STC. Ideally, it would be useful to obtain a measurement at the time of breakthrough symptoms. This is often difficult to achieve, especially if nighttime symptoms occur, however, this will become easier with the new analytical techniques.[29]

The time of the peak STC depends on the route, formulation, and method of administration. For parenteral administration with bolus doses infused over 15–20 minutes, the peak STC occurs after completing the infusion. It is recommended that sufficient time be allowed for distribution to reach equilibrium, and since theophylline distribution is rapid, a peak STC can be measured 15 minutes after terminating the infusion. In this situation, the pre-dose measurement is the lowest or trough concentration. Similarly, for rapidly absorbed oral solutions and tablets, the peak concentration is usually one to two hours after the dose and the lowest concentration occurs prior to the dose. The difference between peak and trough STC may be significant in patients with short elimination half-lives. These measurements may indicate the necessity to increase the dose, the frequency of administration, or a combination of both.

For sustained-release theophylline (SRT) formulations, the time for peak and trough concentration is dependent on the formulation and the dosage interval. It is usually recommended that the peak concentration can be measured four hours after an administered dose. With the availability of new formulations and recommended dosing intervals, this guideline must be qualified. With recognized twice daily SRT formulations demonstrating relatively consistent rates and extent of absorption (for example, TheoDur, Key Pharmaceuticals; Slo-Bid, William H. Rorer, Inc.)., the four-hour post-dose concentration following the morning dose is usually the highest concentration for the day. The STC obtained four hours after the evening dose, however, is not the highest STC. In fact, it may represent the lowest STC of the day.[27,28]

Obtaining an STC measurement four hours after a dose of a once-daily SRT preparation (for example, Theo-24, G. D. Searle & Co. Chicago, Illinois 60680; Uniphyl, The Purdue-Frederick Co. Norwalk, Connecticut 06854) may be misleading. The peak STC actually occurs 8–12 hours following the dose. The predose STC in this situation is actually the lowest STC of the 24-hour period. For these preparations, the percent variation in the lowest to highest STC increases as the patient's elimination half-life decreases (unpublished observations). These observations are significant in the proper use of STC measurements for evaluation of potential toxicity and dosage adjustments to improve clinical response.

Dosage Adjustment Based on Concentration Measurements

Optimal utilization of STC for dosage adjustment requires an understanding of conditions that may alter theophylline disposition. The following is a brief summary of an approach to the interpretation of STC measurements.[30]

Theophylline concentrations less than 5 µg/ml

Before adjusting the dose based on this measurement, determine whether the prescribed dose, sampling time, and compliance are adequate. Clinical response should be the primary determinant for evaluating the necessity to increase the dose. It is important to carefully assess patients with low concentrations before altering the dose. It is occasionally assumed that the predose concentration represents the average or steady-state STC. While this may be satisfactory for patients with relatively slow metabolism, it is an erroneous assumption for those patients with accelerated theophylline metabolism, especially for patients receiving rapidly absorbed formulations. An attempt to increase the pre-dose STC above 10 μg/ml in these patients could result in peak STC above 30 μg/ml.[31]

Low STC may also be related to impaired theophylline absorption, accelerated metabolism, or a combination thereof. Rapid metabolism should be considered in young children,[17] adolescents and adults who smoke cigarettes or marijuana,[32-35] and also patients who receive concomitant medications that accelerate theophylline metabolism. Phenytoin, carbamazepine, phenobarbital, and rifampin have the potential to induce theophylline elimination.[36-40] There is also the possibility that any drug that accelerates drug metabolism may also effect theophylline elimination (Table 2-3).

Theophylline concentrations greater than 20 μg/ml

Concentrations consistently approaching or exceeding 20 μg/ml are of special concern because of the associated risk for adverse effects. In this circumstance, it is important to reevaluate the prescribed dose and sampling time. In addition, the possibility of concomitant use of two or more theophylline products, either prescribed or self-administered over the counter preparations, should be examined. Exclusion of these possibilities indicates a need for assessment of conditions associated with impaired theophylline metabolism, such as liver disease, congestive heart failure, viral infections, and drug interactions (Table 2-3).

Inconsistent concentrations

Occasionally, certain patients will have documented inconsistencies in STC despite continuation of the same dosage regimen. This is of particular concern in the management of patients with unsatisfactory clinical response. It is difficult to individualize the dose when some concentrations are subtherapeutic and others exceed 20 μg/ml. Poor compliance with the prescribed regimen is the first consideration in these situations and inconsistencies in the sampling times another possibility. It is also important to examine the possibility of laboratory inaccuracies.[41]

Another source of variability is that associated with inconsistent absorption from sustained-release theophylline preparations. Presentation of average STC data during a single daytime dosing interval in scientific and product literature may be misleading since it minimizes intrapatient variability in STC.[25,26,28] This variability in STC during a dosing interval must be appreciated if the clinician is to properly base dosage adjustments on STC measurements. This phenomenon is more likely to occur in patients with a theophylline half-life less than four hours. The clinician should be particularly cautious in the interpretation of single STC measurements in young children and under conditions where accelerated theophylline metabolism is suspected. A detailed pharmacokinetic evaluation may be useful in verifying this observation.

Pharmacokinetic profile

In situations where STC measurements are inconsistent or persistently low despite relatively high theophylline dosage regimens, such factors as noncompliance, incomplete theophylline absorption, laboratory errors, or rapid theophylline metabolism must be considered. In these circumstances it may be useful to determine the individual patient's theophylline elimination parameters. An STC-time profile is obtained after an intravenous aminophylline dose and used to calculate theophylline clearance, half-life and volume of distribution.[42]

The individual elimination parameters can be compared to available literature data and the patient characterized as a rapid, slow or normal metabolizer of theophylline. The parameters can also be used to calculate a dose necessary to obtain a desired STC.

In addition, it may be useful to evaluate the STC-time profile while the patient is receiving an oral SRT formulation. Samples obtained over serial sampling times, for example, every two hours, over several dosage intervals (24–48 hours) will identify dose-to-dose inconsistencies in STC. This information combined with an intravenous aminophylline study permits assessment of inconsistencies in theophylline absorption.[28]

ADVERSE EFFECTS AND THEIR MANAGEMENT

Undesirable effects related to theophylline therapy involve the gastrointestinal, cardiac, and central nervous systems. In most situations, the incidence of adverse effects is dose, or more properly, serum theophylline concentration related. Although it is recognized that the risk of adverse effects increases as the concentration exceeds 20 μg/ml, a number of patients will observe undesirable effects with concentrations below 20 μg/ml, and others may not experience side effects at higher levels. Indeed, some patients appear to be intolerant of theophylline regardless of the dose administered. These undesirable effects usually consist of gastrointestinal distress, restlessness, and insomnia.

The more concerning adverse effects, such as seizures, are usually related to concentrations exceeding 30 μg/ml. As previously discussed, the adverse effects can be minimized by initiating theophylline at lower doses, then gradually increasing to the recommended dose based on clinical response. In addition, therapeutic regimens should be continuously evaluated for medications or conditions that may alter theophylline disposition.

Of concern at the present time in the care of pediatric patients are case experiences suggesting that theophylline may have effects on behavior and memory.[43,44] Additional studies are needed to assess the significance of these effects on long range development. In addition, similar studies should be conducted with other medications used in the treatment of asthma.

Dose related theophylline toxicity can occur as a result of intentional overdose or an alteration in theophylline elimination. It is important to obtain information on the total dose ingested, dosage form (liquid, tablet, sustained-release), time of ingestion, and other drugs ingested. If a sustained-release product is ingested, it is necessary to determine whether the tablet was crushed or chewed, since this will result in destruction of the delivery system and rapid theophylline absorption. Once it is decided that the patient is at risk for theophylline toxicity, immediate induction of emesis is indicated.

Since severe theophylline toxicity, including seizures, may reportedly occur with minimal evidence of other signs of toxicity, a measurement of serum theophylline concentration is essential to analyze the degree of risk. Emesis in the conscious patient or gastric lavage with a sufficiently large orogastric tube should be instituted to remove available theophylline tablets. To prevent further theophylline absorption activated charcoal should be administered in a dose of 30 Gm along with a saline cathartic such as magnesium sulfate, irregardless of the alleged time of ingestion. This is particularly important with SRT preparations since absorption can occur for 12 hours and longer after a dose.

Additional management should include serial measurements of STC to evaluate the rate of theophylline elimination, the efficacy of treatment, and the potential for continuing absorption from orally administered preparations. STC measurements along with clinical signs and symptoms will be most helpful in decisions regarding further treatment. Besides gastric evacuation, activated charcoal and a cathartic, a careful evaluation must include the risk-benefit of other methods to remove theophylline. Available procedures include peritoneal dialysis, hemodialysis, and hemoperfusion. While peritoneal dialysis is readily available, it is the least effective of the three identified. It appears that albumin collodian activated charcoal hemoperfusion is the most efficacious and has limited risk for thrombocytopenia, anemia, and hypocalcemia.

A practical, safe, easy, and apparently effective method of treatment, has been described that involves the administration of multiple oral doses of activated charcoal.[45] This system, referred to as *gastrointestinal dialysis,* is useful but not as effective as the hemoperfusion method. The repeated administration of oral activated charcoal (every 2–3 hours) may enhance theophylline clearance approximately twofold.[45] Clinical experience, however, suggests that it is more likely to be effective when STC is less than 50 µg/ml. Patients with STC greater than 50 µg/ml often vomit the oral activated charcoal.[46]

Suggested guidelines for the initiation of more aggressive measures, including hemodialysis or hemoperfusion, are based on the patient's age and clinical condition. In general, hemoperfusion should be considered in adult patients with STC exceeding 60 µg/ml and in pediatric patients with STC greater than 80 µg/ml, 2–4 hours after ingestion,[47,48] and at lower STC in patients less than one month, or greater than 60 years of age. Additional conditions prompting aggressive management include patients with a theophylline half-life greater than 24 hours, significant liver disease, congestive heart failure, refractory seizures or arrhythmias, evidence of ingestion of other toxic drugs, history suggestive of chronic overdose, and inability to correct metabolic disturbances. The risk-benefit of the procedure, including the experience of the treatment team, must be assessed. It is also suggested that hemoperfusion, combined with frequent administration of oral activated charcoal, if tolerated, may provide an additive effect.

With each method, STC should be measured every 1–2 hours initially. A graphic summary is extremely useful in estimating the rate of elimination and the approximate time to reach safe concentrations (i.e., less than 20 µg/ml).

INTERACTIONS WITH OTHER DRUGS AND CHOICE OF CONCOMITANT AGENTS

Specific interactions were described in relation to the effect of other medications on theophylline elimination (Table 2-3). Phenytoin, carbamazepine, phenobarbital, and rifampin may increase theophylline metabolism. Cimetidine, macrolide antibiotics (erythromycin and troleandomycin), and oral contraceptives may decrease theophylline elimination.[49–53] A detailed summary of reported drug interactions, interpretation, and recommendations for management were recently compiled by Jonkman and Upton,[54] and Hendeles and Weinberger.[55]

Another consideration is the effect of theophylline on other medications. In patients receiving lithium, serum lithium concentration may decrease upon initiating theophylline therapy.[56] It is not clear whether this effect persists with continuing theophylline administration. The mechanism is attributed to the diuretic effect of theophylline and consequent increase in lithium renal clearance. Theophylline also has an effect on decreasing serum phenytoin levels.[57] In this circumstance, it is suggested that theophylline inhibits phenytoin absorption when both are administered simultaneously. Both lithium and phenytoin interactions can be avoided through the use of alternative antiasthma medications, such as cromolyn, β_2-adrenergic agonists or inhaled corticosteroids.

Several past investigations identified the effect of food on theophylline elimination. Prolonged administration of high protein–low carbohydrate diets enhance theophylline elimination, while low protein-high carbohydrate diets tend to decrease theophylline metabolism.[58] Changes from high methylxanthine to low methylxanthine diets result in an increase in theophylline disposition.[59] Unfortunately, in both circumstances the changes in diet were over prolonged study periods and at the present time it is not known whether immediate effects may occur from short-term dietary changes, for example, a single high protein-low carbohydrate meal or a single day of high caffeine ingestion. The quantitative dose-related effect of caffeine ingestion on theophylline elimination has not been elucidated.

Of recent concern is the effect of food on theophylline absorption, particularly in relation to SRT preparations. Pedersen[60] first identified the effect of food on the rate of theophylline absorption from an SRT formulation. Since it did not affect the extent of theophylline absorption and the preparation was not utilized in the United States, the significance of this interaction was not appreciated. Interest regarding the food-theophylline absorption interaction was enhanced by investigations related to two SRT preparations available for use in the U.S. Pedersen and Moller-Petersen[61] identified the effect of food, and specifically the water content of such, on the rate and extent of theophylline absorption from Theo-Dur Sprinkle (Key Pharmaceuticals Miami, Florida 33169), a preparation designed for use in pediatric patients. This interaction can apparently be minimized by administering the medication on an empty stomach, at least five minutes before a meal. Since these studies were performed with single doses, information on absorption during multiple dose therapy, consistent with actual clinical conditions, should be obtained.

The previous interactions identified the effect of food on decreasing the rate or extent of theophylline absorption from the SRT preparations evaluated. Of greater concern is the observation of Hendeles et al.[62] on the effect of food on the absorption of theophylline from a once daily formulation, Theo-24 (Searle Pharmaceuticals). Administering this formulation after a specific meal resulted in a significant increase in the rate and extent of absorption during single dose studies. Investigations are in progress to identify the conditions contributing to this effect (i.e., timing of meal, food composition, etc.). These studies will likely define conditions that will minimize this effect, but these observations have raised questions regarding the effect of food on the rate and extent of theophylline absorption from all SRT products. The consistency of both the rate and extent of theophylline absorption are significant determinants in the resultant STC-time profiles, and thus important in the application of therapeutic drug monitoring in individualizing theophylline dosage regimens.

PROSPECTUS

There is no doubt that significant progress has resulted in the safe and effective use of theophylline in the treatment of respiratory disorders. The advantages in ease of administration, rapid onset of action, long duration of action and ability to individualize dose, have contributed to the popularity of theophylline.

Questions for the future center around the effects of theophylline on behavior and memory. In addition, with the numerous sustained-release formulations available and the recent issues regarding the effect of food on theophylline absorption, attention will be focused on methods of medication administration and selection.

Disadvantages of theophylline include the relatively low margin of safety and the severity of adverse effects. Attempts have been made to develop other xanthine derivatives, however, a suitable alternative is not presently available. The most promising derivative is enprofylline; however, its rapid elimination and consequent necessity for frequent administration, balance proposed advantages of reduced risks for life-threatening adverse effects. Until a suitable dosage form is developed for enprofylline or another analog derived, theophylline will continue to maintain a primary position in the treatment of reactive airways disease and recurrent apnea in the newborn.

ACKNOWLEDGMENT

Supported in part by grant HL 30513 from the National Heart, Lung, and Blood Institute. The secretarial assistance of Helga Cole in manuscript preparation is greatly appreciated. Dr. Szefler is in The Ira J. and Jacqueline Neimark Laboratory of Clinical Pharmacology in Pediatrics.

REFERENCES

1. Bergstrand H: Phosphodiesterase inhibition and theophylline. Eur J Respir Dis 61 (Suppl 109):37–44, 1980
2. Rall TW: The Xanthines. In: Gilman AG, Goodman LS, Gilman A. eds. The pharamcological basis of therapeutics. 6th ed New York, Macmillan, 592–607, 1980
3. Lunell E, Svedmyr N, Andersson KE et al: A novel bronchodilator xanthine apparently without adenosine receptor antagonism and tremorogenic effect. Eur J Respir Dis 64:333–339, 1983
4. Murciano D, Aubier M, Lecocguic Y, et al: Effects of theophylline on diaphragmatic strength and fatigue in patients with chronic obstructive pulmonary disease. N Engl J Med 311:349–353, 1984
5. Supinski GS, Deal EC, Kelsen SG: The effects of caffeine and theophylline on diaphragm contractility. Am Rev Respir Dis 130:429–433, 1984
6. McWilliams BC, Menendez R, Kelly HW, et al: Effects of theophylline on inhaled methacholine and histamine in asthmatic children. Am Rev Resp Dis 130:193–197, 1984
7. FDA Drug Bulletin: IV dosage guidelines for theophylline products. 10:4–6, February 1980
8. Weinberger M: The pharmacology and therapeutic use of theophylline. J Allergy Clin Immunol 73:525–540, 1984
9. Weinberger M, Ginchansky E: Dose-dependent kinetics of theophylline disposition in asthmatic children. J Pediatr 91:820–824, 1977
10. Aranda JV, Grondin D, Sasyniuk BI: Pharmacologic considerations in the therapy of neonatal apnea. Ped Clin N Amer 28:113–133, 1981
11. Aranda JV, Sitar DS, Parsons WD, et al: Pharmacokinetic aspects of theophylline in premature newborns. N Engl J Med 295:413–416, 1976

12. Eyal F, Alpan G, Sagi E, et al: Aminophylline versus doxapram in idiopathic apnea of prematurity: a double-blind controlled study. Pediatrics 75:709-713, 1985
13. Alexander MR, Dull WL, Kasik JE. Treatment of chronic obstructive pulmonary disease with orally administered theophylline. JAMA 244:2286-2290, 1980
14. Eaton ML, Green BA, Church TR, et al: Efficacy of theophylline in 'irreversible' airflow obstruction. Ann Intern Med 92:758-761, 1980
15. Jenne JW: Theophylline in chronic obstructive lung disease, In: Jonkman JHG, Jenne JW, Simons FER. (eds) Sustained release theophylline in the treatment of chronic reversible airways obstruction. Amsterdam: Excerpta Medica, 164-172, 1984
16. Giacoia G, Jusko WJ, Menke J, et al: Theophylline pharmacokinetics in premature infants with apnea. J Pediatrics 89:829-832, 1976
17. Ellis EF, Koysooko R, Levy G: Pharmacokinetics of theophylline in children with asthma. Pediatrics 58:542-547, 1976
18. Loughnan PM, Sitar DS, Ogilvie RI, et al: Pharmacokinetic analysis of the disposition of intravenous theophylline in young children. J Pediatr 88:874-879, 1976
19. Ginchansky E, Weinberger M: Relationship of theophylline clearance to oral dosage in children with chronic asthma. J Pediatr 91:655-660, 1977
20. Gibaldi M, Levy G: Pharmacokinetics in clinical practice. 1. Concepts. JAMA 235:1864-1867, 1976
21. Gibaldi M, Levy G: Pharmacokinetics in clinical practice. 2. Applications. JAMA 235:1987-1992, 1976
22. Koup JR: Principles of therapeutics, In: Middleton E, Reed CE, Ellis EF (eds) Allergy: Principles and Practice. St. Louis: CV Mosby, 485-501, 1983
23. Lillehei JP: Aminophylline: oral vs rectal administration. JAMA 205:118-121, 1968
24. Segal MS, Weiss EB, Carta C: Rectal aminopylline (blood levels with concentrated solutions). Ann Allergy 29:135-138, 1971
25. Dederich RA, Szefler SJ, Green ER: Intrasubject variation in sustained-release theophylline absorption. J Allergy Clin Immunol 67:465-471, 1981
26. Pollack GM, Baswell B, Szefler SJ, et al: Comparison of inter- and intra-subject variation in oral absorption of theophylline from sustained-release products. Int J Pharmaceut 21:3-16, 1984
27. Scott PH, Tabachnik E, MacLeod S, et al: Sustained-release theophylline for childhood asthma: Evidence for circadian variation of theophylline pharmacokinetics. J Pediatr 99:476-479, 1981
28. Rogers RJ, Kalisker A, Wiener MB, et al: Inconsistent absorption from a sustained-release theophylline preparation during continuous therapy in asthmatic children. J Pediatr 106:496-501, 1985
29. Conboy C, Ellis EF, Jenne J, et al: Evaluation of a whole blood theophylline test requiring no instrument. J Allergy Clin Immunol 75:128, 1985 (abstract)
30. Szefler SJ: Practical considerations in the safe and effective use of theophylline. Ped Clin N Amer 30:943-954, 1983
31. Szefler SJ: Using serum measurements to tailor theophylline therapy. J Respir Dis 4(5):13-23, 1983
32. Hunt SN, Jusko WJ, Yurchak AM: Effect of smoking on theophylline disposition. Clin Pharmacol Ther 19:546-551, 1976

33. Jenne J, Nagasawa H, McHugh R, et al: Decreased theophylline half-life in cigarette smokers. Life Sci 17:195-198, 1975
34. Jusko WJ, Schentag JJ, Clark JH, et al: Enhanced biotransformation of theophylline in marijuana and tobacco smokers. Clin Pharmacol Ther 24:406-410, 1978
35. Powell JR, Thiercelin JF, Vozeh S, et al: The influence of cigarette smoking and sex on theophylline disposition. Am Rev Respir Dis 116:17-23, 1977
36. Marquis, JF, Carruthers SG, Spence JD, et al: Phenytoin-theophylline interaction. N Eng J Med 307:1189-1190, 1982
37. Rosenberry KR, Defusco CJ, Mansmann HC, et al: Reduced theophylline half-life induced by carbamazepine therapy. J Pediatr 102:472-474, 1983
38. Landay RA, Gonzalez MA, Taylor JC. Effect of phenobarbital on theophylline disposition. J Allergy Clin Immunol 62:27-29, 1978
39. Hauser AR, Lee C, Teague RB, et al: The effect of rifampin on theophylline disposition. Clin Pharmacol Ther 33:254, 1983 (abstract)
40. Robson RA, Miners JO, Wing LMH, et al: Theophylline-rifampicin interaction: non-selective induction of theophylline metabolic pathways. Br J Clin Pharmac 18:445-448, 1984
41. Bonham A, Hendeles L, Vaughan L, et al: The reliability of serum theophylline determinations from clinical laboratories. Am Rev Respir Dis 122:829-832, 1980
42. Georgitis JW, Szefler SJ, Baswell B, et al: Use of pharmacokinetic profile in evaluating patients with repeatedly low theophylline concentrations. Ann Allergy 53:231-235, 1984
43. Furukawa CT, Shapiro GG, DuHamel T, et al: Learning and behaviour problems associated with theophylline therapy. Lancet i:621, 1984
44. Furukawa CT, Shapiro GG, Bierman CW, et al: A double-blind study comparing the effectiveness of cromolyn sodium and sustained-release theophylline in childhood asthma. Pediatrics 74:453-459, 1984
45. Berlinger WG, Spector R, Goldberg MJ, et al: Enhancement of theophylline clearance by oral activated charcoal. Clin Pharmacol Ther 33:351-354, 1983
46. Sessler CN, Glauser FL, Cooper KR: Treatment of theophylline toxicity with oral activated charcoal. Chest 87:325-329, 1985
47. Park GD, Spector R, Roberts RJ, et al: Use of hemoperfusion for treatment of theophylline intoxication. Amer J Med 74:961-966, 1983
48. Gaudreault P, Wason S, Lovejoy FH: Acute pediatric theophylline overdose: A summary of 28 cases. J Pediatr 102:474-476, 1983
49. Reitberg DP, Bernhard H, Schentag JJ: Alteration of theophylline clearance and half-life by cimetidine in normal volunteers. Ann Intern Med 95:582-585, 1981
50. LaForce CF, Miller MF, Chai H: Effect of erythromycin on theophylline clearance in asthmatic children. J Pediatr 99:153-156, 1981
51. Prince RA, Wing DS, Weinberger MM, et al: Effect of erythromycin on theophylline kinetics. J Allergy Clin Immunol 68:427-431, 1981
52. Renton KW, Gray JD, Hung OR: Depression of theophylline elimination by erythromycin. Clin Pharmacol Ther 30:422-426, 1981
53. Weinberger M, Hudgel D, Spector S, et al: Inhibition of theophylline clearance by troleandomycin. J Allergy Clin Immunol 59:228-231, 1977
54. Jonkman JHG, Upton RA: Pharmacokinetic drug interactions with theophylline. Clin Pharmacokin 9:309-334, 1984

55. Hendeles L, Weinberger, M: Theophylline: a "state of the art" review. Pharmacotherapy 3:2–44, 1983
56. Thomsen K, Schou M: Renal lithium excretion in man. Am J Physiol 215:823–827, 1968
57. Hendeles L, Wyatt R, Weinberger M, et al: Decreased oral phenytoin absorption following concurrent theophylline administration. J Allergy Clin Immunol 63:156, 1979 (abstract)
58. Kappas A, Anderson KE, Conney AH, et al: Influence of dietary protein and carbohydrate on antipyrine and theophylline metabolism in man. Clin Pharmacol Ther 20:643–653, 1976
59. Caldwell J, Lancaster R, Monks TJ, et al: The influence of dietary methylxanthines on the metabolism and pharmacokinetics of intravenously administered theophylline. Br J Clin Pharmacol 4:637–638, 1977
60. Pedersen S: Delay in the absorption rate of theophylline from a sustained-release theophylline preparation caused by food. Br J Clin Pharmac 12:904–905, 1981
61. Pedersen S, Moller-Petersen J: Erratic absorption of a slow-release theophylline sprinkle product. Pediatrics 74:534–538, 1984
62. Hendeles L, Weinberger M, Milavetz G, et al: Food induced "dose-dumping" from a once-a-day theophylline product as a cause of theophylline toxicity. Chest 87:758–765, 1985

Lynn M. Marshall

3

Cromolyn Sodium and Other Mast-Cell-Stabilizers

The mast cell is defined as a connective tissue element, which possesses cytoplasmic granules that stain metachromatically under ordinary conditions. It is a fixed cell containing a wide range of potent, biologically active substances, or mediators, which when released from the cell, cause havoc with the surrounding tissue, by generating both immediate and late phase allergic reactions. The mast cells are widely distributed throughout the body, and are found in all organs rich in connective tissue and in mucosal membranes: the submucosa of the respiratory and gastrointestinal tracts, skin, lymphoid organs, bone marrow, serous membranes, and tissue surrounding the eyes.

The normal function of the mast cell in man is not fully understood. It has been implied by Pepys that they may have a vital physiological function in the homeostatic control of connective tissue metabolism and protection against tissue damage by noxious agents. The mediators contained within the mast cell granules are vasoactive agents such as histamine, serotonin, SRS-A (leukotrienes C, D, and E), prostaglandins, chemotactic factors, heparin, bradykinins, and platelet activating factor (Table 3-1). Some are preformed in the cell and others are new mediators generated by actions of primary or preformed mediators on target tissues.

Mast cell degranulation or release of mediators can be triggered by many factors such as IgE/Antigen complex, food antigens, chemical irritation, physical injury, infective agents, and complement components. The mediators released by the degranulation of the mast cell are chemically and biologically

DRUGS FOR THE RESPIRATORY SYSTEM Copyright © 1986 by Grune & Stratton, Inc.
ISBN 0-8089-1818-4 All rights of reproduction in any form reserved.

Table 3-1
Mediators Released by the Mast Cell

Mediator	Actions
A. Pre-formed mediators: rapidly released	
Histamine	Smooth muscle contraction; increased vascular permeability; stimulate sensory receptors; mucous secretion; prostaglandin synthesis; affects eosinophil migration
ECF-A	Attracts eosinophils & neutrophils
NCF-A	Attracts eosinophils & neutrophils
B. Pre-formed mediators: slowly released	
Heparin	Anticoagulation
Trypsin-chymotrypsin	Proinflammatory
Inflammatory factor	Generation of late-phase allergic reactions
C. Newly generated mediators: generated by pre-formed mediators	
SRS-A (leukotrienes C, D & E)	Smooth muscle contraction; increased vascular permeability
Prostaglandins	Control bronchomotor tone
Bradykinin	Smooth muscle contraction; vasodilation
Serotonin	Smooth muscle contraction
PAF	Platelet aggregation & degranulation

diverse, and are discharged over a period of time. They can generate both the immediate and late-phase allergic reaction, and thereby induce all the pathophysiologic changes seen in asthma such as bronchoconstriction, mucous secretion, edema, and inflammation.[1]

Since it is unlikely that therapeutic agents can be found to combat all of these mast cell mediators individually, the advent of mast cell stabilizers to prevent mast cell degranulation has become a well recognized therapeutic approach to the treatment of asthma and other conditions involving the release of mast cell mediators such as allergic rhinitis and conjunctivitis. Currently, the only drug categorized as a mast cell stabilizer approved for use in the U.S. is cromolyn sodium. Other drugs are being tested presently, and some of these will be discussed.

CROMOLYN SODIUM

Cromolyn was discovered in 1965 after a decade of search for an improved bronchodilator agent, and is derived from khellin (a naturally-occurring chro-

Cromolyn Sodium and Other Mast-Cell-Stabilizers

mone derivative with smooth muscle relaxant properties, extracted from the plant Ammi visnaga). Cromolyn sodium, whose molecular structure is depicted in Figure 3-1, was the most active of the bis-chromones synthesized. When inhaled at various intervals before antigen challenge, it also proved to be effective in protecting against the asthmatic response to specific antigen in man.

Cromolyn sodium is thought to modulate the release of mast cell mediators by preventing the degranulation of mast cells triggered by a variety of immunological and nonimmunological mechanisms.[2] A second mode of action has also been described; cromolyn sodium appears to be able to block nonimmunologic challenge through a neurophysiologic pathway.[3]

Although used extensively in Great Britain, cromolyn was primarily labeled a *steroid-sparing drug* and generally utilized as the "last resort," to be used only after corticosteroids had already been added to the patients' regimen. It is unfortunate that, when it was first introduced in the United States, its effectiveness did not reach the level of most physicians' expectations, so that cromolyn sodium quickly fell from the pedestal on which many had placed it. Investigation and experience has shown, however, that cromolyn was simply placed incorrectly on the treatment ladder.

The safety of cromolyn sodium in long-term use is one of its most salient features and this, together with its clinical efficacy,[4-8] makes it an eminently acceptable drug for the treatment and prophylaxis of asthma. In view of its extremely low toxicity, a therapeutic trial should be considered in patients with asthma whether or not allergic factors can be demonstrated.[9] Thus, it should probably be tried in both allergic and non-allergic asthmatics when chronic symptoms persist in perennial or seasonal asthma, as well as prior to exercise in suspected exercise-induced bronchospasm (EIB) or exposure to lung irritants. Clearly, then, there has been a conceptual switch from using cromolyn in the most severe asthmatics to beginning cromolyn as a first-line drug in the newly diagnosed asthmatics.

Mode of Action

Cromolyn sodium was originally thought to have one specific mode of action, mast cell stabilization. Recently, however, understanding of this agent's

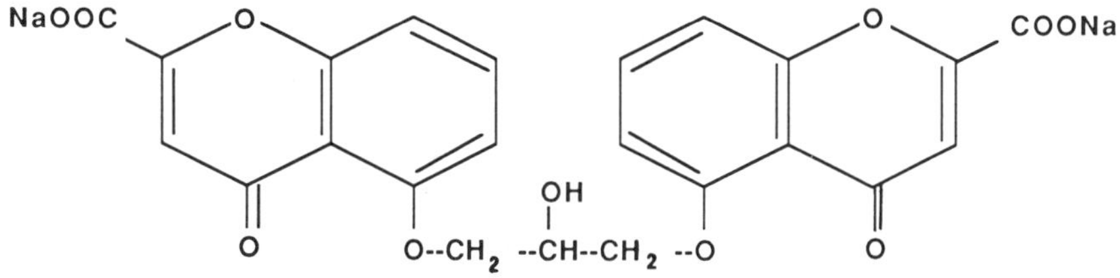

Fig. 3-1 The molecular structure of cromolyn sodium. Cromolyn sodium is the disodium salt of 1, 3 bis (2-carboxychromon-5-yloxy)-2-hydroxypropane. Cromolyn sodium has a molecular weight of 512.34. Cromolyn sodium is soluble in water.

mechanism of action has become more complicated because a second mode of action has been demonstrated; the drug can apparently modulate several types of reflex-induced asthma that are generally presumed to have no relationship to mast cell activity.

Mast Cell Stabilizer

Early animal studies demonstrated that cromolyn was able to specifically inhibit IgE antibody/antigen mechanisms,[10] and as such, represented a novel agent for the treatment of allergic asthma. This action of the drug is the best understood, and involves its ability to stabilize the mast cell, and prevent the liberation of mediators of anaphylaxis from sensitized and nonsensitized mast cells after immunologic (antigen) or nonimmunologic (Compound 48/80) challenge (Figure 3-2). The mechanism underlying its ability to stabilize the mast cell membrane has not been conclusively explained. Most investigators hypothesize that the drug affects the "calcium gate"[11] or calcium regulation by enhancing the phosphorylation of a large molecular weight protein that may be a blocker of calcium transport.[12]

Recently, Diaz et al showed that symptom scores decreased significantly, and that morning and evening peak expiratory flow rates improved, while the percentages of bronchial mucous eosinophils and bronchoalveolar lavage eosinophils, as well as levels of house dust mite specific IgE fell in patients receiving cromolyn sodium.[13] Thus, cromolyn, by stabilizing lung mast cells, would appear to inhibit the release of the eosinophil chemotactic factor of anaphylaxis and other eosinophilotactic agents, thereby reducing eosinophil infiltration.[13]

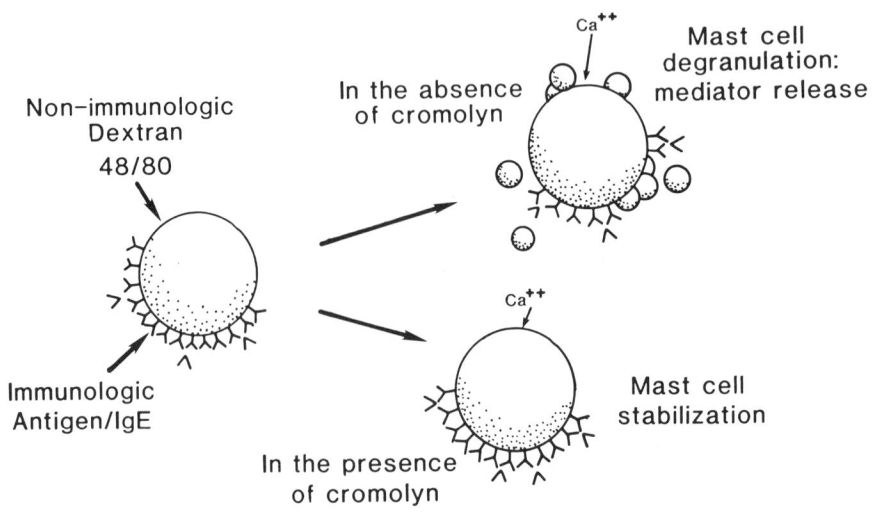

Fig. 3-2 Cromolyn sodium: mast cell stabilization.

This agent's ability to stabilize the mast cell also results in a reduction of bronchial hyperreactivity; it has the unique ability to block both the immediate and late asthmatic response after a variety of bronchoprovocations.[14] Since the late asthmatic reaction is associated with an increase in bronchial hyperreactivity,[15] the long term effect of reducing bronchial hyperreactivity is probably an indirect consequence of its ability to block the late asthmatic reaction. Thus, cromolyn, by blocking the late reaction in asthma and reducing hyperreactivity, works to "cool down" the airways and makes the patient's disease easier to control.

The link between the late asthmatic response and bronchial hyperreactivity is almost certainly bronchial inflammation. Leukotrienes and other secondary mediators that are released by the mast cell cause a local accumulation of the cell types that constitute the inflammatory reaction. Inflammation causes local tissue damage particularly to the bronchial epithelium, and the airway irritant receptors or other sensory receptors, which are mostly situated below the epithelial cells, become exposed and hypersensitive.

Modulator of Reflex-Induced Asthma

Although it was thought that it was the mast cell stabilizing properties of cromolyn that were crucial, it has been shown that other compounds many hundred times more potent at preventing mast cell degranulation than cromolyn sodium are clinically ineffective.[16] Recent reports have suggested that cromolyn may act on other aspects of bronchial hyperreactivity, independent of the mast cell.[17-21] Thus, cromolyn has been shown to prevent reflex-induced obstruction due to (1) chemicals, such as sulfur dioxide[17] and toluene diisocyanate;[18] (2) ultrasonically nebulized water;[19] (3) cold air;[20] and 4 exercise.[21] Similarly a non-mast cell effect of inhibition by cromolyn of histamine aerosol-induced airway constriction of vagal reflex origin has been demonstrated in dogs. It is likely that vagal reflex mechanisms are important in some or all of these responses, although mediator release from mast cells may be involved in the bronchoconstrictor response, particularly to exercise. In any case, it is clear that not all of the actions of cromolyn can be explained on the basis of mast cell stabilization. As suggested by Dixon et al,[22] cromolyn sodium may suppress the excitatory effects of "C" fibers, unmyelinated vagal sensory nerve endings that cause reflex bronchoconstriction in dogs. If it can be shown that activation of "C" fibers in man results in bronchoconstriction, then this neuropharmacological action of cromolyn may explain its ability to inhibit reflex-induced bronchoconstriction in man.

Thus, it would appear that cromolyn can block or reduce release of mediators and interrupt the resultant sequence of events that lead to inflammatory changes and cell damage in immediate hypersensitivity reactions such as bronchial asthma. In turn, it may prevent an increase in bronchial mucosal permeability, or opening of tight junctions in the epithelium of the airways,[23] and limit access of allergens and nonspecific stimuli to sub-epithelial mast cells and others such as nerve and respiratory smooth muscle cells. In addition, it appears to block reflex-induced bronchoconstriction through a neuro-pharmacological action, which may, in fact, be its most important therapeutic effect (see Figure 3-3).

Indications

The various forms of cromolyn that are available and their indications are shown in Table 3-2.

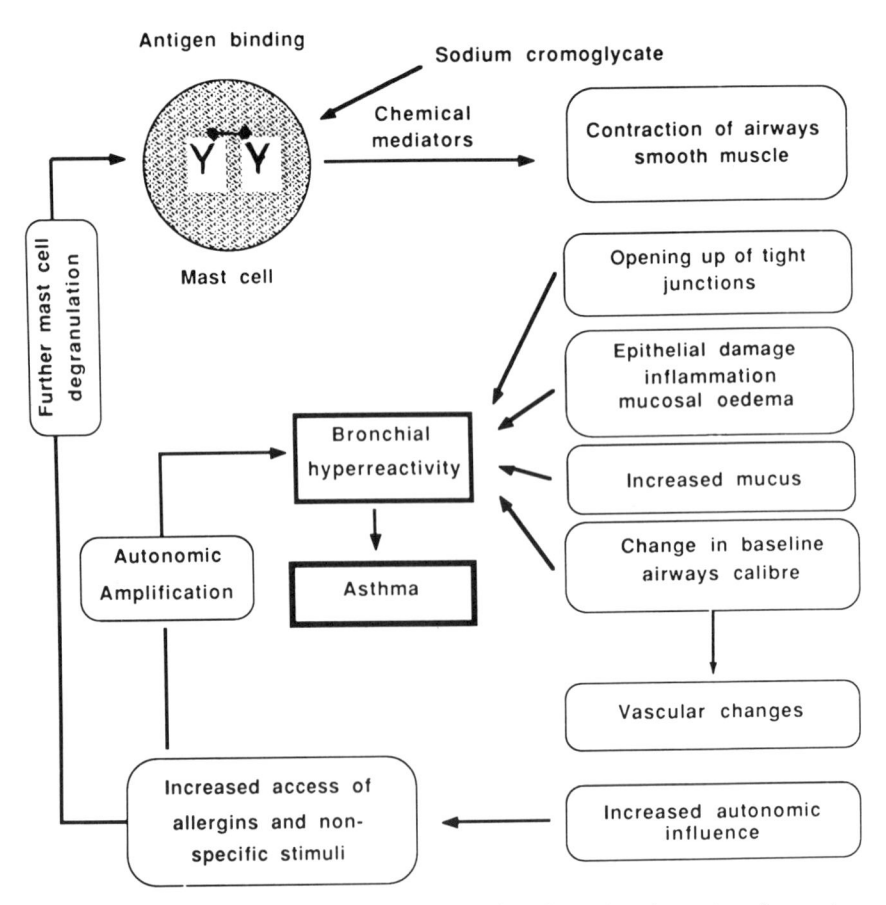

Fig. 3-3 Factors which may be involved in allergic asthma. A major action of cromolyn sodium is to block mediator release and thus to prevent the cascade of events which leads to the symptoms of asthma.

Table 3-2
Forms of Cromolyn Sodium

	Description:	Indications:	Dosage:
Intal Capsules:	Each capsule contains 20 mg cromolyn sodium & 20 mg lactose for inhalation via Spinhaler. A water-soluble, odorless, white, hydrated crystalline powder, tasteless at first, leaving a slightly bitter aftertaste.	A prophylactic agent in the management of bronchial asthma & in prevention of the acute bronchoconstriction due to exercise, TDI, and environmental pollutants.	1 cap QID, which can be tapered down to TID & sometimes BID. For acute exposures—1 cap prior to exposure.
Intal Nebulizer Solution:	Each glass ampule contains 20 mg cromolyn in 2 ml purified water administered via a power-operated nebulizer having an adequate flow rate. Clear, colorless, sterile and has a pH of 4.0–7.0.	Management of bronchial asthma and in prevention of the acute bronchoconstriction due to exercise, TDI, and environmental pollutants.	1 amp QID, which can be tapered down to TID & sometimes BID.
Nasalcrom:	Each milliliter contains 40 mg cromolyn in purified water with BKC 0.01% & EDTA 0.01% added to stabilize & protect the solution. pH of 4.5–6.5. Is a 4% cromolyn solution.	Prevention and treatment of seasonal and perrenial allergic rhinitis.	1 spray in each nostril 5–6 times daily, then tapering to 3–4 times daily.
Opticrom:	Each milliliter of this 4% ophthalmic solution contains 40 mg cromolyn in purified water with 0.4% phenylethyl alcohol, 0.01% BKC, 0.01% EDTA to preserve & stabilize. Clear, colorless, sterile solution, pH of 4.0–7.0 intended for topical administration to the eye.	Treatment of certain allergic ocular disorders: vernal keratoconjunctivitis, vernal conjunctivitis, giant papillary conjunctivitis, vernal keratitis, & allergic keratoconjunctivitis.	1–2 drops in each eye 4–6 times daily. One drop contains 1.6 mg cromolyn sodium.
Intal Metered Dose Inhaler:	Each actuation of the inhaler contains 1 mg of cromolyn sodium	Prevention & management of bronchial asthma & prevention of acute bronchoconstriction due to exercise, TDI, and environmental pollutants.	2 puffs QID. Prior to acute exposures, 2 puffs prior to exposure.

Indications for Long-term Therapy

Perennial asthma. Cromolyn is indicated for patients with either antigen-induced or intrinsic asthma, both adults and children, when they have chronic symptoms that are not satisfactorily controlled by p.r.n. bronchodilators. In patients with severe asthma, there was no correlation between changes in attack severity or frequency, pulmonary function or disability resulting from cromolyn therapy and the patient's age.[9,24] Children may respond to treatment more rapidly, but this is presumably because the extent of chronic inflammation is less than that in the adult chronic asthmatic. As indicated earlier, cromolyn attenuates both the immediate and late asthmatic response following exposure to a variety of antigens, [25-27] and it also apparently inhibits the reduction in mucociliary transport[28] which is frequently associated. The safety of its long-term administration is one of its attractive features.[7] Furukawa et al recently reported that cromolyn was as efficacious as theophylline in treating asthma, and superior to theophylline in decreasing bronchial hyperreactivity, and in side effects.[29] Since its efficacy in chronic asthma is comparable to that of theophylline and produces fewer adverse effects, its use as a first-line drug in chronic asthma is recommended.

Chronic cough. Inhaled bronchodilators on a p.r.n. basis are often effective in those who cough infrequently. However, it has been demonstrated that there is an association between chronic cough without wheezing and exercise-induced airway hyperreactivity,[30,31] and cromolyn may be the drug of choice for those individuals in whom the cough is present most of the time.

Exercise induced bronchospasm. Patients with EIB who are very active and require continuous protection, should take cromolyn round the clock. Some patients demonstrate a late asthmatic reaction following exercise and cromolyn has been shown to provide greater protection against this reaction than theophylline and either oral or inhaled metaproterenol.[32]

Hyperreactive airways. Cromolyn has been shown to reduce bronchial hyperresponsiveness or "twitchy lung" in many patients. In atopic patients given cromolyn during their allergy season, there was a reduced responsivity to inhalation challenges with histamine, antigen, and thermal stimuli after several weeks of therapy.[33-35] When cromolyn therapy was stopped, responsivity once again increased.[35]

Occupational asthma. Cromolyn is indicated in occupational asthma when industry controls are insufficient, or the removal of the worker from the environment is not feasible, or the employee insists on continuing to work. Numerous studies have indicated the efficacy of cromolyn in occupational asthma in cattle farmers[36] and wheat farmers,[37] as well as that associated with wheat and flour,[38,39] Western Red Cedar,[40] animal dander,[25] and chemical dusts and gases such as solder flux fumes and toluene diisocyanate.[41,18] The use of cromolyn can allow some individuals with asthma to continue in their occupation while simultaneously minimizing the morbidity of their disease.

During immunotherapy. Aeroallergen immunotherapy may offer potential benefits to some allergic patients with asthma. Cromolyn may be beneficial during immunotherapy because: (1) there is a latent period of 3–12 months before the immunotherapeutic response becomes maximal; (2) patients may be sensitive to more aeroallergens than those for which they are receiving immunization; (3) non-immunologic triggers of the asthmatic reaction are at least as important as immunologic triggers in most asthmatics. Thus, the use of cromolyn during immunotherapy may allow realization of the goal of general desensitization of the patient to specific allergens. While immunotherapy provides systemic hyposensitization, cromolyn may provide local desensitization by topical application to the target organ where it can stabilize the mast cell. A number of clinical reports tend to support the complementary effect of the two therapies.[26,42,43]

Allergic rhinitis. Mast cells are very prevalent in the mucosa and submucosa of the nose as well as in the lungs. Because of its ability to stabilize mast cells, cromolyn, in the form of a nasal spray, can be particularly effective in the treatment of perennial and seasonal allergic rhinitis.

Dosage for Long-Term Therapy

In general, the longer cromolyn therapy is taken, the less frequently it must be inhaled. The initial dosing of cromolyn for the long-term treatment of chronic symptoms in children and adults is inhalation of 20 mg q.i.d. In mild to moderate asthmatics, when the symptoms are well controlled, cromolyn can be titrated down to t.i.d.[29] and often to b.i.d. In addition, it is important to provide all patients with ancillary treatment for breakthrough attacks (β-agonists, prednisone and if tolerated, theophylline).

If the environment worsens or patients begin to develop increased symptoms after lowering the dose of cromolyn, the dose should be increased back to q.i.d. until good control has once again been achieved. It must be stressed that if possible the patient should not stop inhaling cromolyn when a breakthrough occurs or if an upper respiratory infection occurs, because this is when increased protection is needed. All therapies should be intensified and precipitating factors treated. When chest tightness is present, the bronchodilator should be inhaled properly first and followed by cromolyn if the powdered capsule or metered dose form is used. Otherwise the bronchodilator can be added in with the nebulized solution of cromolyn.

In allergic rhinitis the 4 percent cromolyn solution preparation should be sprayed once in each nostril every 3-4 waking hours; when less control is needed, dosing may be reduced to every 5-6 waking hours.

Indications for Short-term Therapy

Short-term exercise. A single dose of cromolyn (20 mg) a few minutes before exercise generally prevents EIB in many individuals.[44] In others, the combination of cromolyn and a β-agonist may be necessary to prevent EIB. McFadden found that pretreatment with cromolyn did not absolutely prevent bronchospasm associated with exercise or isocapnic hyperventilation of freezing air, but rather shifted the stimulus-response curve rightward in a manner similar to that seen following sympathomimetic and anticholinergic agents.[33] Cromolyn and β_2 agents had different effects at various times in the same individual depending on the severity of the challenge. A treatment regimen using both drugs can therefore, be beneficial, particularly when performing heavy exercise on a cold day.

The mechanism by which cromolyn prevents EIB or cold-induced airway obstruction in asthmatics and normal individuals is unknown, but it is thought that: (1) mast cell derived mediators are involved;[44] and/or (2) cromolyn reduces the degree of airway cooling by probably reducing the water loss during periods of high ventilation, thus preventing a reflex-induced bronchoconstriction.[33]

Antigen exposure. A single dose of cromolyn can afford protection from anticipated short-term exposure to known antigens such as grass or pollen when mowing the yard or taking a nature walk, and can also be effective in preventing an attack of asthma triggered by an exposure to animal dander.

Irritant exposure. Cromolyn is effective in providing protection from anticipated exposure to chemicals such as toluene diisocyanate and/or irritants such as smoke or cold air and SO_2.

Seasonal asthma. Studies showing cromolyn's ability to block both the immediate and late reactions to allergen challenge provide logic for utilization of cromolyn for seasonal asthma.[45-47] Crockcroft et al have shown that it is the late reaction that is associated with an increase in bronchial hyperreactivity,[15] so that when the late reaction is allowed to develop, it acts by positive feedback and further accentuates the effect of the next challenge. Cromolyn given for a sufficient length of time can raise the threshold of airways to histamine (i.e., reduce airway hyperreactivity), and foster tolerance to pollen, mold or histamine levels that previously would have provoked bronchospasm.

Dosing for Short-term Therapy

A single dose of 20 mg or 40 mg of cromolyn sodium taken no more than one hour (preferably several minutes) prior to the anticipated exposure usually provides adequate protection against bronchoconstriction for an estimated two hours. In patients with asthma who are seasonally allergic, cromolyn therapy (20 mg q.i.d.) should be initiated several days to one week prior to the onset of their particular season. If the drug is started during the troublesome season, the decrease in symptomatology will take longer because the patients will have already developed increased bronchial responsiveness. When good control of the asthma has been instituted, as in long-term treatment, the dose of drug generally can be reduced to t.i.d. and sometimes to b.i.d., with the proviso that it should be increased to q.i.d. if the condition worsens.

CONTRAINDICATIONS

Cromolyn would appear to be contraindicated only in those patients who have shown a hypersensitive reaction to the drug, which is manifested by a skin rash or sustained bronchial tightness.

SIDE EFFECTS AND THEIR MANAGEMENT

There is a very low incidence of side effects with cromolyn sodium usage (about 2 percent of patients),[7,29,48,49] and these are generally minor and disappear when the drug is discontinued[8] and no deaths have been reported. Cough and transient bronchospasm are the most frequent side effects and they generally occur following inhalation of the powder. This irritation can be minimized by adherance to a proper inhalation technique with the spinhaler, or by having the patient inhale bronchodilator prior to inhalation of the powder. Some patients complain of pharyngeal irritation by the powder, and this can be obviated by drinking water immediately before and after the inhalation. The nebulizer solution of cromolyn does not appear to be irritating, so that these side effects may not be a problem, nor are they troublesome when the cromolyn metered-dose inhaler (MDI) is used.

There have been a few isolated reports of apparent allergic reactions to cromolyn including urticaria, angioedema, and maculo-papular rashes. Pulmonary infiltrates with eosinophilia have also been reported, although a cause and effect relationship with cromolyn has not been established.

INTERACTIONS WITH OTHER DRUGS AND CHOICE OF CONCOMITANT AGENTS

Cromolyn sodium does not interact adversely with any other drug. It has been extensively studied in combination with commonly used medications for asthma. Thus, all of the agents utilized in the treatment of the asthmatic patient can be used concomitantly with cromolyn sodium. It has been shown that the combination of theophylline and cromolyn can decrease the usage of albuterol[50] and that cromolyn may obviate the need for theophylline completely.[51]

Patients with asthma who are receiving corticosteroids, should continue to take concomitant corticosteroids, as well as bronchodilators, following the introduction of cromolyn. If improvement occurs, gradual tapering of the corticosteroids should be begun and an alternate day regimen instituted if at all possible. It is important that the dose be reduced slowly, and close supervision of the patient be maintained to avoid an exacerbation of asthma.

Other Mast Cell Stabilizers

Many investigators have been working on cromolyn-like compounds, searching for agents that have greater potency and absorptive properties, but progress has been very slow.

Some compounds such as doxantrazole, nivimedone, bufrolin, proxicromil, and probicromil[16,52] have shown initial promise, all being more potent than cromolyn sodium by 30–1500 times, but all have been discarded because of toxicity, or lack of clinical efficacy *in vivo,* or as in the case of doxantrazole, because they do not attenuate the late phase asthmatic reaction.

The reason for difficulty in developing new agents may be three-fold: (1) the absence of suitable animal models; (2) the dubious relationship between human challenge experiments and clinical efficacy; and (3) difficulties in the therapeutic evaluation of antiallergic compounds.

KETOTIFEN

Ketotifen is the first oral, nonbronchodilating drug that may have a prophylactic role in the treatment of bronchial asthma, but it has not yet been approved for use in the United States. Known elsewhere as Zaditen, this compound may have some mast-cell stabilizing properties, but its primary mode of action is as a histamine H_1 receptor antagonist. It has been shown to have antiallergic activity in some animal studies, and selectively inhibits the release of SRS-A from human chopped lung tissue, but its clinical effectiveness varies considerably.[52]

Ketotifen is prescribed orally in doses of 1–2 mg b.i.d. Short-term treatment or even a single dose of ketotifen has been shown to inhibit bronchoconstriction following provocation by antigen, histamine, and aspirin, but it does not prevent bronchospasm induced by inhalation of acetylcholine and its effect on EIB is inconsistent.[53] Long-term administration of ketotifen, however, may reduce bronchial hyperreactivity, and may prevent or reverse a reduced β-adrenoceptor sensitivity[54] which may be important if the latter plays a role in the progression of asthma.

Ketotifen is absorbed through the GI (gastrointestinal) tract and excreted in the urine and its most noteworthy side effect is sedation. As with antihistamines in general, there can be increased appetite and weight gain, dizziness, headaches, dry mouth, and nausea.[53]

NEDOCROMIL SODIUM

Nedocromil sodium, Tilade®, (Fisons, Bedford, Massachusetts 01730) is the disodium salt of a novel pyranoquinoline dicarboxylic acid, which is delivered by pressurized aerosol. Safety studies in animals show the drug to have a low order of toxicity and to be well tolerated, even at doses several times higher than that proposed for clinical use (4 mg by inhalation two to four times daily). It has been shown to exert a protective effect against allergen and non-allergen induced bronchoconstriction when given as a single dose prior to challenge,[55,56,57,58] and to reduce allergen-induced increase in bronchial hyperreactivity when given at a regular dosage during the grass pollen season.[59] In double-blind trials it has been shown to be effective in patients with chronic asthma who were maintained on bronchodilator or inhaled steroid therapy.[60,61,62]

Nedocromil sodium is currently undergoing long-term safety and acceptability studies in asthmatic patients, and no significant untoward effects have been reported. Initial expectations are that nedocromil sodium may have a useful place in the management of reversible obstructive airways disease where airway inflammation and bronchial hyperresponsiveness are implicated.

LODOXAMIDE

Lodoxamide (Upjohn, Kalamazoo, Michigan 49001) has the ability to block histamine release from rat peritoneal mast cells challenged with compound 48/80 *in vitro* and is reported to be 2500 times as potent as cromolyn sodium. It can inhibit exercise and allergen-induced bronchoconstriction, although no effect on the late reaction has been demonstrated. A number of unpleasant, dose-related side effects, have been reported particularly when taken by the oral route. These include sensations of body warmth (flushing), urethral burning, nausea, headache, infrequent vomiting, and increased blood pressure.[52]

ZAPRINAST

Zaprinast (M&B-22948) is an azaxanthine derivative and has also been shown to inhibit exercise and antigen-induced bronchospasm in asthmatics.[16,53] This agent probably derives its antiasthmatic activity mainly through phosphodiesterase inhibition, although it also appears to possess antiallergic properties. It apparently induces phosphorylation of the same high molecular weight (78,000 dalton) protein as cromolyn sodium.

WY-41195

Wy-41195 (Wyeth, Philadelphia, Pennsylvania 19101) is a sodium salt that is about 520 times as potent as cromolyn sodium, as reflected by the rat passive cutaneous anaphylaxis test. It can be administered orally and is effective in inhibiting histamine-induced reflex bronchoconstriction in the dog. Like cromolyn sodium, it also reverses the hyperreactivity to methacholine induced by sulphur dioxide in the conscious dog.[52]

SUDEXANOX

Sudexanox (Hoechst-Roussel, Somerville, New Jersey 08876) is a tromethamine salt from the xanthone category and has been shown to be orally active by the rat passive cutaneous anaphylaxis test. It also partially inhibits the IgG-mediated reaction and anaphylactic bronchoconstriction in the rat, indicating a mode of action similar to cromolyn sodium. It has been shown to be effective in about 66 percent of children and adults who suffer from extrinsic asthma.[52]

REFERENCES

1. Holgate ST, Kay AB: Mast cells, mediators and asthma. Clinical Allergy 15:221–234, 1985
2. Orr TSC: Mode of action of disodium cromoglycate. Acta Allergol 32(13):S9–27, 1977
3. Altounyan REC: Review of the clinical activity and modes of action of sodium cromoglycate, in Pepys J and Edwards AM (eds): The Mast Cell—Its Role in Health and Disease. Davos, Pitman Medical, London, 199–216, 1979
4. Morrison Smith J and Pizarro YA: Observations on the safety of sodium cromoglycate in long-term use in children. Clinical Allergy 2:143–151, 1972
5. Chai H: The long-term efficacy and safety of Intal therapy in asthmatic children and Intal in bronchial asthma—8th International Congress allergol: Sectional meeting on

disodium cromoglycate. (eds) Pepys J and Yamamura Y, Tokyo, Oct. 17:55-64, 1973
6. Godfrey S, Balfour-Lynn L, Konig P: The place of cromolyn sodium in the long-term management of childhood asthma based on a 3 to 5 year follow-up. J Ped 87:465-473, 1975
7. Toogood JH: Multi-center surveillance of long-term safety of sodium cromoglycate. Acta Allergologica 32(13):44-52, 1977
8. Settipane GA, Klein DE, Boyd GK, et al: Adverse reactions to cromolyn. JAMA 241:811-813, 1979
9. Toogood JH, Lefcoe NM, Wonnacott TM, et al: Cromolyn sodium therapy: Predictors of response. Adv Asthma All Pulm Dis 5(1):2-15, 1978
10. Cox JSG: Disodium cromoglycate (FLP 670) (Intal): A specific inhibitor of reaginic antibody-antigen mechanisms. Nature, (London) 216:1328-1329, 1967
11. Mazurek N, Berger G, Pecht I: A binding site on mast cells and basophils for the anti-allergic drug cromolyn. Nature 286:722-723, 1980
12. Theoharides TC, Seighart W, Greengard P, et al: Antiallergic drug cromolyn may inhibit histamine secretion by regulating phosphorylation of a mast cell protein. Science 207:80-82, 1980
13. Diaz P, Galleguillos FR, Gonzalez MC, et al: Bronchoalveolar lavage in asthma: The effect of disodium cromoglycate on leukocyte counts, immunoglobulins, and complement. J Allergy Clin Immunol 74(1):41-48, 1984
14. Pepys J, Hargreave FE, Chan M, et al: Inhibitory effect of disodium cromoglycate on allergen inhalation tests. Lancet 2:134-137, 1968
15. Cockcroft DW, Ruffin RE, Dolovich J, et al: Allergin-induced increase in non-allergic bronchial reactivity. Clinical Allergy 7:503-513, 1977
16. Stokes TC, Morley J: Prospects for an oral Intal. Br J Dis Chest 75:1-14, 1981
17. Harries MG, Parkes PEG, Lessof MH: Role of bronchial irritant receptors in asthma. Lancet 1:5-7, 1981
18. Butcher BT, Karr RM, O'Neil CE, et al: Inhalation challenge and pharmacologic studies of toluene diisocyanate (TDI)-sensitive workers. J Allergy Clin Immunol 64:146-152, 1979
19. Allegra L, Bianco S: Non-specific bronchoreactivity obtained with an ultrasonic aerosal of distilled water. Envr J Respir Dis 61:S166-175, 1980
20. Breslin FJ, McFadden ER, Ingram RG: The effect of cromolyn sodium on the airway response to hyperpnea and cold air in asthma. Am Rev Respir Dis 122:11-16, 1980
21. Godfrey S, Konig P: Suppression of exercise-induced asthma by salbutamol, theophylline, atropine, cromolyn and placebo in a group of asthmatic children. Pediatrics 56:930-936, 1975
22. Dixon M, Jackson DM, Richards IM: The action of sodium cromoglycate on "C" fibre endings in the dog lung. Br J Pharmacol 80:11-13, 1980
23. Hogg JC: Bronchial mucosal permeability and its relationship to airways hyperreactivity. J Allergy Clin Immunol 67:421-425, 1981
24. Toogood JH, Lefcoe NM, Rose DK, et al: A double-blind study of disodium cromoglycate for prophylaxis of bronchial asthma. Am Rev Respir Dis 104:323-330, 1971

25. Gross NJ: Allergy to laboratory animals—epidemiologic, clinical, and physiologic aspects, and a trial of cromolyn in its management. J Allergy Clin Immunol 66:158-165, 1980
26. Engstrom I: Evaluation of Iomudal (Intal) treatment in children. Scan J Resp Dis 101:S49-56, 1977
27. Altounyan REC: Inhibition of experimental asthma by a new compound—disodium cromoglycate (Intal). Acta Allergol 22:487-489, 1967
28. Wanner A: The role of mucociliary dysfunction in bronchial asthma. Am J Med 67:477-485, 1979
29. Furukawa CT, Shapiro GG, Bierman CW: A double-blind study comparing the effectiveness of cromolyn sodium and sustained-release theophylline in childhood asthma. Pediatrics 74:453-459, 1984
30. Konig P: Hidden asthma in childhood. Am J Dis Children 135:1053-1055, 1981
31. Cloutier NM, Loughlin GM: Chronic cough in children: A manifestation of airway hyperreactivity. Pediatrics 67(1):6-12, 1981
32. Feldman CH, Fox J, Draut E: Exercise induced asthma (EIA): Treatment for early and late responses. Am Rev Respir Dis 125:191, 1982
33. Griffin MP, MacDonald N, McFadden ER: Short and long term effects of cromolyn sodium on the airway reactivity of asthmatics. J Allergy Clin Immunol 71:331-338, 1983
34. Altounyan REC: Review of clinical activity and mode of action of sodium cromoglycate. Clin Allergy 10:S481-489, 1980
35. Dickson W: One year's trial of Intal compound in 24 children with severe asthma, in: Pepys M, Frankland AW (eds): Disodium cromoglycate in allergic airways disease. Butterworths
36. DeHaller R: Round-table discussion on prevention and treatment, in Proc. 45th International Symp. "Aspergillosis and Farmers' Lung in Man and Animals." (eds) DeHaller R, Suter F, Hans Huber, Vienna:300-302, 1974
37. Finch PS: Wheat farmers' asthma in Australia. Med J Australia 2:1102-1105, 1983
38. Schultze-Werninghaus G, Schwarting HH: Effect of disodium cromoglycate on allergen inhalation tests in occupational asthma of bakers. Pneumologie 151:115-126, 1974
39. Gaffuri E: Respiratory effects of biological detergents. Br Med J 4:52-57, 1970
40. Chan-Yeung M, Barton GM, MacLean Lonia et al: Occupational asthma and rhinitis due to Western Red Cedar. Am Rev Respir Dis 108:1094-1102, 1973
41. Pepys J: The role of industrial agents in the etiology of asthma. Adv Asthma, Allergy and Pulm Dis 3(1):1-8, 1976
42. Koutsoukos AG: Use of disodium cromoglycate during the course of specific desensitizing treatment in asthmatic patients. Acta Allergol 28:62-67, 1973
43. Svanborg N: Desensitization during Lomodal treatment. Acta Allergol 30(12):106-112, 1975
44. Altounyan REC: Disodium cromoglycate clinical pharmacology in obstructive airways disease, in: Orie NGM, Van Der Lende R (ed): 3rd International Symp. "Bronchitis," Groningen, 346-353, 1970
45. Pepys J, Hutchcroft J: Bronchial provocation tests in etiologic diagnosis and analysis of asthma. Am Rev Respir Dis 112(6):829-859, 1975

46. Booij-Noord H, Orie NGM, DeVries K: Immediate and late bronchial obstructive reactions to inhalation of housedust and protective effects of disodium cromoglycate and prednisolone. J Allergy Clin Immunol 48:344–354, 1971
47. Godfrey S, Konig P: Inhibition of exercise-induced asthma by different pharmacological pathways. Thorax 31:137–143, 1976
48. Bernstein IL, Siegel SC, Brandon ML, et al: A controlled study of cromolyn sodium sponsored by the drug committee of the American Academy of Allergy and Immunology. J Allergy Clin Immunol 50:235–245, 1972
49. Dickson W, Cole M: Severe asthma in children—a 10 year follow-up, in: Pepys J, Edwards AM (eds): *The Mast Cell—Its Roles in Health and Disease*. Turnbridge Wells, England: Pitman Medical Publishing Co., 343–352, 1979
50. Newth CJL, Newth CV, Turner JAP: Comparison of nebulized sodium cromoglycate and oral theophylline in controlling symptoms of chronic asthma in pre-school children: A double blind study. Aust NZ J Med 12:232–238, 1982
51. Hilman B, Hyte MK, Vekovius A, et al: Safety and efficacy of nebulized cromolyn sodium in asthmatic children. Ann Allergy 47:118, 1981
52. Suschitsky JL, Sheard P: The search for antiallergic drugs for the treatment of asthma—problems in finding a successor to sodium cromoglycate. Progress in Medicinal Chemistry 21:1–60, 1984
53. Craps LP: Ketotifen in the oral prophylaxis of bronchial asthma: A review. Pharmatherapeutica 3:18–35, 1981
54. Craps LP, Ney UM: Ketotifen: Current views on its mechanism of action and their therapeutic implications. Resp 45:411–421, 1984
55. Youngchaiyud P, Lee TB: Effect of nedocromil sodium on the immediate response to antigen challenge in asthmatic patients. Clinical Allergy 16(2), 1986
56. Dahl R, Pedersen B: The influence of nedocromil sodium on the dual asthmatic reaction after allergen challenge: a double-blind crossover study. Proc 4th Cong Eur Soc Pneumol (SEP):Stresa (Milan), Sept. 1985
57. Shaw RJ, Kay AB: Nedocromil, a mucosal and connective tissue mast cell stabilizer, inhibits exercise-induced asthma. Br J Dis Chest 79:385–389, 1985
58. Altounyan REC, Cole M, Lee TB: Inhibition of sulphur dioxide-induced bronchoconstriction by nedcromil sodium in non-asthmatic atopic subjects. Annals Allergy 55 (Part II):398, 1985
59. Altounyan REC, Cole M, Lee TB: Effects of nedocromil sodium on changes in bronchial hyperreactivity in non-asthmatic atopic rhinitic subjects during the grass pollen season. Prog Resp Res 19:397–400, 1985
60. Fyans P, Chatterjee P, Chatterjee SS: Double-blind group comparative clinical trial of nedocromil sodium and placebo in bronchial asthma. Respiration, 46(Suppl 1):102, 1984
61. Lal S, Malhotra S, Gribben D, et al: Nedocromil sodium: a new drug for the management of bronchial asthma. Thorax 39(11):809–812, 1984
62. van As A, Kemp J, Townley R, et al: The efficacy and safety of inhaled nedocromil sodium in asthma. Chest 88 I(Special Issue):33 S, 1985
63. van As A, Kemp J, Townley R, et al: The efficacy and safety of inhaled nedocromil sodium in asthma. Chest 88 I(Special Issue):33 S, 1985

Robert A. Bethel
Charles G. Irvin

4

Anticholinergic, Antimuscarinic Drugs (Atropine Sulfate, Ipratropium Bromide)

Anticholinergic, antimuscarinic drugs have been rediscovered in recent years to be effective bronchodilators. The use of these drugs in present day medicine is one example of effective pharmacotherapy that is derived from herbal medicine. The medical literature of India three centuries ago recommends smoking the leaves of *Datura stramonium,* which contain antimuscarinic drugs, for respiratory disorders.[1-4] Several plants contain antimuscarinic drugs including *Atropa belladonna* (deadly nightshade),[1] *Datura stramonium* (jimson weed, locoweed, stink weed, thorn apple, and devil's apple),[1,2] *Hyocyamus niger* (henbane), and *Scopolia carniolica*. The smoking, inhaling, chewing, and drinking of these herbs was widely used to treat asthma throughout Europe and North America in the nineteenth century. Even today these herbs are used in much of the world due to their low cost and ready availability.[2,5] The adverse effects of these herbs, including tachycardia, urinary retention, and dysphoria, were recognized. In this century, when adrenergic drugs were demonstrated to effectively dilate airways, the antimuscarinic drugs fell into disuse.

In recent years a number of investigational studies have reestablished the efficacy of antimuscarinic drugs in relieving bronchoconstriction.[6,7] The chemical purity of the drugs used, atropine and atropine sulfate, makes dosing with these drugs more reliable than with herbs, but adverse effects once again have limited the usefulness of these drugs. Perhaps more important in the recent enthusiasm for the use of antimuscarinic drugs as bronchodilators has been the development of quaternary ammonium antimuscarinic drugs.[6,7] These latter

DRUGS FOR THE RESPIRATORY SYSTEM
ISBN 0-8089-1818-4

Copyright © 1986 by Grune & Stratton, Inc.
All rights of reproduction in any form reserved.

drugs, unlike the tertiary ammonium compounds atropine and atropine sulfate, are absorbed poorly and also cross the blood-brain barrier poorly. They appear to be almost free of adverse effects in therapeutic doses and are effective bronchodilators.

As airway mucous glands are innervated by cholinergic nerves, the anticholinergic, antimuscarinic drugs are being studied to determine whether these drugs decrease secretions in disorders such as bronchitis. Whether it is wise to try to decrease secretions in such disorders and whether antimuscarinic drugs do so is uncertain.

MECHANISM OF ACTION

Parasympathetic Nervous System

The action of anticholinergic drugs can be fully appreciated only with a clear understanding of the anatomy and physiology of the parasympathetic arm of the autonomic nervous system (Fig 4-1). Parasympathetic nerves arise from either the brainstem or the sacral segments of the spinal cord. They have long preganglionic fibers that synapse in peripheral ganglia located within the organs innervated. From these ganglia arise a second postganglionic fiber that innervates the effector organ (e.g., smooth muscle or mucous gland of the tracheal-bronchial tree). Parasympathetic innervation to the lungs begins in the vagal nuclei of the brainstem and travels to the lungs via the vagus nerves.

The vagal nuclei generate a constant neural tone to airway smooth muscle so that when this tone is interrupted, as by anticholinergic drugs, smooth muscle relaxes and bronchodilation occurs.[8,9] The vagal nuclei receive neural input from higher central nervous system centers through which emotion may affect airway tone. The vagal nuclei also receive sensory neural input from several areas of the body, including the lung itself. Stimulation of irritant nerve endings located between the cells of the respiratory epithelium by such agents as smoke, fumes, etc. can cause bronchoconstriction through vagal reflexes (Fig 4-1). Stimulation of irritant nerve endings in other areas of the body such as the nose, pharynx, larynx, and esophagus have also been implicated in causing bronchoconstriction through vagal reflexes. The final step in vagal stimulation of airway smooth muscle is the release of acetylcholine from the parasympathetic nerve ending at the neuromuscular junction. It is at this final step that atropine and the other antimuscarinic drugs work as competitive inhibitors of acetylcholine.

Junctional Transmission of the Neural Impulse

When the neural action potential reaches the nerve ending, the following events are thought to occur[10,11] (Fig 4-2). Depolarization of the membrane of the axon terminal causes an influx of calcium, which promotes the fusion to the cell

Anticholinergic, Antimuscarinic Drugs

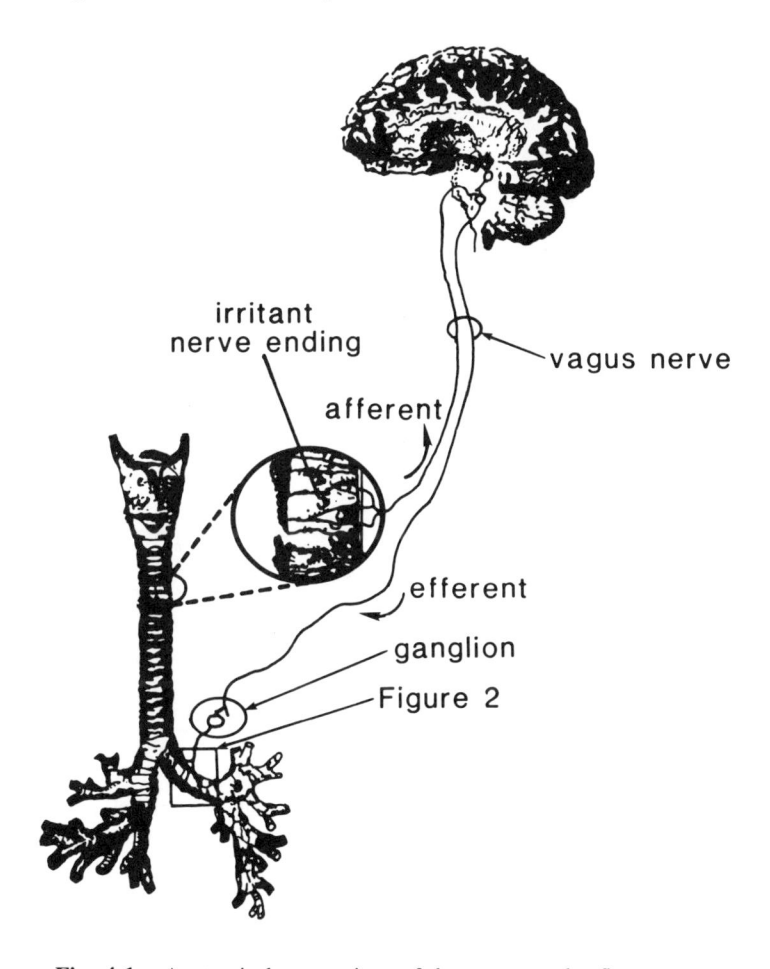

Fig. 4-1. Anatomical connections of the vago-vagal reflex arc. The sensory receptor most often implicated is the irritant or rapidly adapting nerve ending located between cells of the airway epithelium (insert). Both afferent and efferent nerve fibers travel in the vagus nerve trunk. The central synapse occurs in the dorsal motor nucleus of the midbrain and can be influenced by higher centers. Peripheral ganglia are located within airway walls. Events at the neuromuscular junction are presented in Figure 2.

membrane of small, clear, agranular vesicles containing acetycholine. These vesicles then discharge their contents into the synaptic cleft through exocytosis. The acetylcholine from one vesicle diffuses across the junctional cleft (80–200 nm) and combines with acetylcholine receptors on the postjunctional membrane. Binding of acetylcholine to a receptor only slightly depolarizes the postsynaptic membrane; however, if enough of these events (quanta) occur, the entire membrane depolarizes resulting in the propagation of the signal. These events are

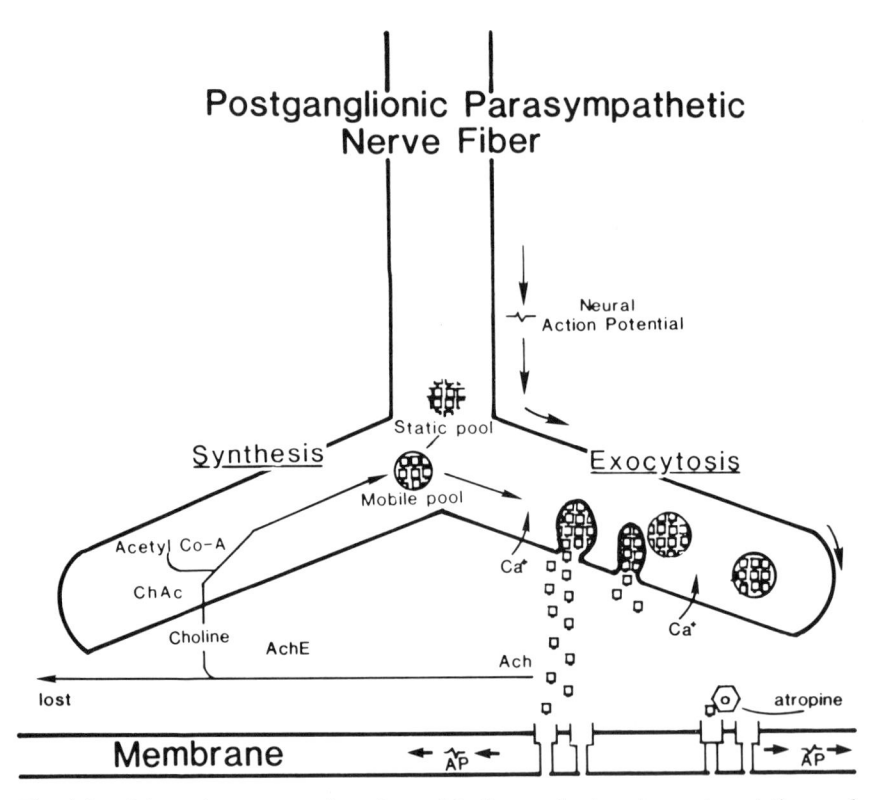

Fig. 4-2. Schematic representation of acetylcholine synthesis, release, degradation, and reuptake at the neuromuscular parasympathetic junction. Choline acetylase (ChAc) catalyzes the combination of Acetyl Co-A and choline to form acetylcholine (Ach). Ach is stored both within vesicles (mobile pool) and outside vesicles (static pool). A neural action potential initiates calcium influx into the nerve ending which in turn initiates exocytosis of Ach from its vesicles. The Ach diffuses across the neuromuscular junction and attaches to an Ach receptor on the muscle membrane where a muscle action potential (AP) is induced. Competitive inhibitors of Ach, such as atropine, usually have one moiety that fits the Ach receptor attached to a bulkier moiety. The Ach in the neuromuscular junction is degraded by acetylcholinesterase (AchE) and the liberated choline is largely retaken up by the nerve ending and reused in Ach synthesis.

continuous in bronchial muscle since there is always a degree of nervous traffic along the vagus. Blocking the parasympathetic nervous system with atropine results in smooth muscle relaxation and a decrease in airflow resistance even in healthy persons.[8,9]

Acetylcholine

Acetylcholine (Fig 4-3) is a principle neurotransmitter of all the main animal phyla. In humans, it functions as a neurotransmitter in synapses of the central nervous system, in the sympathetic and parasympathetic ganglia, in the skeletal

Anticholinergic, Antimuscarinic Drugs

AGONISTS

Acetylcholine

$$H_3C-\underset{CH_3}{\underset{|}{\overset{CH_3}{\overset{|}{N^+}}}}-CH_2-CH_2-O-\overset{O}{\overset{\|}{C}}-CH_3$$

Muscarine

ANTAGONISTS

Tertiary Ammonium Compound

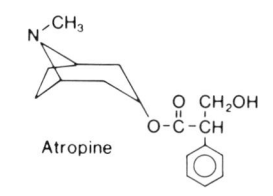

Atropine

Quaternary Ammonium Compounds

Atropine Methonitrate $+ NO_3^- \cdot H_2O$

Ipratropium Bromide $\cdot Br^- \cdot H_2O$

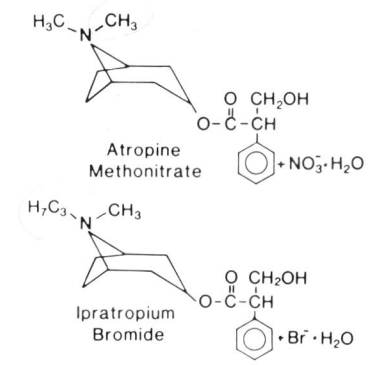

Fig. 4-3. Chemical structures of muscarinic agonists and antagonists. Antagonists have additions to the nitrogen of the tropic acid subunit: atropine—one methyl addition, atropine methonitrate—two methyl additions, and: ipratropium bromide—one methyl and one isopropyl additions.

neuromuscular junction, and in the postganglionic parasympathetic junction. There are four types of acetylcholine receptors: central nervous system receptors, such as are found in the limbic system; neuromuscular receptors, such as are found on skeletal muscle; ganglionic receptors, such as are found in both the sympathetic and parasympathetic ganglia; and postganglionic parasympathetic receptors, such as are found on bronchial smooth muscle and mucous glands.[12] Each type of receptor has an associated class of blocking agents. Ganglionic and smooth muscle receptors are also named nicotinic and muscarinic (Fig 4-3) respectively, for the selective agonists that stimulate them. Atropine and other anticholinergic drugs we will discuss (Fig 4-3) are preferentially muscarinic, acetylcholine blockers; although in some cases (quaternary ammonium compounds) these drugs also have ganglionic (nicotinic) blocking effects.

Acetylcholine is formed by the transfer of an acetyl group from acetylcoenzyme A to choline[12,13] (Fig 4-2). The enzyme acetyltransferase catalyzes this reaction. Newly formed acetylcholine is stored within small agranular vesicles found predominantly along the presynaptic membrane, a location from which they are readily released. There is at least one other storage level of acetylcholine, termed the stationary or static pool, that is not so readily mobilized and probably is not stored within vesicles. After the release of acetylcholine into the synaptic cleft through exocytosis, the action of acetylcholine is terminated by the enzyme acetylcholinesterase. The action of acetylcholinesterase is antagonized by physostigmine which increases concentrations of acetylcholine in the synaptic cleft and is sometimes used to reverse atropine poisoning. Acetylcholinesterase hydrolyzes acetylcholine into acetyl-A and choline. Thirty-five to 50 percent of the liberated choline is retaken up by the nerve ending in a process so efficient as to keep pace with stimulation rates as high as 20 per second.[14]

Antimuscarinic Drugs

Of all the receptors for neurotransmitters, the nicotinic and muscarinic are the most extensively studied. While there is a great deal known about these two receptors, there is still much to be learned. It has been recently suggested,[15,16] for instance, that muscarinic receptors may have subclasses (M_1 and M_2) and that the receptor for atropine, while similar to the acetylcholine receptor, is nonetheless different. However, both of these contentions have yet to be widely accepted. Currently, the acetylcholine receptor is thought to have two parts, one part that protrudes above and one part that penetrates through the plasma membrane into the interior of the cell. A channel passing through the length of the receptor is thought to be the site of ion transport that initiates and propagates the action potential. Atropine combines competitively with this receptor but, unlike acetylcholine, closes the channel, preventing depolarization of the postsynaptic membrane.[17]

Other drugs currently used to antagonize the effects of acetylcholine on airway smooth muscle are all antimuscarinic (Fig 4-3). Their site of action is the muscarinic receptor on the postsynaptic membrane of the parasympathetic neuromuscular junction. Like atropine, they bind competitively to the acetylcholine receptor. In general, anticholinergic drugs are derived from acetylcholine by the replacement of the acetyl group with a more bulky subunit. In the prototypic antimuscarinic drug, atropine, several substitutions have been made (Fig 4-3). Atropine methonitrate (Fig 4-3), a quaternary ammonium derivative of atropine, has a second methyl group added to the nitrogen of the tropic acid subunit. Ipratropium bromide, another quaternary ammonium derivative of atropine, has an isopropyl group added to the same nitrogen on the tropic acid subunit. These small changes to the atropine molecule alter the absorption of these drugs from mucosal surfaces and alter their ability to cross the blood-brain barrier.[18]

INDICATIONS

Bronchoconstriction

Antimuscarinic drugs effectively relieve bronchoconstriction in a variety of clinical circumstances. The two drugs that have been most widely studied and

Anticholinergic, Antimuscarinic Drugs

used as bronchodilators are atropine sulfate (a tertiary ammonium compound well absorbed from mucosal surfaces) and ipratropium bromide (a quaternary ammonium compound poorly absorbed). Both drugs relieve bronchoconstriction in chronic bronchitis and emphysema as well as in asthma.[19] Both are best administered by inhalation when used to treat bronchoconstriction.

At the time of this writing, the U.S. Food and Drug Administration has not approved any antimuscarinic drug for treatment of bronchoconstriction. Atropine sulfate, however, is available for other indications and is fairly widely used as a bronchodilator. Nevertheless, the narrow margin between the dose of atropine sulfate that induces bronchodilation and the dose that causes significant adverse effects limits the usefulness of this drug as a bronchodilator. Ipratropium bromide, which is better tolerated because it is poorly absorbed, is being considered for approval by the U.S. Food and Drug Administration. At present, it is available in the United States only for investigational use, but is available in several other parts of the world for general clinical use.

Antimuscarinic drugs are most useful as bronchodilators in persons who have chronic bronchitis and emphysema.[19] In this disorder, atropine sulfate[20] and ipratropium bromide[21] dilate airways as well as, or better than β-adrenergic bronchodilators and often have a longer duration of action. Many persons who have chronic bronchitis and emphysema respond well with bronchodilation to antimuscarinic drugs but not at all to β-agonists.[20,22] As noted above, frequent adverse effects to atropine sulfate limit its use, but ipratropium bromide or other nonabsorbable antimuscarinic drugs will probably be widely used in the future as bronchodilators in persons who have chronic bronchitis and emphysema.

Antimuscarinic drugs are also useful as bronchodilators in persons who have asthma[23,24] (Table 4-1). However, in asthma, β-agonists often dilate airways more effectively than antimuscarinic drugs.[19] Pretreatment with antimuscarinic drugs diminishes the bronchoconstriction induced by inhaled gases, dusts, and irritants, by inhaled antigen, and by exercise, hyperventilation, and cold air. Pretreatment with beta agonists, however, is generally more effective in diminishing the bronchoconstriction induced by these stimuli. Nevertheless in some circumstances, antimuscarinic drugs may be preferred to β-agonists in the treatment of asthma. In person who have concomitant heart disease and tolerate poorly the tachycardia induced by β-agonists and methylxanthines, ipratropium bromide may be preferred. Similarly, in persons in whom tremor is a major complication of β-agonist therapy, antimuscarinic drugs avoid this adverse effect. Patients in whom bronchospasm has been precipitated by β-blockers often respond poorly to β-agonists and usually respond better to antimuscarinic drugs. Similarly, antimuscarinic drugs may be preferred to treat bronchoconstriction induced by anticholinesterase therapy. Psychogenic exacerbation of asthma is thought to be largely mediated through vagal cholinergic stimulation of airway smooth muscle. If this is true, antimuscarinic drugs theoretically would specifically inhibit this bronchoconstrictor response. The bronchodilator effect of ipratropium bromide is additive to that of β-agonists and appears to prolong the

Table 4-1
Summary of Efficacy of Anticholinergic Agents Against Specific Bronchospastic Stimuli

Stimulus	Efficacy of Anticholinergic Agents	Efficacy of Adrenergic Agents Relative to Anticholinergic Agents
Cholinergic agents	Fully protective	
Histamine	Partially protective at most	More effective
Various mediators, PGF$_{2\alpha}$ serotonin, bradykinin	Partially protective at most	
Beta blockade	Effective reversal	Much less effective
Gases, dust, irritants	Variable, usually some protection	
Antigens	Variable, from none to excellent	More effective
Exercise, hyperventilation, cold air	Moderately effective, possibly more so in large doses	Invariably more effective
Psychogenic factors	Good protection	Probably less effective

From: Gross NJ, Skorodin MS.[19] Anticholinergic, antimuscarinic bronchodilators. Am Rev Resp Dis 1984; 129:856–870. By Permission.

response.[25,26] It may be a useful adjunct to β-agonists in the treatment of asthma. (See Interactions with Other Drugs, below.)

Why antimuscarinic drugs are relatively more effective as bronchodilators in persons who have chronic bronchitis and emphysema than in those who have asthma is unclear. Cholinergic receptors are more plentiful in central than in peripheral airways, whereas adrenergic receptors are more plentiful peripherally than centrally.[19] The finding that antimuscarinic drugs are more effective bronchodilators than β-agonists in persons who have chronic bronchitis and emphysema suggests that in this disorder there is greater obstruction centrally than peripherally. For emphysema though, this generally is not thought to be the case. The finding that β-agonists are more effective bronchodilators than antimuscarinic drugs in asthma suggests that peripheral airway obstruction is more prominent in this disorder.

Bronchorrhea

Atropine sulfate may reduce massive bronchorrhea. Atropine sulfate decreases mucous secretion and transmucosal ion flux *in vitro* and decreases ciliary activity and mucous transport rates *in vivo*. Ipratropium bromide, which was actually selected for development from among its congeners because of a

Anticholinergic, Antimuscarinic Drugs

high ratio of bronchodilator to secretion inhibitory effects, does not alter any of these functions. Neither drug alters mucous viscosity. Data on whether inhaled atropine sulfate and ipratropium bromide decrease the volume of secretions in patients who have asthma or chronic bronchitis are conflicting.[19] Nevertheless, atropine has been found to decrease secretions in patients who have massive bronchorrhea and is probably worth trying in the rare patient with this symptom.[27,28]

Prophylaxis Against Vaso-Vagal Reactions

Subcutaneous atropine sulfate is regularly given to prevent vaso-vagal hypotension before a number of procedures of pulmonary medicine: bronchoscopy, thoracentesis, pleural biopsy, and chest tube insertion.

CONTRAINDICATIONS

Atropine sulfate and other tertiary ammonium antimuscarinic drugs, which are absorbed from the tracheobronchial tree, are contraindicated in patients who have nonpulmonary disorders exacerbated by blockade of parasympathetic innervation. In angle closure glaucoma, gastric outlet obstruction, bladder outlet obstruction, and some heart disease, atropine sulfate is contraindicated. In patients who have angle closure glaucoma, the mydriasis induced by atropine sulfate may precipitate acute attacks of glaucoma. In those who have gastric outlet obstruction the loss of parasympathetic tone to the stomach may precipitate gastric retention. In prostatic hypertrophy or bladder outlet obstruction due to other causes, atropine sulfate may cause urinary retention. In patients who have heart disease who cannot tolerate the increase in heart rate induced by parasympathetic blockade, atropine sulfate is contraindicated. On the other hand, quaternary ammonium antimuscarinic drugs, such a ipratropium bromide and atropine methonitrate, are only minimally absorbed from mucosal surfaces and, therefore, are not contraindicated in any of the above disorders.[19]

It has long been feared that antimuscarinic drugs may adversely affect patients who have asthma and chronic bronchitis by altering airway secretions. Atropine sulfate does decrease mucous secretions, transmucosal electrolyte and water flux, ciliary motility, and mucous transport, but ipratropium bromide does not affect any of these functions. Neither drug affects sputum viscosity. Most studies have shown that neither drug affects the volume of sputum produced in either chronic bronchitis or asthma.[19] Therefore, on the basis of the present evidence, the fear of causing inspissation of mucous in asthma or chronic bronchitis should probably not contraindicate the use of these drugs.

DOSAGE

To choose an appropriate dose of inhaled atropine sulfate, one needs to know one's nebulization system well. The dose of atropine sulfate placed in a nebulizer is usually considerably greater than the dose tolerated by parenteral administration. Nevertheless, as atropine sulfate is well absorbed, the fact that patients tolerate the larger nebulizer dose merely indicates that only a fraction of the nebulized dose reaches the oral, pharyngeal, airway, and gastrointestinal surfaces where it is absorbed. Much of the nebulized dose precipitates on the surfaces of the nebulization system, and much is exhaled by the patient as an observable mist. The marked difference in nebulizers, pressure generating systems, delivery tubing, and mouthpieces or facemasks explains the marked difference in delivery of atropine doses. Some investigators have given 15 mg of atropine sulfate by nebulization to patients, without adverse effects, whereas other investigators have induced dysphoria and urinary hesitancy after giving only 2 mg of atropine sulfate. The former investigators reported the dose of atropine sulfate placed in their nebulization system, the latter investigators calculated the delivered dose by weighing their nebulizer before and after use.

The size of particles generated by a nebulizer also affects the delivery of the drug and the dose of drug retained. Larger particles impact on the surfaces of the mouth, pharynx and central airways, while smaller particles are carried more peripherally. Very small particles may not impact at all and may be exhaled. A large proportion of any inhaled dose of atropine sulfate probably acts on the airways after absorption from the mouth, pharynx, and gastrointestinal tract, and delivery to the airways by the circulation.

Having cautioned against the blind acceptance of recommended doses of inhaled atropine sulfate, we suggest treating adults by placing in the nebulizer 0.5–2.0 mg of atropine sulfate diluted in saline to a volume of 3 ml. If the initial dose does not cause the desired bronchodilator effect or significant adverse effects, the dose may be increased. Optimal bronchodilation is said to occur at a dose of 0.05 mg/kg in children and 0.025 mg/kg in adults. It is worth reiterating that the therapeutic margin for atropine is minimal and that adverse effects are common at therapeutic doses.

Ipratropium bromide is usually administered from a metered-dose inhaler that delivers 20 μg per puff. The conventional dose is 40–80 μg. Optimal bronchodilation in stable asthma is obtained with a dose of 40–80 μg. In status asthmaticus, however, the bronchodilator response increases through cumulative doses of up to 500 μg. This dose is tolerated without adverse effects. In chronic bronchitis and emphysema, doses above 125 μg give no incremental bronchodilation.

The onset of the bronchodilator effect of both atropine sulfate and ipratropium bromide is almost immediate, but is probably not as rapid as that of β-agonists. Patients need to know that the bronchodilator effect will be somewhat

Anticholinergic, Antimuscarinic Drugs

delayed to avoid taking repeated doses while awaiting the drug effect. Peak effects do not occur until 30–60 minutes and bronchodilator effects last at least four hours. In stable patients three or four times daily dosing is usually sufficient.

To prevent vaso-vagal reactions during a pulmonary procedure 0.6–0.8 mg of atropine sulfate is usually given to adults subcutaneously 30–60 minutes before the procedure.

ADVERSE EFFECTS AND THEIR MANAGEMENT

Adverse effects to inhaled atropine sulfate are common at therapeutic doses and limit broader use of this particular drug as a bronchodilator. On the other hand, adverse effects to inhaled ipratropium bromide and atropine methonitrate, which are poorly absorbed from mucosal surfaces, are rare except for dry mouth and a bad taste. The lack of adverse effects of these latter drugs augers well for their wider use in the future.

The adverse effects of antimuscarinic drugs are dose-related and involve various organ systems at different doses (Table 4-2).[18] As is true for most drugs, individuals vary in response to a given dose. The adverse effects due to antimuscarinic drugs include dryness of the mucous membranes, dysphagia, difficulty talking, thirst, blurry vision due to loss of accommodation, photophobia, mydriasis, hot, dry, flushed skin, increased body temperature, rapid pulse, palpitations, hypertension, urinary retention, and abdominal distention. Central nervous system symptoms are common and include first, restlessness, excitation, confusion, and dyscoordination. At higher doses mania, hallucinations, and

Table 4-2
Effects of Atropine in Relation to Dosage

Dose	Effects
0.5 mg	Slight cardiac slowing; some dryness of mouth; inhibition of sweating
1.0 mg	Definite dryness of mouth; thirst; acceleration of heart, sometimes preceded by slowing; mild dilation of pupil
2.0 mg	Rapid heart rate; palpitation; marked dryness of mouth; dilated pupils; some blurring of near vision
5.0 mg	All the above symptoms marked; speech disturbed; difficulty in swallowing; restlessness and fatigue; headache; dry, hot skin; difficulty in micturition; reduced intestinal peristalsis
10.0 mg and more	Above symptoms more marked; pulse rapid and weak; iris practically obliterated; vision very blurred; skin flushed, hot dry, and scarlet; ataxia, restlessness, and excitement; hallucinations and delirium; coma

From: Weiner N.[18] Atropine, scopolamine, and related antimuscarinic drugs. In Gilman AG, Goodman LS, and Gilman A, editors: The Pharmacologic Basis of Therapeutics. ed 6, New York 1980, MacMillan Publishing Co. By Permission.

delirium occur and at still higher doses central nervous system depression and coma develop. At a dose of 0.5 mg, atropine sulfate causes dry mouth and dry skin, at 1.0 mg, thirst, increased heart rate and mydriasis. At 2.0 mg it causes palpitations and loss of visual accommodation. With 5.0 mg, speech is disturbed, and there is dysphagia, restlessness, hot, dry skin, and difficulty with urination. At 10 mg atropine sulfate causes ataxia, excitement, hallucinations, delirium, and coma. Since atropine is hydrolized by the liver and is excreted unchanged by the kidneys, both hepatic and renal insufficiency may result in toxicity at doses that are otherwise well tolerated.

The treatment of adverse effects of antimuscarinic drugs is chiefly symptomatic, allowing time for clearance of the drug, which may take several days. Symptomatic therapy should include measures to decrease body temperature, and to moisten mucous membranes. Bladder catheterization may be required. Agitation and seizures may require appropriate drug therapy. If the antimuscarinic drug has been taken orally, which is unlikely to be the case in treatment of pulmonary diseases, gastric lavage should be performed and activated charcoal given. If the patient has coma, life threatening arrhythmias, severe hallucinations, or severe hypotension, the anticholinesterase inhibitor physostigmine may partially reverse symptoms. Death due to antimuscarinic toxicity is rare and there are no sequelae in those who recover.

Ipratropium bromide in therapeutic doses has been found to have no effect on pupil size, ocular accommodation, intraocular pressure, heart rate, or urinary flow.[19] In a manner analogous to that seen with β-agonists, however, it has been reported at times to cause a paradoxical decrease in airflow.

Also in a manner analogous to that seen with β-agonists, antimuscarinic drugs at times increase alveolar-arterial oxygen difference while causing bronchodilation.[29] β-agonists presumably increase the oxygen difference by altering ventilation-perfusion matching, and antimuscarinic drugs presumably have the same effect. This effect is considerably smaller with antimuscarinic drugs than with β-agonists, but one needs to be wary of a potential large effect in occasional patients.

INTERACTION WITH OTHER DRUGS, CHOICE OF CONCOMITANT AGENTS

Antimuscarinic bronchodilators interact both favorably and unfavorably with other drugs. They interact favorably with adrenergic bronchodilators.[30,31] The bronchodilator effect of antimuscarinic drugs is independent and additive to that of adrenergic drugs in the treatment of both asthma and chronic bronchitis and emphysema. When maximal bronchodilation has been obtained with either adrenergic or antimuscarinic drugs, the addition of the other type of drug causes further bronchodilation. The combination of an antimuscarinic plus an adrenergic drug may have a more prolonged duration of action than either drug alone. Thus, the combination of antimuscarinic and adrenergic drugs may be beneficial in three ways: (1) the duration of action may be prolonged; (2) the use of two drugs in smaller dosage may cause fewer adverse effects than the use of one drug in a larger dose; and (3) when maximal dosage of a drug of one type does not produce sufficient bronchodilation, addition of a drug of the other type should cause greater bronchodilation. To our knowledge, unfavorable interaction between antimuscarinic drugs and either adrenergic or xanthine bronchodilators has not been reported.

The tertiary ammonium antimuscarinic drugs, which are absorbed from mucosa and thus have systemic effects, may interact unfavorably with other drugs. Atropine sulfate may add to the adverse effects of other drugs having anticholinergic actions: antiParkinsonian drugs (Cogentin, Artane), tricyclic antidepressants, antihistamines, glutethimide (Doriden), meperidine (Demerol), and propantheline (ProBanthine). Also, by delaying gastric emptying, atropine sulfate may alter the absorption of other drugs. Delayed gastric emptying increases the degradation of 1-dopa and phenothiazines within the stomach and thus decreases small intestinal absorption. Addition of atropine sulfate to a medication regimen may decrease serum concentrations of 1-dopa and phenothiazines, and removal of atropine sulfate may increase serum concentrations of these drugs. In a different manner, delayed gastric emptying increases dissolution of nitrofurantoin within the stomach and increases subsequent small intestinal absorbtion. Thus atropine sulfate may increase or decrease absorption of other drugs.

REFERENCES

1. The Dispensary of the United States of America, 25th Edition, Osal, A and Farrar GE (eds). Philadelphia, JB Lippincott Company, 1955
2. Charpin D, Orehek J, Velardocchio JM: Bronchodilator effects of antiasthmatic cigarette smoke (Datura stromonium). Thorax 34:259–261, 1979
3. Gandevia B: Historical review of the use of parasympatholytic agents in the treatment of respiratory disorders. Postgraduate Med J, Suppl (7) 51:13–20, 1975
4. Hertz CW: Historical aspects of anticholinergic treatment of obstructive airways disease. Scand J Resp Dis, Suppl 103:105–109, 1979
5. Herxheimer H: Atropine cigarettes in asthma and emphysema. Brit Med J 2:167–171, 1959
6. Scandinavian Symposium on Chronic Obstructive Airways Disease. Scan J Resp Dis Suppl 103:1–223, 1979
7. The place of parasympatholytic drugs in the management of chronic obstructive airways disease, in Hoffband BI, (ed): Proceedings of an international symposium. Postgraduate Med J (Suppl 7) 51:1–161, 1975

8. DeTroyer A, Yernault JC, Rodenstein D: Effect of vagal blockade on lung mechanics in normal man. J Appl Physiol 46:217–226, 1979
9. Douglas NJ, Sudlow MF, Flenley DC: The effect of an inhaled atropine-like drug on airway function in normal subjects. J Appl Physiol 46:256–262, 1976
10. Mayer SE: Neurohumoral transmission and the autonomic nervous system, in Gilman AG, Goodman LS, Gilman A. (eds): The Pharmacological Basis of Therapeutics. MacMillan Publishing Company, New York, 1980, pp 56–90
11. Birks RI, MacIntosh FC: Acetylcholine metabolism at nerve endings. Brit Med Bull 13:157–161, 1957
12. Taylor P: Cholinergic agonists, in Gilman AG, Goodman LS, Gilman A (eds): The Pharmacological Basis of Therapeutics. 6th Edition, New York, MacMillan Publishing Company, 1980, pp 91–99
13. Szentivanyi A, Krzanowski JJ, Polson JB: The autonomic nervous system, in Middleton E Jr, Reed CE, Ellis EF (eds): Allergy: Principles and Practice. 2nd Edition, St. Louis, The CV Mosby Company, 1983, pp 317–320
14. Potter LT: Synthesis, storage and release of acetylcholine, in Bourne, GH (ed): The Structure and Function of Nerve Tissue. Vol. 4, New York, Academic Press, Inc. 1972
15. Hammer R, Berrie CP, Birdsall NJM, et al: Pirenzepine distinguishes between different subclasses of muscarinic receptors. Nature 283:90–92, 1980
16. Vickroy TW, Watson M, Yamamura HI, et al: Agonist binding to multiple muscarinic receptors. Fed Proc 43:2785–2790, 1984
17. Changeux JP, Devillers-Thiery A, Chemouilli P: Acetylcholine receptor: an allosteric protein. Science 225:1335–1345, 1984
18. Weiner N: Atropine, scopolamine, and related antimuscarinic drugs, in: Gilman AG, Goodman LS, Gilman A (eds), The Pharmacologic Basis of Therapeutics, 6th Edition, New York, MacMillan Publishing Company, 1980, pp 120–137
19. Gross NJ, Skorodin MS: Anticholinergic, antimuscarinic bronchodilators. State of the Art. Am Rev Resp Dis 129:856–870, 1984
20. Klock LE, Miller TD, Morris AA, et al: A comparative study of atropine sulfate and isoproterenol hydrochloride in chronic bronchitis. Am Rev Resp Dis 112:371–376, 1975
21. Baigelman W, Chodosh S: Bronchodilator action of the anticholinergic drug, ipratropium bromide (SCH 1000), as an aerosol in chronic bronchitis and asthma. Chest 71:324–328, 1977
22. Marini JJ, Lakschminarayan S: The effect of atropine inhalation in "irreversible" chronic bronchitis. Chest 77:591–596, 1980
23. Altounyan REC: Variation of drug action on airway obstruction in man. Thorax 19:406–415, 1964
24. Snow RW, Miller WC, Blair HT, et al: Inhaled atropine in asthma. Ann Allergy 42:286–289, 1979
25. Bruderman I, Cohen-Aronovski R, Smorzik J: A comparative study of various combinations of ipratropium bromide and metaproterenol in allergic asthmatic patients. Chest 83:208–210, 1983
26. Ullah MI, Newman GB, Saunders KB: Influence of age on response to ipratropium and salbutamol in asthma. Thorax 36:523–529, 1981

27. Lopez-Vidriero MT, Costello J, Clark TJH, et al: Effect of atropine on sputum production. Thorax 30:543–547, 1975
28. Wick MM, Ingram RH: Bronchorrhea responsive to aerosolized atropine. JAMA 235:1356, 1976
29. Field GB: The effects of posture, oxygen, isoproterenol and atropine on ventilation-perfusion relationships in the lung in human asthma. Clin Sci 32:279–288, 1967
30. Lightbody IM, Ingram CG, Legge JS, et al: Ipratropium bromide, salbutamol and prednisolone in bronchial asthma and chronic bronchitis. Br J Dis Chest 72:181–186, 1978
31. Wilson RHL, Battaglia PJ, Wilson NL: Crossover study with nebulized bronchodilators and atropine. Chest 73 (Suppl):998–1000, 1978

Shih-Wen Chang
Talmadge E. King

5

Corticosteroids

Among the drugs used in treating respiratory disorders, corticosteroids are unique in several respects. They are endogenous substances released by the adrenal cortex and have important physiologic effects on many organs. Deficiency causes symptoms of adrenal insufficiency and may result in death. Many of the undesirable effects of pharmacological doses of corticosteroids are simply the amplification of their normal physiological actions. A unique side effect, that of hypothalamic-pituitary-adrenal suppression, is associated with the rapid withdrawal of corticosteroid after prolonged administration. They are nonspecific in their action, and are the most powerful agents available for the treatment of a variety of respiratory diseases including asthma, bronchitis, and some interstitial lung diseases. This nonspecificity fosters their usefulness in a wide variety of respiratory disorders ranging from asthma to fat emboli. However, the nonspecificity of action also leads to two potential problems in the therapeutic use of corticosteroids: (1) the normal mechanism for containing an infectious agent is suppressed, thus increasing the likelihood of acquiring serious infections; (2) corticosteroid therapy is "palliative" and suppresses symptoms, therefore, the underlying cause of the disease may not be addressed by the physician or the patient. For example, in patients with allergic asthma, removing pets from the home or discontinuing exposure to other environmental irritants may not be rigorously pursued if the patient's symptoms are well-controlled on corticosteroids.

Correct and appropriate use of corticosteroids requires a full understanding of the physiologic effects, clinical pharmacology, and disease-drug interactions of the various corticosteroid preparations. When used improperly, the

DRUGS FOR THE RESPIRATORY SYSTEM
ISBN 0-8089-1818-4

Copyright © 1986 by Grune & Stratton, Inc.
All rights of reproduction in any form reserved.

corticosteroid-induced change in body habitus, personality, and other chronic sequelaes may alter the patient's life style and self-image irreparably. For some patients, the treatment may be worse than the disease. On the other hand, some physicians may be so wary of the side effects of corticosteroids as to undertreat the patients, thus depriving them of the chance to lead a symptom-free existence.

MECHANISM OF ACTION

Corticosteroids can be classified according to their actions as either glucocorticoids or mineralocorticoids, both of which are synthesized from cholesterol by the adrenal cortex. Cortisol is the major endogenous glucocorticoid, while aldosterone is the major endogenous mineralocorticoid. The glucocorticoids have powerful and diverse effects on cellular metabolism, while the mineralocorticoids are important in the regulation of extracellular fluid volume and potassium concentration.

Cortisol is synthesized and secreted by the adrenal cortex under the stimulatory action of adrenocorticotropic hormone (ACTH) from the anterior pituitary gland. When the corticosteroid level falls to a low point, the hypothalamus is activated to release corticotropin releasing factor (CRF), which stimulates the release of ACTH from the pituitary. This complex set of interactions comprises the hypothalamic-pituitary-adrenal (HPA) system. In the normal individual about 15–30 mg of cortisol is secreted each day. There is a marked diurnal pattern of cortisol secretion that reaches a peak at about 8:00 AM and a trough at about 4:00 PM. Under stresses such as infection, surgery, or hypoglycemia, the adrenal cortex can increase the synthesis and secretion of glucocorticoids as much as 10-fold. More than 90 percent of the circulating plasma cortisol is bound to plasma proteins, of which the most important are cortisol-binding globulin and albumin. Only the unbound fraction of the plasma cortisol is physiologically active. Cortisol is metabolized by the liver into inactive metabolites, which are then excreted by the kidney.

In comparison to cortisol, aldosterone is secreted in much smaller amounts and the basal plasma concentration of aldosterone is correspondingly lower. Although ACTH can stimulate aldosterone secretion, the major control mechanism for aldosterone release is through the renin-angiotensin system. Aldosterone stimulates renal sodium reabsorption and potassium excretion and is, therefore, an important regulator of the extracellular fluid volume and plasma potassium concentration.

All synthetic corticosteroids exhibit varying proportions of glucocorticoid and mineralocorticoid activity.[1] In general, the desired antiinflammatory effect of a corticosteroid preparation correlates well with its glucocorticoid potency, whereas the undesirable effects of fluid retention and potassium loss are due to its mineralocorticoid properties. Thus, except in replacement therapy for adrenal insufficiency, the corticosteroid preparations with predominant glucocorticoid effects are preferred over those with significant mineralocorticoid effects.

Table 5-1 summarizes the major pharmacological actions of the corticosteroids. Only the actions that are pertinent to their use as therapeutic agents will be reviewed. These actions of corticosteroids include modulation of cellular metabolism, suppression of immune and inflammatory responses, potentiation of β-adrenergic agonist effects and other miscellaneous effects.

Effects on Cellular Metabolism

The exact cellular mechanism of corticosteroid action is still poorly understood. Much of the metabolic effects of the glucocorticoid hormones can be explained by the corticosteroid receptor hypothesis.[2] In target tissues, cortisol diffuses across the cell membrane and binds to cytoplasmic receptors. The hormone-receptor complex then moves into the cell nucleus and alters the transcription process from DNA to RNA. This ultimately results in a change in the rate of protein synthesis in the cell. It is unclear whether this receptor-mediated mechanism adequately explains all the pharmacological effects of the glucocorticoids and other hypotheses that have been proposed including stimulation of

Table 5-1
Mechanism of Action of Corticosteroids

Effect on Cellular Metabolism
    Stimulate hepatic gluconeogenesis
    Decrease peripheral utilization of glucose
    Increase protein catabolism
    Increase lipolysis
    Exert a "permissive effect" for the metabolic action of other hormones.
Immunosuppressive and Anti-inflammatory Effects
    Effect on cellular elements
        Lymphopenia, leukocytosis, eosinopenia
        Inhibits delayed hypersensitivity reactions
    Vasoconstriction in inflamed vessels
    Effect on lipid mediators—decreased synthesis of prostaglandins, and leukotrienes
    Inhibition of chemotaxis at suprapharmacologic concentrations
Effect on Adrenergic Receptor
    Abolish the tachyphylaxis to beta-adrenergic agents
Miscellaneous Effects
    Inhibit fibroblast growth and collagen synthesis
    Decreased reticuloendothelial clearance of antibody-coated cells
    Mild decrease in immunoglobulin levels but no decrease in specific antibody production
    Decrease in lysosomal release and stabilization of lysosomal membranes at suprapharmacologic concentrations

intracellular cyclic 3'5' adenosine-monophosphate (cAMP) production or direct lysosomal membrane-stabilization.[2]

In general, the actions of glucocorticoids on carbohydrate, protein, and lipid metabolism are opposite to those of insulin. In a predisposed individual, prolonged excessive glucocorticoid action can lead to a diabetes-like state with hyperglycemia and glucosuria. Muscle wasting, skin thinning, and osteoporosis reflect the catabolic effect of glucocorticoids on tissue protein. The glucocorticoids also increase lipolysis and stimulate the release of free fatty acids and glycerol from fat stores. The differential sensitivity of central and peripheral fat tissues to the glucocorticoids leads to a redistribution of fat stores toward a more central location. Thus, prolonged glucocorticoid therapy induces the features of Cushing's syndrome including the "moon face" and the "buffalo hump."

In addition to these direct actions, the glucocorticoids exert a "permissive effect" on the cellular action of many hormones.[2] For example, in the absence of physiological amounts of glucocorticoids, the actions of epinephrine on gluconeogenesis and lipolysis are markedly impaired. Other substances for which the permissive effect of glucocorticoids is important include norepinephrine, glucagon, thyrotropin, and prostaglandin E. The importance of this permissive effect is seen in patients with adrenal insufficiency. These patients can function adequately under normal conditions, but during periods of stress and reduced availability of exogenous nutrients such as starvation, infection or surgery, they are unable to maintain the stable homeostatic environment essential for survival.

Immunosuppressive and Anti-Inflammatory Effects[3]

Glucocorticoids affect virtually every step in both the immune response and inflammation, and because there is great overlap in their mechanisms, these effects of glucocorticoids will be reviewed together.

Effects on Cellular Elements

In some animals, glucocorticoids have a powerful lympholytic action, but human lymphocytes are much more resistant. Lymphopenia (both T- and B-cells) is observed 4–6 hours after a single dose of prednisone or hydrocortisone,[3,4] primarily because of a temporary redistribution of the circulating T lymphocytes from the intravascular compartment to the lymphoid tissues, mainly the bone marrow. In addition, the T-cell lymphopenia is due to a decrease in the T_4 (helper-inducer) subset of cells. The precise mechanism of this redistribution of lymphocytes is unknown, but an alteration of cell surfaces and effects on the microvascular endothelium have been postulated. Long-term alternate day corticosteroid administration produces a transient lymphopenia in corticosteroid-dependent asthmatics very similar to that produced by a single dose in normals, and may occur even after years of prednisone ingestion. An exaggerated rebound of the lumphocyte count occurs in 50 percent of these patients at 24 hours after the dose was given. This phenomenon is not seen in patients given short-term corticosteroid administration.

Glucocorticoids also alter lymphocyte-mediated responses, predominantly T-cell mediated immune responses. An example of the effect of glucocorticoids on cell-mediated immune reactions, is the well known inhibition of cutaneous delayed hypersensitivity (e.g. tuberculin response).[5,6]

Antibody production is not usually suppressed by conventional glucocorticoid therapy, and occasionally it is increased.[3] However, mild decreases in serum immunoglobulins, especially IgG, will occur in some patients and presumably results from increased catabolism rather than suppression of production.

The monocyte-macrophage system can be profoundly affected by glucocorticoids. Monocytopenia like lymphopenia results from the redistribution of cells from the intravascular compartment to lymphoid tissue and is proportionately of greater severity than the lymphopenia.[3] Other effects on monocyte-macrophage function include: inhibition of phagocytosis and killing of microorganisms, inhibition of pyrogen production and secretion of collagenase, elastase, and plasminogen activator. Monocyte-macrophages are key cells in the chronic inflammatory process because of both direct local action and recruitment of other cell types. Consequently, corticosteroid alteration of the monocyte-macrophage migration, activity, and secretion will profoundly affect the inflammatory response.

Glucocorticoids produce a peripheral leukocytosis both acutely following a single dose (peak at 4–6 hours) and chronically in patients receiving long-term prednisone therapy (maximal levels occur within two weeks and then decline but not to pretreatment levels.[7] The glucocorticoid-induced neutrophilic leukocytosis results from accelerated release of mature neutrophils from the bone marrow reserves and a decrease in neutrophil egress from the blood. In this regard, excessive numbers of immature leukocytes (a left-shift in the cell differential) is unusual with corticosteroid therapy, and should alert the physician to search for possible infectious etiologies.[7]

The net effect is suppression in the accumulation of cells (both neutrophils and monocyte-macrophages) at inflammatory loci. This is probably the major antiinflammatory mechanism of glucocorticoids and explains in part the reduction in host defenses that occur in patients on long-term therapy. Glucocorticoids also interfere with neutrophil chemotaxis, and *in vitro* data suggest that they interfere with neutrophil phagocytosis and intracellular killing of microorganisms when given in suprapharmacologic concentrations.

Circulating eosinophils and basophils also decrease after glucocorticoid administration primarily as a result of the redistribution out of the intravascular compartment to other tissues. The effect of corticosteroids on their cellular function is not known. Patients treated with commonly used doses of prednisone do not have significant alterations in platelet function. Corticosteroids have no apparent effect on mast cells at pharmacological doses, but inhibition of histamine release and stabilization of cell or lysosomal membranes has been described at suprapharmacologic levels.

Effects on Blood Vessels

Glucocorticoids cause vasoconstriction and oppose the increase in capillary permeability at the site of inflammation, so that extravasation of cells and fluids into the inflamed tissues is reduced. The vasoconstrictive effect appears to be specific for inflamed vessels, since in other vascular beds glucocorticoids can cause vasodilation.[3] The mechanisms for these effects of glucocorticoids are unknown but may include the inhibition of lipid mediator(s) production or decrease in kinin activation.[2]

Effects on Lipid Mediators[8]

One of the most important amplification systems in the inflammatory response involves the arachidonic acid metabolites.[9] Arachidonic acid, a 20 carbon fatty acid with four double bonds, is a normal component of membrane phospholipids. Both immunologic and nonimmunologic stimuli can trigger the release of arachidonic acid from the cell membrane by activating the enzyme phospholipase A_2. Free arachidonic acids can then be metabolized by the cyclooxygenase enzymes into various products including prostaglandins and thromboxane. One of the prostaglandins, PGD_2, is a potent bronchoconstrictor and stimulates neutrophil and eosinophil random migration. Thromboxane A_2 causes vasoconstriction and bronchoconstriction, whereas other prostaglandins such as PGI_2 cause vaso- and bronchodilation. In addition, thromboxane A_2 and PGI_2 are important regulators of platelet and leukocyte aggregation and adhesion to endothelial cells.

Alternatively, arachidonic acid can be metabolized by enzymes of the lipoxygenase pathway into another group of powerful inflammatory mediators: the leukotrienes. Leukotriene B_4 is a powerful chemotactic factor for neutrophils and eosinophils. Leukotriene C_4, D_4, and E_4, together known as slow reacting substances of anaphylaxis (SRS-A), cause bronchoconstriction, vasoconstriction, increased venopermeability and increased airway secretion.[9] SRS-A is thought to be an important mediator of asthma.[10]

Glucocorticoids block the release of free arachidonic acid from membrane lipids, by mediating synthesis of the protein's lipomodulin and macrocortin that inhibit the action of phospholipase A_2.[11,12] Lipomodulin is isolated from neutrophils and macrocortin from macrophages. It has been suggested that macrocortin is a phosphorylated fragment of lipomodulin. By decreasing the availability of free arachidonic acid, glucocorticoids decrease the formation of prostaglandins, thromboxane and leukotrienes, thus effectively depriving the body of a potent mechanism for amplifying inflammatory responses.

More recently, another powerful inflammatory mediator has been identified. This is platelet activating factor (PAF), which at extremely low concentrations causes platelet aggregation, smooth muscle contraction (including bronchoconstriction), and increased vasopermeability. It has been suggested that phospholipase A_2 may release arachidonic acid and PAF from a common precursor molecule in the cell membrane.[8] By inhibiting phospholipase A_2, glucocorticoids can also inhibit the release of PAF. The suppression of release of these lipid mediators from the cell membrane is a major mechanism accounting for the powerful antiinflammatory and immunosuppressive effect of glucocorticoids.

Effect on Adrenergic Receptors

Chronic administration of β-adrenergic agonists may decrease their bronchodilatory effect in both asthmatics and normal individuals.[13] Glucocorticoids facilitate β-2-agonist effects and can thus abolish this state of tachyphylaxis to the β-adrenergic agonists. The mechanism of this glucocorticoid effect is not completely understood, but is thought to be due to both the stimulation of an increase in the number of β-adrenergic receptors as well as potentiation of cAMP synthesis once the receptor is activated. Some studies have also suggested that glucocorticoids may inhibit the activity of phosphodiesterase and thus decrease the degradation of cAMP, but this is not generally accepted. The net effect of glucocorticoids is to increase the intracellular cAMP in response to β-adrenergic agents. The increase in cAMP not only can lead to relaxation of airway smooth muscles, but can modulate leukocyte function by inhibition of release of mediators or lysosomal enzymes.

Miscellaneous Effects

Glucocorticoids have been reported to decrease the release of enzymes from lysosomes *in vitro*. Because extremely high doses are required, this effect is unlikely to be an important mechanism for glucocorticoid action,[2] except in sepsis and shock where extremely high doses of corticosteroids have been advocated.

Glucocorticoids inhibit fibroblast growth as well as collagen synthesis.[14] This is an important effect on chronic inflammation and wound healing and is one of the rationales behind using corticosteroids for the chronic inflammatory and fibrosing lung disorders.

CLINICAL PHARMACOLOGY[1,15-17]

Liver Metabolism

Structural-activity relationship analysis indicates that the antiinflammatory and glucocorticoid effects of corticosteroids require a hydroxyl group on the C11 carbon. Thus, compounds such as prednisone and cortisone, which have a ketone group on C11 carbon require metabolic processing before becoming pharmacologically active. This reduction from ketone to hydroxyl group on C11 occurs in the liver. Prednisone is converted to prednisolone and cortisone to cortisol. Although comparable plasma prednisolone levels are achieved when equipotent doses of prednisone and prednisolone are given to a normal individual, this may not be true in patients with liver impairment.[18] This suggests that one should avoid using oral prednisone or cortisone in patients with marked impairment of liver functions.

The liver is also important in the metabolic disposal of corticosteroids. The microsomal enzymes in the hepatocytes metabolize corticosteroids into inactive compounds that are then excreted by the kidney. The liver metabolism of corticosteroids can be enhanced by hyperthyroidism and drugs such as phenobarbital and ephedrine. Hypothyroidism, cirrhosis, or concomitant use of erythromycin or troleandomycin (TAO) (see later) lead to decreased hepatic clearance of the corticosteroids.

In patients with active hepatocellular disease and low serum albumin concentration, significantly more of the plasma prednisolone circulates in the unbound form.[18] Since only the free form of circulating corticosteroid is pharmacologically active, one would expect a greater degree of corticosteroid effect in patients with hypoalbuminemia. This effect, combined with the decrease in metabolism of corticosteroids by the diseased liver, suggests that prednisolone dosage may need to be reduced in patients with severe liver disease and hypoalbuminemia.

Plasma and Physiologic Half Life

Corticosteroids have been arbitrarily classified into short-, intermediate- and long-acting preparations based on the length of time ACTH is suppressed after a single dose of corticosteroid administration[19] (Table 5-2). The short-acting corticosteroids, including hydrocortisone, prednisone, and methylprednisolone inhibit plasma ACTH activity for up to 24–36 hours. The intermediate-acting corticosteroids, such as triamcinolone, inhibit ACTH activity for up to 48 hours, and the long-acting corticosteroids such as dexamethasone and betamethasone for over 48 hours. However, the actual plasma half-lives of the corticosteroids are much shorter (Table 5-2), and range from 30 minutes for cortisone to 115–252 minutes for prednisolone and 110–210 minutes for dexamethasone.[1] There is no correlation between the plasma half-life and the physiologic action for a given preparation, and corticosteroids with similar plasma half-lives (i.e., prednisolone and dexamethasone) differ greatly in the duration of physiologic action in terms of ACTH suppression.

Table 5-2
Comparison of the Clinical Properties of Commonly Used Corticosteroid Preparations

Duration of Action*	Glucocorticoid potency**	Equivalent dosage (mg)	Mineralocorticoid potency†	Requires liver activation	Approximate plasma half-life (min)
Short-acting					
cortisol (hydrocortisone)	1	20	1	No	90
cortisone	0.8	25	0.8	Yes	30
prednisone	4	5	0.8	Yes	60
prednisolone	4	5	0.8	No	200
methylprednisolone	5	4	0–0.5	No	180
Intermediate-acting					
triamcinolone	5	4	0	No	300
Long-acting					
betamethasone	25	0.75	0	No	200
dexamethasone	30	0.75	0	No	200

*Modified from Harter[19]
**The values are relative. Cortisol is arbitrarily assigned a value of one.[1]
†Mineralocorticoid effects are dose related and usually detectable only as supraphysiologic doses.

Preparations of Corticosteroids

Table 5-2 shows the commonly used corticosteroids, their relative glucocorticoid and mineralocorticoid potencies, and equivalent dosages for a given level of antiinflammatory effect. Corticosteroids can be administered in a variety of ways: oral, intravenous, intramuscular, and topical (including inhalation). Cortisol and most of the synthetic corticosteroids are effective by mouth. Water-soluble esters of corticosteroids can be given intravenously or intramuscularly, whereas ester conjugates with poor water-solubility are useful for topical therapy where systemic absorption would be undesirable. Some general points may help in the selection of a particular preparation for clinical use:

1. As noted earlier, prednisone and cortisone require activation by the liver and thus the therapeutic efficacy of these two preparations may be unreliable in patients with severe liver disease.
2. Cortisol and cortisone have a relatively high ratio of mineralocorticoid to glucocorticoid effect, so one can expect more problems with fluid retention and hypokalemia. Thus, for prolonged therapy, cortisol and cortisone should not be used except as replacement therapy for adrenal insufficiency.
3. Dexamethasone and betamethasone are powerful glucocorticoids with virtually no mineralocorticoid activity. It has been suggested that dexamethasone may have less potentiating action on the bronchodilator effect of isoproterenol than methylprednisolone making it relatively less useful in the treatment of asthma. Moreover, because of the long period of HPA suppression after dexamethasone or betamethasone, these agents should not be used for alternate day therapy and should be avoided in situations where eventual alternate day therapy is anticipated.

Method of Administration

In general, oral corticosteroids should be given as a single dose early in the morning. In most studies, the efficacy of single dose corticosteroid given daily is equivalent to several divided doses during the day.[20] Although single dose therapy does not decrease the likelihood of developing Cushing's syndrome, it appears to reduce the likelihood and severity of HPA suppression.

ALTERNATE DAY THERAPY

In patients who require prolonged therapy with corticosteroids, every attempt should be made to treat the patient with alternate day therapy, which is as effective as a similar dose given in divided doses every day.[19] Moreover, the side effects of corticosteroid therapy and degree of HPA suppression are markedly reduced with alternate day therapy. Alternate day therapy is associated with less or no suppression of fever, white blood cell counts, or delayed-type hypersensitivity skin tests. For alternate day therapy to be maximally effective, a short-acting corticosteroid such as prednisone or methylprednisolone should be used. The use of long-acting preparations such as dexamethasone in high doses may lead to HPA suppression even when given every 48 hours.[21] In patients who have been on prolonged corticosteroid therapy every day, the change to alternate day therapy should be gradual to prevent the emergence of adrenal insufficiency. It is important to realize that in patients with preexisting HPA suppression, adrenal insufficiency can develop on the "OFF" day of the alternate day therapy. One method for the conversion from daily corticosteroids to alternate day therapy is a gradual decrease of corticosteroid dosage on the odd days, while increasing the corticosteroid dosage on the even days, until twice the original dose is taken on the even days and none on the odd days. In some patients, 3-4 times the normal daily dose may be required initially. After the patient is on an alternate day regimen, the corticosteroid dosage should be gradually decreased to the lowest dose of corticosteroid compatible with an optimal level of function (see later).

CORTICOSTEROID AEROSOL[22,23]

Corticosteroid aerosol was proposed for treatment of asthma as early as the 1950s. Early studies using water-soluble corticosteroids such as hydrocortisone or dexamethasone phosphate were either unimpressive or showed no advantage over oral corticosteroids in systemic side-effects. Subsequent preparations with improved topical antiinflammatory potency and reduced systemic absorption have been shown to be highly effective with minimal systemic side effects, and thus have become a major therapeutic modality in the treatment of asthma and allergic rhinitis.

Preparation and Dosages

Currently, three different preparations of corticosteroid aerosols are available in the United States (Table 5-3). Each meter dose inhalation of Beclomethasone dipropionate (BDP) delivers 42 mcg. The usual adult dose of BDP is 400 mcg, which is said to be comparable in efficacy against asthma as 5-10 mg of oral prednisone, but 1000 mcg per day may be required in some patients. Mild adrenal suppression may be seen at doses greater than 1600 mcg per day. BDP is recommended to be given in divided doses 3-4 times each day although in patients with mild asthma twice a day dosage may be just as effective.[23]

Triamcinolone acetonide and flunisolide have recently also become available in the United States.[22] The recommended daily dose of Triamcinolone is 2 puffs (one puff delivers approximately 100 mcg) 3-4 times a day. Flunisolide is approximately equal to triamcinolone in antiinflammatory potency. The recom-

Table 5-3
Corticosteroid Aerosol Preparations

Drug	Trade Name	Amount per Inhalation	Recommended Dosage (Adult)
Beclomethasone dipropionate	Vanceril Beclovent	42 mcg	2 inhal. tid up to 20 inhal. per day
Triamcinolone acetonide	Azmacort	100 mcg	2 inhal. tid up to 16 inhal. per day
Flunisolide	Aerobid	250 mcg	2 inhal. bid up to 8 inhal. per day

mended starting dose of flunisolide is two puffs twice a day with each puff delivering about 250 mcg to the airway.

The primary indications for corticosteroid aerosol are in the treatment of patients with chronic asthma, whose symptoms are not adequately controlled by β-adrenergic drugs and theophylline, and in allergic rhinitis that is not controlled by antihistamines, decongestants, and/or cromolyn. In patients not receiving steroid therapy, corticosteroid aerosol can improve pulmonary function and decrease the symptoms of asthma. In corticosteroid-dependent asthmatics, the addition of corticosteroid aerosol can help in the conversion to an alternate day therapy and in some cases, replace oral corticosteroids completely. Acute exacerbations of asthma, however, should be treated with systemic corticosteroids and the corticosteroid aerosol resumed after the attack resolves. Very few studies have examined the efficacy of corticosteroid aerosols in diseases other than asthma and allergic rhinitis, but they were found to be of no value in the management of patients with chronic bronchitis and sarcoidosis.[23,24]

CORTICOSTEROID WITHDRAWAL[1,25,26]

The most common indication for corticosteroid withdrawal is the physician's judgment that the underlying disease for which the corticosteroid was prescribed has remitted sufficiently so that corticosteroid therapy is no longer necessary. A second indication is the development of unacceptable side-effects, such as poorly-regulated diabetes mellitus, severe Cushingoid features, gastrointestinal bleeding secondary to peptic ulceration, or poor post-operative wound healing. In most instances the physician can dictate the pace of corticosteroid withdrawal, which should be individualized for each patient. Acute withdrawal (i.e., within 1–2 days) is rarely indicated, except in such situations as acute corticosteroid psychosis and disseminated herpes simplex virus infection.

During the withdrawal from corticosteroid therapy, the acute corticosteroid withdrawal syndrome, signs and symptoms of HPA suppression (see adverse effects) and exacerbation of the underlying disease may occur. The frequency of these adverse consequences depend on the duration of therapy, the dosage schedule, the specific corticosteroid preparation, the underlying disease and other poorly defined patient-related factors. In patients who have received only a brief (less than two weeks) course of corticosteroid therapy and who were not previously on corticosteroids, HPA suppression is unlikely to occur, and the corticosteroids can be abruptly discontinued provided the underlying disease is not likely to flare, (e.g., the patient with stable chronic obstructive pulmonary disease (COPD) who has not responded to a trial of corticosteroid therapy).

In the majority of patients who have received pharmacological doses of corticosteroids for more than two weeks, one can assume that HPA suppression has occurred and the taper should be slow especially when the dose is reduced below the physiologic level. There is no evidence that the administration of ACTH can prevent or reverse the development of glucocorticoid-induced HPA suppression.[1]

Protocol for Withdrawal

Many specific corticosteroid withdrawal protocols have been devised,[25-27] but the physician must realize that these are only guidelines to help design individual protocols.

In patients with documented or presumed HPA suppression the reduction from a pharmacologic to physiologic dose of corticosteroid is limited by the status of the underlying disease whereas the reduction below the physiologic dose is limited by the signs and symptoms of HPA suppression. Therefore, when the underlying disease is potentially life threatening, the initial taper should be relatively slow.

In patients receiving a dose-range of 15-40 mg of prednisone or equivalent daily, the dose can be reduced by 2.5 to 5 mg every 3-7 days until a physiologic dose, approximately 5 mg/day of prednisone, is reached. In those patients receiving more than 40 mg/day of prednisone, the taper down to 40 mg can be relatively rapid, but should be followed by the slower withdrawal schedule described above. After the physiologic dose of corticosteroid is reached, the patient can then be switched to a single morning dose of 20 mg hydrocortisone daily. Subsequently, the hydrocortisone dose can be reduced by 2.5 mg each week until a level of 10 mg/day is reached. During this stage the patient should be clearly informed regarding the importance of compliance, and the need for supplemental corticosteroids for acute stress or illness. If for some reason, oral medication cannot be given during their episodes of stress, the corticosteroids should be administered intravenously or intramuscularly. During minor stresses, such as viral infections or bacterial pharyngitis, the patient should receive an additional 100 mg of hydrocortisone orally in two divided doses. For major stresses such as trauma or surgery, 100 mg of hydrocortisone every 6-8 hours should be given parenterally. When the stress is resolved, the corticosteroid dosage can be quickly tapered down to the previous level.

When the patient reaches 10 mg/day of hydrocortisone, then measurement of 8:00 AM plasma cortisol level can guide the physician in deciding subsequent therapy. A level of greater than 10 mcg/dl indicates recovery of basal functioning of the HPA system and hydrocortisone can be discontinued. However, it is important to realize that corticosteroid coverage for major stresses may be necessary for up to 16 months after complete corticosteroid withdrawal.

INDICATIONS

Asthma[10,28]

Corticosteroids, by their antiinflammatory action and their ability to decrease the release of lipid mediators in areas of inflammation, can be expected to ameliorate the clinical manifestations of asthma.[29-31] In addition, corticosteroids can abolish tachyphylaxis that may develop to both inhaled and subcutaneous β-adrenergic agonists, thus potentiating the effects of β-adrenergic agonists on bronchial smooth muscles. Unfortunately, the usefulness of chronic corticosteroid therapy in asthma is limited by the frequent side-effects that occur.

Status Asthmaticus

Status asthmaticus refers to a severe attack of bronchospasm that is prolonged and relatively resistant to treatment with the usual bronchodilators. Corticosteroids should be given to patients who are refractory to standard bronchodilator therapy, especially those who require hospitalization or have received corticosteroids within the preceding year since adrenal insufficiency may be present.[30] Hydrocortisone hemisuccinate 4-8 mg/kg intravenously every 4-6 hours is a reasonable initial dose. Methylprednisolone has less sodium retaining effect and is often used in equivalent doses. Within the first 2-3 days of therapy, provided clinical improvement is observed, patients can be switched to oral prednisone or prednisolone (60-80 mg) given as a single dose in the morning. The subsequent rate of corticosteroid taper depends on factors such as the rapidity of clinical and physiologic improvement, the level of corticosteroid therapy prior to the asthma attack, and the frequency and severity of recent asthma attacks. In patients who have not required corticosteroids in the past year and who responded to treatment rapidly, it would be possible to taper the corticosteroid completely within 1 week. On the other hand, patients with prolonged, severe attacks, or patients who had frequent exacerbations of asthma in the previous months may need to be discharged on corticosteroid and tapered slowly as an outpatient. It is important to remember that corticosteroid therapy is only one of the many modalities required by patients in status asthmaticus, others include: hydration, controlled flow oxygen therapy, intravenous theophylline, inhaled sympathomimetic amines, bronchial hygiene and antibiotics.

Chronic Asthma

Long term systemic corticosteroid therapy should only be prescribed after appropriate administration of β-agonists, theophylline, anticholinergic agents, and cromolyn have proven to be inadequate to maintain optimum function. A brief course of high dose corticosteroid therapy is associated with minimal side-effects, whereas chronic corticosteroid therapy, even at a relatively low dose, can lead to many adverse effects. Before starting corticosteroids, adequate theophylline dosage should be documented with serum levels, and patients properly instructed on the correct technique of inhalational therapy involved. In some patients, the addition of inhaled corticosteroids may be adequate to render some patients symptom-free. If a patient is severely obstructed, high-dose oral corticosteroids (equivalent to 60 mg of prednisone) should be prescribed. The initial high dose may need to be maintained for 5-10 days to be followed by a tapering regimen. It is extremely important that the physician document the physiologic response to corticosteroid therapy. In fact, the patient should record the FEV_1 regularly and peak flow several times/day during the corticosteroid trial.

If a patient must be maintained on chronic corticosteroid therapy, every attempt should be made to prescribe alternate day therapy at the lowest possible dose. Inhaled corticosteroid may be a useful adjunct in the patients with milder disease or when corticosteroid taper is attempted (see earlier section). Further, in some patients, macrolide antibiotics may facilitate reduction of corticosteroid therapy (see later).

Allergic Bronchopulmonary Aspergillosis (ABPA)[32]

ABPA, a hypersensitivity reaction of the lung to antigens of Aspergillus species, occurs most commonly in patients with severe asthma.[33] Clinically, ABPA is characterized by bronchospasm, cough productive of mucus plugs, peripheral eosinophilia and transient migratory infiltrates on chest x-ray. Diagnosis is made by the above clinical signs, an elevated serum IgE concentration and evidence of hypersensitivity to Aspergillus antigen by skin test or precipitating antibodies.

Corticosteroids are the treatment of choice for ABPA.[34] One recommended protocol is to begin prednisone at 0.5-1.0 mg/kg daily as initial therapy for flare of the disease.[35] After 2 weeks, if the patient improves clinically, prednisone is given as 0.5 mg/kg every other day for the next three months, during which there should be radiographic improvement as well as substantial reduction in the total serum IgE. Prednisone can then be tapered and discontinued over the following 3 month period. During the taper, serum IgE should be measured monthly, as increases in serum IgE can be a sensitive marker for subsequent clinical exacerbations.[35] Some patients with ABPA may require chronic low-dose corticosteroids to suppress the activity of the disease.

Chronic Obstructive Pulmonary Disease (COPD)[36,37]

COPD includes the pathologic entity of emphysema as well as the clinical-pathologic entity chronic bronchitis. Patients with emphysema would not be expected to respond to corticosteroids, but those with chronic bronchitis have varying degrees of airway inflammation, bronchial gland hyperplasia, and airway obstruction with edema or mucus; and they may be improved by the antiinflammatory action of corticosteroid. In practice, it is extremely difficult and sometimes impossible to classify COPD patients into either a strictly bronchitic or strictly emphysematous type, so we will discuss the use of corticosteroids in COPD patients as a group. Management goals and strategy differ depending on whether the patient is treated during an acute exacerbation or during the stable, chronic state.

Stable Patients

Published results of corticosteroid treatment in stable COPD patients vary from no effect to significant improvement in 30 percent of the patients treated[24,36,38] Clinical features that have been proposed as important predictors include history of atopy, presence of blood or sputum eosinophilia, marked day to day variation in airway obstruction, and significant improvement in lung function after inhaled bronchodilator.[24,39] Although the most reliable feature appears to be a 15–20 percent improvement in FEV_1 after inhaled β-adrenergic agonists (isoproterenol and metaproterenol), up to 40 percent of corticosteroid-responsive patients do not improve significantly with inhaled bronchodilators.[40,41] Consequently, the lack of a 15 percent or greater response should not be considered to be an absolute contraindication to a trial of corticosteroids.

All COPD patients with symptomatic and/or progressive disease despite smoking cessation, maximal therapy with oral theophylline, inhaled bronchodilators, physical rehabilitation, oxygen etc. should receive a short-term (less than four weeks) clinical trial of corticosteroid therapy. A reasonable regimen is 40 mg of prednisone given as a single dose each day for two weeks. Patients should be monitored with spirometric measurements (FEV_1) prior to and following the corticosteroid trial. If improvement in FEV_1 is not observed, then the corticosteroid should be tapered rapidly. If improvement is observed, the corticosteroid should be tapered gradually, to the lowest dose which maintains the FEV_1 at the maximum level.

Another approach would be to start the patient on 80 mg of prednisone (or equivalent dosage of another corticosteroid preparation) every other day for two weeks. Although the decrease in corticosteroid side effects with every other day therapy is not a significant factor in the first two weeks, the corticosteroid-responsive patients can easily have their corticosteroid dosage tapered while remaining on every other day therapy.

No matter which approach is chosen, it is extremely important that the physician (and patient) undertake a defined trial with objective measurements before and after the institution of corticosteroids (vital capacity and FEV_1 measurements). These spirometric measurements are important for both patient-selection and in determining the lowest effective corticosteroid dose. Furthermore, it lessens the likelihood that patients who "feel better" on corticosteroids without measurable benefit will be subjected inappropriately to the many risks of this therapy.

Acute Exacerbation of COPD

There are conflicting data about the usefulness of corticosteroids as treatment for acute exacerbations of COPD.[36] Albert recently demonstrated that intravenous methylprednisolone (0.5 mg/kg every six hours for 72 hours) in addition to the usual treatment (oxygen, inhaled bronchodilator, intravenous antibiotic, and theophylline) was associated with a more rapid decrease in airway obstruction than was seen with placebo,[42] although it is not clear whether hospital stay or mortality was reduced, or lung function on discharge improved.

We feel that patients hospitalized for exacerbations of COPD except for those with obvious infections, such as pneumonia or sepsis, should receive a course of corticosteroids. The standard regimen of supplemental oxygen, antibiotic, inhaled and intravenous bronchodilators should be instituted. A reasonable dosage regimen is methylprednisolone 0.5 mg/kg intravenously every 6 hours for the first 72 hours. Sequential spirometry, arterial blood gas, and frequent clinical assessment should be performed. Because many patients seek help late in the course of their exacerbation, respiratory failure may occur before the therapy becomes effective. Thus, careful attention to the patient's ventilatory status and appropriate intervention with intubation and mechanical ventilation are essential for a favorable outcome.

Since such patients generally have very little respiratory reserve, it is prudent to maintain them on a reasonable morning dose of oral corticosteroid daily, and gradually taper the drug after discharge, monitoring spirometry regularly to detect any deterioration in lung function.

Chronic Allergic Rhinitis[43]

Corticosteroids are indicated in the management of severe allergic or vasomotor rhinitis and rhinitis medicamentosa when these are not controlled by conventional antihistamine and sympathomimetic therapy, or in the case of allergic rhinitis, by intranasal cromolyn or immunotherapy. In seasonal allergic rhinitis it is recommended that intranasal corticosteroids be given during acute attacks in a rapidly tapered course of 4–5 weeks duration. Often the topical corticosteroids are given as one spray four times a day for one week, three times a day for one week, twice a day for a week, and once daily for a week, with the drug being discontinued if improvement has been documented. In perennial allergic rhinitis the therapeutic regimen consists of avoidance of the allergens and immunotherapy. Immunotherapy can be helpful in treating specific IgE-mediated disorders, but it is only an adjunctive therapy and not a substitute for other forms of therapy traditionally used for the treatment of these diseases. The severity and duration of the disease, the response to environmental control and conventional medication are the key determining factors that identify the need for immunotherapy. Topical corticosteroids can be administered as defined above during periods of exacerbations. It should be remembered that 1-2 weeks may be required before the full benefits of topical corticosteroids are noticed. Systemic corticosteroid therapy may be indicated in patients with severe allergic rhinitis who have not responded to the previously described regimen. In such patients a dose of 1-2 mg/kg/day of prednisone for 5-7 days may be adequate, followed by the addition of intranasal corticosteroids.

Patients with rhinitis medicamentosa are becoming more frequent because of the prolonged and excessive use of phenylephrine or other topical vasoconstrictors, and the increasing abuse of intranasal cocaine. In severe cases, a brief course of topical corticosteroids may permit reasonable withdrawal from the offending agent.

Finally, intranasal corticosteroids may be of value in the management of nasal polyps, which are usually found in patients with intrinsic asthma, allergic rhinitis, aspirin hypersensitivity, or cystic fibrosis. If obstructing polyps produce symptoms of nasal congestion, rhinitis, difficulty in breathing, and sinus infection, chronic intranasal corticosteroids may be required. It must be remembered that corticosteroids are contraindicated in the presence of viral or fungal nasal infections.

Connective Tissue Diseases[44-46]

Systemic Lupus Erythematosus[47,48]

The pleuropulmonary manifestations of systemic lupus erythematosus (SLE) are (1) pleurisy with and without effusion, (2) atelectasis, (3) acute lupus pneumonitis, (4) diffuse interstitial lung disease, (5) uremic pulmonary edema, (6) diaphragmatic dysfunction with loss of lung volume and, (7) infections. SLE has a striking predilection for women and varies from mild episodic disease to rapidly fulminant processes. Interstitial pneumonitis involves less than 5 percent of patients and occurs in two forms: acute interstitial pneumonitis with tachypnea, dyspnea, high fever, cyanosis, and pulmonary hemorrhage, which can be fatal; and chronic interstitial pneumonia characterized by dyspnea, nonproductive cough, pleuritic chest pain, hypocapnia, impaired diffusing capacity and a restrictive ventilatory defect.[49]

In general, patients with mild disease are well controlled with nonsteroidal antiinflammatory agents, however corticosteroids are often required for severe manifestations. When required, corticosteroids should be used aggressively to prevent irreversible organ failure. The generally accepted indications for corticosteroid therapy in patients with SLE are: nephritis, pericarditis, myocarditis, pleuritis, interstitial lung disease, myositis, hemolytic anemia, thrombocytopenia, and central nervous system involvement. Most patients respond to a prednisone dose of 1 mg/kg/day, often in divided doses (Table 5-4). Therapy may be needed for long periods of time and often at very high doses (i.e., 80–100 mg per day) to produce an adequate clinical response. Intravenous "pulse" methylprednisolone therapy has been shown to be efficacious in the treatment of renal SLE. It is not known whether this high dose intravenous therapy is useful in the management of the pulmonary complications of SLE. Two other oral immunosuppressive drugs have been tried, azathioprine and cyclophosphamide, both in

Table 5-4
Corticosteroid Therapy Protocol

Initial and Maintenance Therapy
1. Oral prednisone, 1 mg/kg/day (usually not exceeding 100 mg/day) for 4 to 6 weeks.*
2. Patient is monitored for signs of improvement, i.e. clinical response, chest roentgenogram, physiologic studies.
3. If stable or improved, taper prednisone over next 6 weeks to 0.25 mg/kg/daily, usually at rate of 1 to 5 mg/week.
4. Maintain prednisone at this dose and follow clinical parameters at 3 to 6 month interval. Most patients require 9 to 12 months of therapy before it can be stopped completely.**

Prednisone Failure
1. If the lung disease does not respond to the initial regimen or if the disease progresses on low doses of prednisone:
    high-dose prednisone may be restarted, or cyclophosphamide or azathioprine may be added.
2. Cyclophosphamide should be given orally, 2 mg/kg/day. Intravenous administration in the same doses can be given to patients who cannot tolerate oral medication.† If fulminant disease exist then 4 mg/kg/day can be given for 48–72 hours followed by conversion to the lower dose.†
3. Azathioprine (2 mg/kg/day) may be added to the regimen in those patients who cannot tolerate cyclophosphamide.
4. Therapy usually is continued for 6 to 9 months while monitoring clinical progress.

*To control the most fulminant disease manifestations 1 mg/kg/day of prednisone may be given in divided doses for 7 to 10 days or intravenous "pulse" hydrocortisone 3 to 4 mg/kg every 6 hours for 24 to 72 hours (depending on clinical response) with conversion to oral prednisone as described.
**In most cases this is suppressive therapy and the treatment cannot be terminated until the disease process has burnt itself out. Thus, one must accept that suppressive therapy may have to continue indefinitely.
†Must monitor the WBC count and maintain between 3000 and 3500 cells per mm^3 or neutrophil count between 1000 to 1500 cells per mm^3 (measure at least biweekly)[49].

combination with low or high doses of corticosteroids. It has been suggested that single drug oral immunosuppressive treatment combined with prednisone is most beneficial in lupus patients with renal disease. This form of therapy has not been adequately evaluated in pulmonary disease.[50]

Rheumatoid Arthritis

The pleural and pulmonary complications associated with rheumatoid arthritis are (1) pleurisy with and without effusion, (2) usual interstitial pneumonitis, (3) necrobiotic nodules (nonpneumoconiotic intrapulmonary rheumatoid nodules) with or without cavities, (4) Caplan's syndrome (rheumatoid pneumoconiosis), and (5) pulmonary hypertension secondary to rheumatoid pulmonary vasculitis. Most patients with pleuropulmonary involvement have clinical evidence of rheumatoid arthritis and high titer rheumatoid factor. However, the lung disease may precede the clinical manifestations of rheumatoid arthritis.

Treatment of rheumatoid lung disease is notoriously unsatisfactory and there are no alternative therapies to prednisone (Table 5-4). In addition, oxygen and vasodilators are often required for patients with diffuse interstitial fibrosis and pulmonary hypertension. Patients with pleuritis, with or without effusions, usually do not require treatment. However, when persistent pleuritic pain or large effusions occur analgesics and thoracentesis are usually the first mode of treatment, but many patients will require corticosteroid therapy (Table 5-4). Frequently, pain and fluid accumulation will recur once the therapy is stopped. Rarely are surgery, decortication, and pleurodesis, necessary to correct the problem. Parenchymal rheumatoid nodules often present a diagnostic dilemma and their management may be a problem. Treatment is usually only necessary in patients who develop persistent hemoptysis or a bronchopleural fistula. The rheumatoid nodules will usually decrease in size with the corticosteroid therapy. Pulmonary vasculitis is best managed with prednisone and cyclophosphamide. The response to cytotoxic drugs may be slow and monitoring for the side-effects of both prednisone and cyclophosphamide is important. Most of the time this therapy is required for a year or more after the signs of clinically active vasculitis have remitted. Prednisone therapy is occasionally required to manage the complications of other therapies used to treat rheumatoid lung disease, as for example in gold hypersensitivity pneumonitis, methotrexate hypersensitivity pneumonitis, and bronchiolitis obliterans and airway obstruction due to penicillamine therapy.

Progressive Systemic Sclerosis (Scleroderma)

Although the exact incidence of pulmonary disease is not known, morphologic studies have demonstrated pleural and pulmonary involvement in 82–90 percent of patients with progressive systemic sclerosis (PSS). The pulmonary complications associated with PSS are (1) diffuse interstitial fibrosis, (2) pulmonary vascular disease, (3) pleural disease, (4) recurrent aspiration pneumonitis, and (5) bronchiolar carcinoma. Diffuse interstitial fibrosis is found in nearly all cases at post-mortem. The interstitial lung disease and pulmonary hypertension associated with scleroderma are strikingly resistant to current modes of therapy. Corticosteroid therapy is used in the fashion described in the standard protocol (Table 5-4). It is generally considered that the interstitial lung disease is a relatively pure "fibrotic" disorder without a significant inflammatory component. However, recent evidence suggests that an inflammatory cell response does precede the fibrotic process so that the identification of the inflammatory stage of this disease may lead to a rational drug therapy in the future.[51]

Sjogren's Syndrome

Sjogren's syndrome occurs as an idiopathic symptom-sign complex characterized by keratoconjunctivitis sicca, xerostomia (oral dryness), and recurrent swelling of the parotid gland. The disease often occurs secondary to another disease, most commonly rheumatoid arthritis or system lupus erythematosus, but is also seen in systemic vasculitis, dermatomyositis, and scleroderma. Pulmonary manifestations occur frequently in Sjogren's syndrome,[45] but, because of the high incidence of rheumatoid disease associated with this disease, it is often difficult to determine if these are specific for Sjogren's.

The pulmonary manifestations of Sjogren's syndrome include (1) pleurisy with or without effusion, (2) interstitial fibrosis (approximately 50 percent of patients) indistinguishable from that found in other connective tissue diseases, (3) dessication of the tracheal bronchial tree secondary to lymphocytic infiltration of the mucous glands, (4) lymphoid interstitial lung disease, which includes pseudolymphoma, histiocytic or lymphocytic lymphoma, and Waldenstrom's macroglobulinemia. The treatment for this disorder is not clearly defined, corticosteroid and cytotoxic therapy has been used with limited success. When corticosteroids are used it is generally for management of the extraglandular disease, not for the glandular form (Table 5-4).

Polymyositis and Dermatomyositis

Polymyositis is a diffuse, inflammatory, and degenerative disorder of striated muscle that causes symmetric weakness and atrophy, principally of the limb girdles, neck, and pharynx. When an erythematous skin rash accompanies the weakness and pain, the disorder is termed dermatomyositis. The pulmonary manifestations seen in polymyositis and dermatomyositis include: (1) usual interstitial pneumonitis (5 percent of patients), (2) aspiration pneumonia caused by esophageal pathology, (3) hypostatic pneumonia secondary to chest wall involvement and hypoventilation and (4) drug-induced hypersensitivity pneumonitis, (e.g., methotrexate). Interstitial pneumonitis has been well documented in patients with polymyositis, but less frequently than in other connective tissue diseases.

Corticosteroids have caused remission with stabilization or improvement in the symptomatic, radiographic, and physiological abnormalities in 40 percent of patients. Other immunosuppressive agents, especially methotrexate, are frequently used to treat this disorder (Table 5-4). It must be remembered that the total treatment may be quite long, lasting two to three years for patients with polymyositis. A problem peculiar to polymyositis is a difficulty in distinguishing between myopathy secondary to the polymyositis and that due to corticosteroid toxicity. Consequently, a very careful examination to document the presence of myopathy is required because it is important to determine whether more or less prednisone is required. Frequently, these patients can be maintained on alternate-day regimens, which should be tried as soon as possible. Since malignancy is an associated complication of polymyositis its occurrence must be monitored frequently during the course.[49,52] It is important to remember that although corticosteroids are widely accepted as the drug of choice in the management of polymyositis and dermatomyositis this is based upon empirical evidence without adequate control studies. In fact, questions remain unanswered about the method of administration of corticosteroids, such as whether patients should receive corticosteroids as a single daily dose, a divided dose, or on alternate days. Methotrexate, cyclophosphamide, azathioprine, and chlorambucil are promising agents that have been reported to be helpful and to produce a corticosteroid-sparing effect in patients treated with a combination of prednisone and one of the above drugs.[53-55]

Mixed Connective Tissue Disease

Mixed connective tissue disease is a syndrome characterized by overlapping clinical features suggestive, but not typical, of SLE, scleroderma, polymyositis, and rheumatoid arthritis. Patients with chronic disease may progress to have serious involvement of many organ systems producing pericarditis, myocarditis, central nervous system disease, severe myositis, and nephritis.[49]

Mixed connective tissue disease is one of the autoimmune diseases most responsive to corticosteroid therapy. Pleural effusions and interstitial lung disease are the most commonly associated lung disorders in mixed connective tissue disease and both of these respond very well to corticosteroid therapy unless features strongly suggestive of scleroderma are prominent components of this disorder (Table 5-4). Often these patients can quite easily be converted to an alternate day regimen. Prolonged remissions off all drugs or with minimal maintenance therapy is not unusual. It is recommended that aggressive corticosteroid therapy during the early phase of the disease might prevent the subsequent development of more severe disease, but control studies have not been done. In milder phases of the disease, salicylates or other nonsteroidal antiinflammatory drugs are used.

Vasculitic Syndromes

The pulmonary vasculitides constitute a heterogeneous group of disorders that have in common the feature of necrotizing inflammation of blood vessels of any size or type and involving virtually any organ system. The major groupings include systemic diseases such as Wegener's granulomatosis, systemic necrotizing vasculitis syndromes, cutaneous vasculitis, Henoch-Schonlein syndrome, and the giant cell arteritides such as temporal arteritis. The vasculitides may occur as primary entities or as secondary components of underlying diseases, including the classic connective tissue diseases, neoplasms, and infection. Many of the vasculitides respond very well to the basic corticosteroid protocol (Table 5-4). If unsuccessful, low dose cytotoxic therapy can be added.

Wegener's Granulomatosis[56]

This disorder is characterized by the triad of: (1) necrotizing granulomatous vasculitides of the upper (profuse rhinorrhea with sinus pain, epistaxis, and saddle nose deformity) and lower (cough, hemoptysis, and nodular, often cavitary densities on chest roentgenogram) respiratory tracts; (2) disseminated leukocytoclastic vasculitis; and (3) glomerulonephritis (azotemia, hypertension and proteinuria). Single or multiple pulmonary nodules with a tendency to cavitation are the primary pulmonary manifestations. Pleural effusions are seen in 20 percent of patients and 15 percent have endobronchial involvement that may cause atelectasis,[56] although bronchoscopic biopsy of the latter usually reveal no specific findings. Lung biopsies usually show granulomas and vasculitis.

It is generally recommended that treatment of Wegener's granulomatosis be with a combination of prednisone and a cytotoxic agent from the very beginning.[57-59] Irreversible organ system dysfunction may occur if less than optimum therapy is attempted, however short the period of treatment may be.[56] The standard corticosteroid protocol is employed (Table 5-4). The dose is gradually tapered to an alternate-day regimen over the second month and maintained at 60 mg on alternate-days during the third month. The alternate-day dose is then tapered to zero over a three to six month period, if the patient shows signs of remission. Cyclophosphamide therapy (2 mg/kg/day orally) is the most important agent in treatment and is started usually at the same time. If the disease is fulminant, 4 mg/kg/day is prescribed for the first 2-3 days, and then reduced to the lower dose. Patients who cannot tolerate this medication are generally started on azathioprine as an alternative. With cyclophosphamide therapy it is particularly important to maintain blood neutrophils at a level of approximately 1000-1500 per mm^3, with a total white blood cell count in the 3000-3500 per mm^3 range. Following the induction of a complete remission, corticosteroid therapy can be reduced and eventually eliminated, while cyclophosphamide alone is carried on for six months to a year. When one uses azathioprine the dosage is 2 mg/kg/day with the same adjustments regarding white cell counts. Intravenous bolus administration of a gram of methylprednisolone daily for 1-3 days has been attempted in the occasional patient with fulminant disease. The efficacy of this regimen has not been established, but it has few side-effects and may induce a more rapid response in some patients. The effect of glucocorticoids is usually relatively rapid with response being seen within the first 3-5 days, whereas a response with cyclophosphamide by the oral route usually takes 2-3 weeks.

Lymphomatoid Granulomatosis

Lymphomatoid granulomatosis is clinically similar to Wegener's granulomatosis.[60,61] However, they differ in that: (1) involved organs are infiltrated by a pleomorphic mass of invasive atypical lymphocytes and plasmacytoid cells, which is accompanied by a granulomatous reaction in an angiocentric and angiodestructive pattern; (2) septal and palatal perforations occur; (3) glomerulitis is rare; (4) there is a tendency to progress to malignant lymphoma in untreated patients; and (5) lesions of the central nervous system and skin are frequent in lymphomatoid granulomatosis. It is unclear whether there is a continuum from the benign lymphocytic angiitis and granulomatosis, to lymphomatoid granulomatosis, and then to frank lymphoma, or whether these processes are indeed separate and should be categorized as such.[62]

The pulmonary manifestations of lymphomatoid granulomatosis include diffuse reticulonodular infiltration of the lungs and nodular densities of varying sizes and distribution, the latter occurring in 80 percent of cases. Cavitation occurs in up to 20 percent of cases and often is associated with life-threatening hemoptysis. In one recent series, 50 percent of the patients showed an evolution of lymphomatoid granulomatosis to frank lymphoma during the follow-up period, with an overall mortality of 53 percent.[62] Cyclophosphamide and corticosteroid therapy can induce long-term remission in some patients, but lymphoma may develop in those who do not respond, and this disease is generally felt to be refractory to treatment.[62] An aggressive combination chemotherapeutic protocol very similar to that for Wegener's granulomatosis is indicated in the early management of these patients (Table 5-4).

Hypersensitivity Vasculitides

Henoch-Schonlein purpura and cryoglobulinemia infrequently involve the lung but are primarily systemic with skin and visceral involvement, and secondary to other underlying conditions, whose list is very long and includes a number of autoimmune processes such as SLE and PSS as well as carcinoma, hepatitis, and inflammatory bowel disease. Consequently, therapy is directed at the primary condition. In those patients requiring therapy, corticosteroid protocol similar to that described above (Table 5-4) is recommended. Usually the dose can be rapidly tapered, since in most patients the vasculitis itself is a self-limited process. In a small number of patients who have severe necrotizing vasculitis, corticosteroid and cytotoxic combinations are required. When patients have chronic exacerbations and remissions, an alternate day therapy program for 4–6 weeks or longer may result in amelioration of the symptoms.

Bronchocentric Granulomatosis

Bronchocentric granulomatosis is a form of pulmonary granulomatosis and angiitis characterized by necrotizing granulomatous reaction centered around both large and small airways.[63] It may, in fact, in some cases represent the end of the spectrum of allergic bronchopulmonary aspergillosis (see above).[64,65] The prognosis of bronchocentric granulomatosis appears to be quite good, with patients responding to both surgical resection and corticosteroid therapy, and some even have spontaneous remission of their disease. The defined regimen for management of this disease is not known, and it is recommended that a protocol similar to that described in Table 5-4 be tried. Removal of the involved lobe often is curative although some patients require corticosteroid therapy postoperatively.[66]

Hypersensitivity Pneumonitis

Hypersensitivity pneumonitis is a disease associated with repeated intense inhalation of organic dust that produces diffuse, patchy interstitial and/or alveolar infiltrates following the formation of antigen-antibody complexes (Arthus reaction).[67-70] Farmer's lung, caused by exposure to moldy hay containing fungal spores of thermophilic actinomycetes, is the prototype, while air conditioner or humidifier lung disease due to fungal overgrowth and aerosolization via the ventilation system is more common in urban areas.

In early cases it is reasonable to wait for spontaneous improvement following the removal of exposure to the antigens. However, this frequently requires a radical change in life style, and often nearly insurmountable problems exist in trying to accomplish removal from the environment that which has caused the disease. Alternatives to a complete removal from the environment include avoidance of obvious sources of heavy exposure, the use of masks, hoods, and filtration devices, and premedication with agents that prevent the reaction.[68,70] Sodium cromolyn will block the immediate and late reactions in some patients with hypersensitivity pneumonitis, whereas corticosteroids block only the late reaction. It is not certain that control of symptoms by these drugs in the presence of continued exposure to the antigen will prevent subsequent development of lung damage. Therefore, the most important approach is to avoid exposure if at all possible and not to rely on preventive therapy with sodium cromolyn or corticosteroids.

When the disease is established and no, or incomplete recovery, has occurred following removal of the exposures, then corticosteroid therapy is indicated. Prednisone therapy, approximately 60 mg daily, either in a single dose or occasionally in divided doses, is continued for 7-14 days, and depending on the response, is tapered over the ensuing 14 days to 20 mg per day. The taper is then continued at 5 mg or less per week over a one to two week interval until the dose is completely discontinued or until relapse occurs. In patients who have chronic hypersensitivity pneumonitis, recovery may take 6-12 months.

Drug-induced Hypersensitivity Pneumonitis

Numerous drugs produce pulmonary disease; asthma is a common manifestation of drug-induced anaphylaxis, while nitrofurantoin is the most common cause of drug-induced hypersensitivity pneumonitis. Other drugs include hydrochlorothiazide, gold salts, bleomycin, or busulfan. Chronic reactions may result in interstitial lung disease with a restrictive ventilatory defect and abnormalities of gas exchange. The key to management is removal of the drug. Corticosteroids may be useful in the management of the acute symptoms but are less effective in chronic restrictive disease. The dose is similar to that described above for hypersensitivity pneumonitis.

Goodpasture's Syndrome

Goodpasture's syndrome or antibasement membrane antibody-induced glomerulonephritis and pulmonary hemorrhage is manifested by dyspnea, cough, hemoptysis, occasionally leading to asphyxiation, and microcytic hypochromic anemia. Therapy of patients with Goodpasture's syndrome includes plasmapheresis, cyclophosphamide, and prednisone. In patients who have life threatening pulmonary hemorrhage, immediate plasmapheresis is mandatory. Daily plasmapheresis is continued until pulmonary hemorrhage subsides. The patients are also begun on corticosteroid and cyclophosphamide therapy (Table 5-4). In some centers azathioprine, 1 mg/kg/day orally is added to this immunosuppressive regimen. Once the acute illness is controlled, long-term therapy with cyclophosphamide and prednisone is often required. The prednisone dose is usually maintained around 15 mg per day orally. Acute flares of pulmonary and/or renal disease will require return to plasmapheresis and full doses of prednisone and cyclophosphamide therapy. Cessation of therapy should not be considered unless the disease has been quiescent for at least a year. Idiopathic pulmonary hemosiderosis is similar to Goodpasture's syndrome but without renal disease. It is managed in a similar fashion, (i.e., plasmapheresis, corticosteroids, cytotoxic and chelating agents).

Loeffler's Syndrome[71]

Loeffler's syndrome, pulmonary eosinophilia of unknown etiology occurring in relatively asymptomatic patients who may or may not have bronchial asthma, is characterized by transient pulmonary infiltrates and eosinophilia in the peripheral blood. Therapy with corticosteroids should be avoided unless absolutely necessary because the disease is benign and often self-limited. When corticosteroid therapy is required, prednisone in a dose of 30 mg/day for 1–2 weeks followed by tapering of dosage by 5 mg per day to complete withdrawal is usually adequate to control the symptoms related to this disease and accelerate the clearance of pulmonary infiltrates. Patients who have associated severe asthma may require prolonged corticosteroid therapy. Some cases of eosinophilic pneumonia and asthma may be associated with "mucoid impaction" of the bronchi and allergic bronchopulmonary aspergillosis.

Chronic Eosinophilic Pneumonia

Unlike most cases of Loeffler's syndrome, most patients with chronic eosinophilic pneumonia present with a clinical picture of high fever, night sweats, weight loss, and severe dyspnea, and a dense pneumonic infiltrate distributed along the periphery of the lung like a photographic negative of the shadows seen in pulmonary edema. Corticosteroid therapy (40–60 mg daily, orally, which is frequently the initial regimen) results in dramatic clinical, radiographic, and functional improvement within several days. Relapses are common after corticosteroid withdrawal and pulmonary lesions reappear in a pattern similar to the original lesions.

Interstitial Lung Diseases

Sarcoidosis

Sarcoidosis is a multi-system, granulomatous disease of unknown etiology with world wide distribution. It commonly affects young adults, 20–30 years of age, presenting most often with bilateral hilar adenopathy, pulmonary infiltrates, skin and/or eye lesions.[72] Approximately 90 percent of patients with sarcoidosis have pulmonary manifestations and 20–25 percent of these patients develop permanent alteration of lung function.

Glucocorticoids have been the chief agents used in the treatment of pulmonary and extrapulmonary sarcoidosis (see Table 5-5). Because of the great variability of the disease and the difficulties in carrying out controlled clinical trials, there are no firm guidelines or evidence to determine whether corticosteroid therapy of sarcoidosis prevents pulmonary fibrosis or is merely symptomatic therapy.[73] Importantly, it is clear that corticosteroids do not cure sarcoidosis, but simply suppress the active phase until the disease burns itself out. Several long-term studies have indicated that in at least two-thirds of the patients with radiographic evidence of sarcoidosis, complete resolution will occur within two years in the absence of any therapy. Consequently, unless there is a specific reason for treatment such as extrapulmonary disease or progressive and substantial shortness of breath, we recommend that patients not be placed on corticosteroid therapy.

Table 5-5
Indications for the Use of Corticosteroids in Sarcoidosis

*1. Ocular sarcoidosis—acute iridocyclitis, chorioretinitis, keratoconjunctivitis, conjunctival follicles. Topical corticosteroids are effective for anterior uveitis.
*2. Abnormal calcium metabolism—hypercalcemia and hypercalciuria.
*3. Myocardial involvement—heart block or cardiac arrhythmia.
*4. Neurosarcoidosis—diabetes insipidus, papilledema and seizures.
*5. Hypersplenism—leading to anemia, leukopenia and thrombocytopenia. Splenectomy may be required.
 6. Hepatic involvement, especially if progressive with significant liver function abnormalities.
 7. Cutaneous lesions—skin rash, erythema nodosum, lupus pernio, scaly plaques and other chronic skin lesions. Methotrexate and chloroquine may be required.
 8. Glandular involvement—particularly if disordered function e.g. dry eyes due to lacrimal gland involvement, or dry mouth due to salivary gland involvement.
 9. Bone and muscle involvement—steroids provide relief of painful, swollen and deforming bone cysts and arthritis. Myositis or myopathy.
 10. Upper respiratory tract—usually indicates chronic, persistent disease needing therapy. Involvement of the pharynx and larynx may cause edema, hoarseness, and stridor due to laryngeal obstruction.
*11. Pulmonary sarcoidosis—see text.

*Indicates those findings where corticosteroid therapy is strongly indicated.

The following points seem pertinent regarding who should and should not be treated with corticosteroids. (1) Patients with bilateral hilar adenopathy (Stage I), without symptoms or extrapulmonary involvement should not be treated with corticosteroid since 66–75 percent of these patients will have spontaneous and complete resolution. Follow-up examinations at 3–6 month intervals are worthwhile. (2) Patients who have breathlessness and are in Stage I of their disease may or may not be begun on corticosteroid therapy. This is a clinical decision and our personal view is that since most of these patients are relatively young, early treatment at this stage may be worthwhile. Even if early spontaneous remission occurs, corticosteroids can be quickly withdrawn with very little harm to the patient. On the other hand, in those destined to develop progressive disease early treatment may be more efficacious and result in prolongation of life and the prevention of late complications. (3) Patients with Stage II sarcoidosis (bilateral hilar adenopathy and parenchymal infiltration) and symptoms such as dyspnea, cough, chest pain, or exercise intolerance, should be treated with corticosteroids. Often they have abnormalities in pulmonary function and elevations in serum angiotensin converting enzyme level, which can be used to monitor the course of the disease. Asymptomatic patients with Stage II disease may be observed for 3 to 9 months to see if there is a progression or regression of the radiographic and pulmonary function abnormalities. If progression is documented, then therapy should be initiated. If the patients remain unchanged, then continued observa-

Corticosteroids

tions would be indicated, although some would recommend treatment at this stage unless the patient is at high risk for side effects from corticosteoid therapy. (4) Patients with Stage III disease (pulmonary parenchymal disease only) should have a complete evaluation. If active disease is suggested, treatment should be initiated even if symptoms are not present. (5) Patients with fibrosis and bullae formation (Stage IV disease) almost always require therapy, although they may not respond. It is especially important to follow closely while on therapy, so that therapy can be discontinued if resolution is not apparent, to avoid any side-effects of the treatment protocol.

It is important to remember that corticosteroids generally improve symptoms but may or may not improve roentgenographic abnormalities or lung functions tests. To be effective, therapy usually requires 3–4 months. Relapses are frequent following withdrawal of corticosteroid therapy. In general, treatment should be based on clinical or laboratory evidence of dysfunction such as severe discomfort or inability to work as a result of dyspnea, fever, fatigue, arthralgia, neuropathy, disfiguring cutaneous disease, or hepatic insufficiency. Treatment of ocular or myocardial sarcoidosis, or hypercalcemia is indicated even when symptoms are slight, because in these incidences severe loss of vision, fatal arrythmias or insidious renal damage may ensue.

The usual starting dose is 30–60 mg of prednisone per day for 14–21 days, followed by gradual reduction to a maintenance level of approximately 0.5 mg/kg/day. Alternate day corticosteroid regimens can be used effectively in certain situations and may result in a reduction in side-effects associated with prolonged daily therapy. Certain findings such as acute uveitis, myocardial involvement, papilledema, and severe hypercalcemia may require higher doses of corticosteroid (up to 60–80 mg of prednisone daily). Local corticosteroids may be given to control low-grade uveitis and may be administered in the form of eye drops or ointment. If the disease progresses, then systemic therapy is recommended.

Occasionally, drugs other than corticosteroids are indicated in the management of certain forms of sarcoidosis. Chloroquine has been found to be useful in lupus pernio and is given at a starting level of 250 mg twice daily for 6 months. Often corticosteroids are continued at a reduced level while this is being administered. Irreversible retinopathy and blindness are complications of chloroquine therapy. Therefore, frequent and careful eye examinations are required. Other drugs used in the management of sarcoidosis when corticosteroids fail include methotrexate, chlorambucil, and azathioprine. Colchicine has been used in the management of arthritis due to sarcoidosis. Prophylactic isoniazid (INH) is recommended in patients with a positive tuberculin test when corticosteroid therapy is instituted.[73,74]

Idiopathic Pulmonary Fibrosis

Idiopathic pulmonary fibrosis (IPF) is a disease characterized by the insidious onset of dyspnea, digital clubbing, interstitial infiltrates on the chest radiograph, pulmonary function tests that reveal a restrictive impairment (decreased static lung volumes), impaired diffusing capacity for carbon monoxide, and arterial hypoxemia, exaggerated or elicited by exercise. The mean survival is 4–6 years, but the clinical course is quite variable. Once the diagnosis of IPF has been made, and the clinical severity established, the majority of patients will require therapy.[75-77]

IPF, like many idiopathic interstitial lung disorders, has no known specific curative therapy. Therefore, drug management is primarily empirical and largely suppressive. Corticosteroids and immunosuppressive therapy are the two major groups of pharmacologic agents that have been used in these patients (Table 5-4). No large, controlled trials have documented efficacy of either of these drugs, although anecdotal experience suggests that such drugs may be helpful in certain cases. It has been suggested from large retrospective studies that about 40–50 percent of patients obtain some subjective improvement of breathlessness and about 15–20 percent obtain objective partial improvement in the chest radiograph and pulmonary function tests. Relatively high doses of oral corticosteroid therapy have been used by our group (1–1.5 mg/kg/day with a maximal dose of 100 mg/day). This is given as a single morning dose. Alternate day therapy is not recommended since anecdotal reports suggest that it is not effective. We recommend that this dose be given for approximately 2–3 months and the patient reevaluated. The responsive patient will report a decrease in symptoms, demonstrate radiographic clearing, physiologic improvement, and/or show no further decline in lung function or other parameters of disease activity. It is often extremely difficult to assess any changes in these patients since the disease is of long duration and improvement may be extremely slow. If the patient is responsive, (i.e., improved or stabilized), the dose of prednisone is tapered 1–2 mg/week to obtain a maintenance dose of approximately 0.5 mg/kg/day, while watching for clinical and physiologic deterioration. If the disease is still stable or improved, prednisone is then maintained at 0.25 mg/kg/day for a total of 6–12 months. Decision on the length of therapy is often difficult, and requires careful follow-up of several subjective and objective parameters. Once the corticosteroid dose has been reduced or stopped the patient should continue to be observed for disease relapse.

Azathioprine and cyclophosphamide are used both as alternatives to corticosteroids and as a form of initial therapy. Both drugs have been shown to be useful in some patients who failed to respond to corticosteroids alone. The dosage regimen used at the present time is 3 mg/kg/day of azathioprine or 2 mg/kg/day of cyclophosphamide as a single daily dose given in conjunction with prednisone at 0.25 mg/kg/day. Little data exists regarding the optimal length of therapy, but we recommend a period of 6–9 months. If stabilization or clinical improvement cannot be documented, therapy should be discontinued since significant adverse reactions can occur.

Recently, pulse corticosteroid therapy has been recommended, although little support exists for its use in IPF. In this form of therapy, treatment is undertaken with intravenous methylprednisolone 2 grams once a week plus 0.25 mg/kg oral prednisone given daily. This regimen has not been demonstrated to alter pulmonary functions or other clinical parameters of disease activity.[79,80]

Eosinophilic Granuloma of the Lung[78,79]

Eosinophilic granuloma of the lung or pulmonary histiocytosis X is a disease whose pathogenesis is unknown, characterized radiographically by diffuse nodular and reticulonodular interstitial infiltrates, and pathologically by infiltration of histiocytes and eosinophils, with characteristic mononuclear phagocytes (referred to as histiocytosis X cells). Spontaneous pneumothorax occurs in about 10 percent of patients. Bone lesions are found in a minority of cases in which there is lung disease, and diabetes insipidus and skin involvement are also uncommon. There is no conclusive evidence that any therapeutic program is effective in patients with eosinophilic granuloma of the lung. Many patients improve without therapy while some show a steady decline despite therapy. The standard therapeutic regimen is to begin corticosteroids as defined in the protocol (see Table 5-4). If the patient has no significant response to therapy or if the disease progresses, then corticosteroid therapy should be discontinued. No realistic alternative exists, although penicillamine in doses of 750-1000 mg/day have been advocated.

Bronchiolitis Obliterans[80,81]

Bronchiolitis obliterans is a lesion that results in partial or complete obstruction of bronchioles by intraluminal granulation tissue and peribronchiolar fibrosis, and has been classified in the following manner: (1) toxic fume bronchiolitis obliterans, (2) post-infectious bronchiolitis obliterans, (3) bronchiolitis obliterans associated with connective tissue disease, (4) localized lesions with bronchiolitis obliterans, and (5) idiopathic bronchiolitis obliterans with organizing pneumonia.[82] Bronchiolitis obliterans associated with aspiration, eosinophilic pneumonia, and allergic alveolitis are excluded from this classification.[82] Corticosteroid therapy has been used in all these settings except localized bronchiolitis which is usually identified after resection. The recent literature has emphasized the association with organizing pneumonia and described a very responsive phase of this disease to corticosteroid therapy.[83,84] Relapses are said to occur as the dose of prednisone is reduced, although control can be reestablished with increasing doses of the prednisone therapy. The interesting finding in these patients is that many of them presented like IPF following a viral pneumonia spanning weeks or a few months, and only after open lung biopsy could they be separated from IPF. Diffuse panbronchiolitis, a term used by Japanese investigators, is apparently a disease of unknown cause characterized by chronic inflammation of respiratory bronchioles without obliteration. Since bronchiolitis obliterans, especially in the presence of organizing pneumonia, has such a favorable prognosis and response to therapy, it is important that it be distinguished from IPF.[83,84] The management is quite similar to that described for IPF in that prednisone is given at 1 mg/kg/day, usually for 1-3 months. The dose is gradually reduced to total discontinuance of the drug, or every other day therapy, but should be continued for at least one year. Some patients require maintenance doses of 10-20 mg every other day indefinitely. Immunosuppressive agents have not been shown to be more useful than corticosteroids. Corticosteroid therapy is also used in the management of fume exposure, post-infectious and connective tissue disease related bronchiolitis obliterans with relatively good results, although the prognosis is not as good in these diseases as it is in bronchiolitis obliterans with organizing pneumonia.[82]

Adult Respiratory Distress Syndrome

The adult respiratory distress syndrome (ARDS) is a serious disorder characterized by severe hypoxemia, noncardiogenic pulmonary edema and a marked decrease in total lung compliance. It commonly follows a variety of pulmonary insults including gastric aspiration, gram-negative sepsis and major trauma. Despite advances in medical and respiratory care, the mortality of ARDS is still about 65 percent.[85] Important issues in the management of ARDS include ventilatory support with positive end-expiratory pressure, judicious fluid management often with monitoring of pulmonary capillary wedge pressure and appropriate recognition and treatment of other medical problems. Whether corticosteroids are beneficial in the treatment or prevention of ARDS is controversial. If corticosteroids are to be used, they should be given as early as possible. Methylprednisolone sodium succinate 30 mg/kg intravenously as a single dose has been used. This dose may be repeated in four hours, but prolonged corticosteroid therapy may be harmful. Patients given corticosteroids must be observed carefully for signs of superinfection so that appropriate treatment for this complication may be initiated.

ARDS Following Sepsis[86]

The presumed mechanism of ARDS following sepsis is that of injury to the alveolo-capillary membrane due to circulating bacterial products, with fluid and protein leaking into the interstitium and alveoli causing noncardiogenic pulmonary edema. Corticosteroids, via their powerful antiinflammatory action, can potentially decrease the amount of injury to the alveolo-capillary membrane and, thus, prevent the development or decrease the severity of ARDS. In experimental studies, methylprednisolone given before or soon after endotoxemia prevented the increase in endotoxin-induced lung vascular permeability in sheep.[87] This suggests that corticosteroids may be useful in preventing ARDS, if given early in the course of endotoxemia.

Older clinical studies of corticosteroid treatment in septic shock and ARDS are encouraging, but not definitive, because of limitation in patient selection and experimental design.[88] These studies did suggest that large doses of corticosteroids (3–4 mg/kg of dexamethasone or 30 mg/kg of methylprednisolone) reduced the degree of pulmonary edema and the mortality from gram-negative shock,[89,90] but more recent studies have not confirmed these beneficial effects of corticosteroids. In fact, there was an increased incidence of superinfection in one study.[91]

ARDS Following Gastric Aspiration

Aspiration of low pH gastric content is a relatively frequent precursor to ARDS. Over the years anecdotal and uncontrolled reports have suggested beneficial effects of corticosteroids in pulmonary aspiration of gastric content. However, several recent studies of larger numbers of patients have found no conclusive data upon which to base the use of corticosteroids in aspiration pneumonia.[91,92] Furthermore, the use of corticosteroids were associated with a higher rate of infection and a higher mortality.[92,93]

Other Respiratory Diseases

Fat Embolism Syndrome

The syndrome of fat embolism is characterized by the clinical triad of confusion, dyspnea and petechiae, 2–3 days following major trauma, and pathological evidence of fat embolism may be found in up to 90 percent of those dying from automobile accidents.[94]

Ashbaugh and Petty were the first to report on the therapeutic efficacy of high dose corticosteroids in the fat embolism syndrome.[95] Since then several uncontrolled studies have suggested decreased mortality in patients with established fat embolism syndrome treated with corticosteroids.[94] Since there is generally a 2–3 day interval between the trauma and the onset of clinical symptoms, one might expect prophylactic corticosteroid therapy to be useful, if a high risk group of patients can be identified.[96,97] Recent data does suggest that prophylactic corticosteroid therapy is of benefit in patients at high risk for developing fat embolism syndrome (i.e. one or more lower-extremity, long-bone fractures without associated major cerebral, thoracic or abdominal injuries).

Although the data for corticosteroid treatment either prophylactically or for established fat embolism syndrome is not firm, we consider corticosteroid treatment in that situation to be reasonable, if there are no major contraindications to the use of corticosteroids. The recommended dose of methylprednisolone is 7.5mg/kg to be administered intravenously every six hours for three days.[97]

Tuberculosis

Miliary tuberculosis. Miliary tuberculosis is an illness produced by hematogenous dissemination of tubercle bacilli, with tiny discrete foci uniformly distributed throughout all lung fields. The keys to management are early diagnosis, the prompt institution of antituberculosis chemotherapy, and appropriate supportive measures. Although controversial, corticosteroids appear to be effective in hastening the reduction in systemic toxicity, the intensity of the inflammatory exudative pulmonary response and the roentgenographic changes. In our experience a brief course of corticosteroid therapy may be beneficial to some patients who are severely ill with disseminated tuberculosis, but because of the potentially severe complications, this therapy should be very carefully reviewed prior to its use.[98]

Extrapulmonary tuberculosis. Although pulmonary involvement is most common, extrapulmonary sites of infection such as meninges, pericardium, peritoneum, and bones account for up to 15 percent of all cases of tuberculosis. Despite adequate antituberculous chemotherapy, certain patients are left with chronic sequelae. Since they can attenuate the inflammatory response and inhibit fibroblast proliferation, corticosteroids have been proposed as important adjuncts to therapy in extrapulmonary tuberculosis, especially the meningeal, pericardial, and peritoneal involvement.

Tuberculous Meningitis[99,100]

From the early 1950s, corticosteroids have been advocated as a useful adjunct in the treatment of tuberculous meningitis to reduce both the acute inflammatory manifestation and the chronic sequelae of obstructive hydrocephalus. Review of the course of over 600 patients with tuberculous meningitis indicated no benefit of the routine use of corticosteroids. Another study has recommended that the presence of signs and symptoms of cerebral edema is the only indication for use of corticosteroids in tuberculous meningitis.[101]

Tuberculous Pericarditis

In well-documented tuberculous pericarditis treated with isoniazid, para-aminosalicylic acid, and streptomycin, prednisone administration was associated with a more rapid decrease in pericardial effusion.[102] In addition, the mortality was lower in the prednisone treated group, although it is unclear whether this difference was entirely due to prednisone therapy.

Tuberculous Peritonitis

The use of corticosteroids as adjunct in the treatment of tuberculous peritonitis is controversial. A randomized study of corticosteroid therapy in tuberculous peritonitis from India showed a lower incidence of late intestinal obstruction in

Corticosteroids

patients treated with prednisone,[103] while another prospective study found excellent outcome in patients treated with antituberculous chemotherapy alone.[104] In view of the low incidence of chronic sequelae in tuberculous peritonitis, we do not recommend routine use of corticosteroids in this condition.

Inhalation Injury[105]

Toxic injury secondary to accidental exposure to high concentrations of irritant gases (e.g., nitrogen dioxide, chlorine, carbon dioxide, phosgene, sulfur dioxide, cyanide, ammonia, and hydrogen sulfide) is becoming a significant problem in our industrialized society. The major clinical manifestations are those associated with acute noncardiogenic pulmonary edema. Management is mainly supportive, and hospitalization is required in any patient with suspected lower respiratory tract injury, because latent periods of up to 12–24 hrs. may occur before the onset of chest symptoms. Furthermore, patients may recover from the acute episode only to develop bronchiolitis obliterans 2–6 weeks later.

The use of corticosteroids in the management of these patients is controversial. In nitrogen dioxide-induced pulmonary disease it is recommended that corticosteroids be started immediately in patients with respiratory failure and pulmonary edema.[106] Prednisone 0.5 mg/kg/day is a reasonable initial daily dose. Therapy may be required for several weeks. In other toxic injuries the role of corticosteroids is not clear.

Thermal Injury and Smoke Inhalation

The major causes of lung injury in smoke inhalation are thermal injury and inhalation of toxic fumes and particulate matter. The complications of smoke inhalation vary temporally but are fairly predictable. Carbon monoxide poisoning occurs early (0–8 hr) and is believed to be the major cause of death at the scene of the fire. Thermal injury causes capillary disruption, mucosal edema, and hemorrhage, which can produce upper airway obstruction (0–8 hr) requiring endotracheal intubation. Stridor is an ominous finding. Toxic fumes (and thermal injury) can cause bronchospasm, stridor, airway plugging (desquamated tissue and secretions), and atelectasis (0–24 hr). Noncardiogenic pulmonary edema (leading to ARDS) is a dreaded complication that usually manifests itself after 24–96 hrs. Finally, pneumonia occurs in a minority of cases, usually after 4–5 days.

Airway management is the first priority with the use of supplemental oxygen in all victims until the situation is accurately defined. Other supportive therapy should be used as indicated. Corticosteroid therapy has not been shown to be of value in management of the respiratory damage from smoke inhalation.

Radiation Pneumonitis

Radiation therapy is widely used for the treatment of malignant disease. Two phases of radiation injury to the lungs occur. The acute phase of radiation pneumonitis is characterized by cough, dyspnea, fever, and chest pain developing 2-6 months after radiation therapy. The late phase of radiation fibrosis usually follows the acute phase by 6 months or more and is characterized by insidious onset of cough and dyspnea. The role of corticosteroids in the management of radiation pneumonitis and fibrosis is unproven. Corticosteroids given prophylactically are not likely to prevent the pneumonitis. In general, prednisone, 60-100 mg daily, is used as soon as the diagnosis is made and results in an objective improvement in many cases, at which time the dose can be reduced cautiously to 20-40 mg daily. Interestingly, the withdrawal of corticosteroids may precipitate or unmask radiation injury in some patients when it has been used as part of the chemotherapy protocol. Therefore, it has been suggested that corticosteroid therapy either not be included in the chemotherapy protocol or that its administration should be continuous.[107]

CONTRAINDICATIONS

There are no absolute contraindications to the use of corticosteroids. Moreover, when corticosteroids are given as a short course, relatively few side effects are expected. In patients with previous history of corticosteroid-induced psycho-

Table 5-6
Potential Complications of Corticosteroid Therapy*

I. Short term, high dose, may be of sudden onset:
   1. Mental and CNS disturbances including mood swings (euphoria to depression), jitteriness, severe psychosis (rare); pseudotumor cerebri (rare).
   2. Sodium and fluid retention.
   3. Impaired glucose tolerance, hyperosmolar non-ketotic coma (especially in presence of parenteral feedings).
   4. Hypokalemic alkalosis, systemic arterial hypertension, glaucoma, pancreatitis, peptic ulceration and gastrointestinal hemorrhage, proximal myopathy (rare).
II. Long term, daily steroids for months or years:
   1. Suppression of the hypothalamic-pituitary-adrenal axis, with adrenal insufficiency.
   2. Cushing's syndrome.
   3. Growth retardation in prepubertal children and in adolescents.
   4. Osteoporosis with vertebral compression and multiple bone fractures, aseptic necrosis of bone.
   5. Proximal myopathy
   6. Increased susceptibility to opportunistic infections.
   7. Impaired wound healing, dermal atrophy.
   8. CNS manifestations—depression, lability of mood, anxiety, seizures.
   9. Posterior sub-capsular cataract formation

*A number of these side-effects are controversial and unproven—see text.

sis or severe diabetes mellitus, attempts should be made to withhold corticosteroids until absolutely necessary, and the dose of corticosteroids should be the lowest dose that is considered efficacious when long-term corticosteroid therapy is contemplated. The major contraindications would include young age, severe diabetes mellitus, generalized osteoporosis, uncontolled peptic ulcer disease, glaucoma, cataract, psychosis, and poor medical compliance.

SIDE EFFECTS AND THEIR MANAGEMENT

Corticosteroid therapy results in adverse reactions in 16 percent of patients.[108] Side effects of corticosteroids are due to either excessive use over a prolonged period, or inappropriately rapid withdrawal. The incidence of side-effects is related to the dose and duration of treatment. Two-thirds of these reactions appear during acute course therapy and high dose therapy causes more problems than lower doses, particularly in psychiatric reactions. Many of the side-effects only occur after prolonged therapy, so that the clinician must always document the continued efficacy of corticosteroid therapy and reduce or ultimately discontinue the drugs, if not proven to be beneficial (Table 5-6).

Side Effects of Excessive and Prolonged Therapy[109]

Iatrogenic Cushing's Syndrome

Iatrogenic Cushing's syndrome differs from spontaneous Cushing's syndrome primarily in that the bilateral adrenal hyperplasia of the latter is associated with an elevated output of ACTH, which causes secretion of adrenal androgens and mineralocorticoids, and accounts for the virilism, acne, menstrual irregularities, and hypertension. Complications that are virtually unique to iatrogenic Cushing's syndrome include benign intracranial hypertension, posterior subcapsular cataract, panniculitis, glaucoma, and pancreatitis. Obesity, psychiatric symptoms, edema, and poor wound healing are equally present in both syndromes.[1] Other signs of the Cushing's syndrome include weight gain, swelling of the face (mooning), central obesity with a buffalo hump over the back of the neck, and stretch marks (striae) over the limbs and trunk. Fat pads may develop in the mediastinum and along the cardiac border resulting in a widening of the mediastinum on the chest x-ray.

Gastrointestinal Disorders

Peptic ulcer and gastrointestinal hemorrhage. The association between corticosteroid therapy and subsequent peptic ulceration and/or gastrointestinal hemorrhage has been the focus of considerable controversy.[109] The incidence of ulcers with corticosteroid therapy is only about 2 percent versus 1 percent of the controls, and is likely associated with higher doses, longer duration of treatment and the presence of predisposing factors such as concurrent use of ulcerogenic drugs (e.g. aspirin), especially in patients with rheumatoid arthritis. Nevertheless, corticosteroids may render an ulcer symptomless and, thus, mask any warning signs of life-threatening hemorrhage or perforation. Esophagitis and/or esophageal perforation is an infrequent complication. Obviously, the drug should be avoided when possible in patients with history of peptic ulcer, gastritis, or esophagitis. If the use of corticosteroids cannot be avoided, the lowest dose that produces the desired effect should be utilized and the patient should be given an aggressive ulcer-prevention program, such as antacids and H-2 blockers. It is not necessary to provide prophylaxis in patients without a history of the disease. All patients should be instructed to check for black or bloody stools, and the presence of anemia in patients receiving corticosteroids should signal the possibility of occult gastrointestinal bleeding.

Other gastrointestinal side-effects include oral candidiasis, nausea, vomiting, and fatty liver.

Acute pancreatitis. Acute pancreatitis appears to be more common in corticosteroid treated patients, especially in children with the nephrotic syndrome, SLE, or organ transplantation. The prognosis in this setting is poor and frequently, the condition is not diagnosed until surgery or autopsy.

Myopathy

Corticosteroids are known to have a catabolic effect on muscles, so not unexpectedly an excessive amount of corticosteroids, whether endogenous or exogenous, can have untoward effects on muscle. Corticosteroid therapy can cause an insidious, painless proximal myopathy characterized by weakness of the pelvic and/or pectoral girdle.[110,111] The pelvic girdle is most frequently involved and the proximal muscles are more severely involved than distal muscles. Atrophy of the type 2B fiber (fast-twitch, glycolytic fibers) is the most consistent finding.[112] The effect of corticosteroids on diaphragm function has not been clearly defined.

Occasionally myalgias, arthralgias and/or an acute fulminating weakness may herald the onset of corticosteroid myopathy. This usually occurs in patients given very high initial dosages or when the dose is rapidly increased from low-dose maintenance levels.[110] However, the most common presenting manifestations are difficulty climbing stairs, getting out of a chair, or combing the hair. Other untoward effects of corticosteroid therapy, especially osteoporosis, are frequently present in patients who develop corticosteroid myopathy. In fact, the absence of other undesirable side effects of corticosteroid therapy is thought to mitigate against the diagnosis of corticosteroid-induced myopathy.

Myopathy is most frequently associated with the use of 9-fluorinated corticosteroids such as triamcinolone or dexamethasone, but have been reported with all forms of corticosteroids used in therapy. Usually high dose, long-term daily therapy is implicated, but it may occur soon after the onset of therapy and be sufficiently severe to prevent ambulation. Low dose prednisone therapy (10 mg or less daily) is not likely to cause myopathy. The pathogenesis is unknown but thought to result from corticosteroid-induced abnormalities in glycolytic and oxidative metabolism that lead to muscle wasting and atrophy.

Corticosteroid myopathy is frequently reversible, therefore, the best management is to reduce or discontinue the drug and to switch to the nonfluorinated steroid preparations. Alternate day therapy may lessen or delay but does not prevent this complication. Phenytoin (Dilantin) and anabolic corticosteroids (norethandrolone or oxandrolone) have been used in an attempt to reverse or reduce the frequency of myopathy, but have not been effective. Muscle strength usually returns to normal within four months after stopping corticosteroid therapy, but this may occasionally take up to one year.

Osteoporosis

It is commonly accepted that patients with endogenous Cushing's syndrome or those receiving long-term supraphysiologic doses of corticosteroid therapy will develop osteoporosis.[113] Corticosteroid therapy is thought to cause osteoporosis by decreasing bone formation and increasing bone resorption. Interestingly, this dual effect on bone loss is quite different from many other skeletal diseases that generally tend to change bone formation and bone resorption in the same direction, although frequently unequally. The mechanism whereby corticosteroid decreases bone formation is likely due to a direct inhibition of osteoclastic functions.[114] On the other hand, bone resorption is the indirect result of corticosteroid-induced inhibition of calcium absorption from the intestine, hypercalciuria, and a compensatory increase in serum parathyroid hormone, which stimulates the activity of osteoclasts and leads to an increase in bone resorption.

The loss of bone density is insidious and predominates in those areas with a high content of trabecular bone, such as ribs and vertebrae. Less dramatic changes occur in areas where cortical bone predominates. As a result, patients usually present with thoracic or lumbar back pain due to vertical collapse. Patients at high risk for the development of osteoporosis, (i.e. postmenopausal women, elderly individuals, or those with restricted physical activity) seem more susceptible to the risk of corticosteroid-induced osteoporosis. Corticosteroid-induced osteoporosis is dose related and appears infrequently in patients treated with 10 mg of prednisolone daily or less.

The diagnosis of corticosteroid-induced osteoporosis is difficult. In patients at high risk photon absorptiometry measurements[115,116] should be performed at the start of corticosteroid therapy and every three to six months thereafter for several years in order to assess the rate of bone loss. Rates of bone loss above the normal suggest the need for preventive measures.[114]

Prevention is the best management for corticosteroid-induced osteoporosis. Evidence of progressive bone loss indicates the need for reduction, and if possible, elimination of corticosteroid therapy. Physical activity appears to stimulate bone formation, therefore, any patient receiving high-dose corticosteroids should be enrolled in a regular exercise program. Also, a rational program of prophylaxis should be instituted. Vitamin D and calcium supplements will correct the depressed enteral calcium absorption, decrease the level of parathyroid hormone and increase the trabecular bone mass. Vitamin D and hydrochlorothiazide in combination will correct hypercalciuria.[114] The latter is relatively easy to recognize, however, it is not clear when prophylaxis is required. Some authors recommend the addition of sodium fluoride (66 to 88 mg per day) to the above regimen, since it appears to stimulate trabecular bone formation. Unfortunately adequate evidence to support the above approach is lacking.

Avascular Osteonecrosis (Aseptic Necrosis)

Avascular osteonecrosis is known to occur in patients with an excessive level of corticosteroids, either as a result of corticosteroid therapy[117,118] or Cushing's syndrome,[119] and is most common in the head of the femur or humerus bilaterally, but can occur at any site. Most often this complication occurs as a result of trauma and in the presence of other diseases that have a higher than expected incidence of avascular necrosis, (e.g. SLE, alcoholism, pancreatitis, fat embolism, and renal transplantation), and in patients with liver disease, hyperlipidemia, diabetes, pancreatitis, polycythemia, hemoglobinopathy (S-S, S-C and others), obesity, gout and hyperuricemia, Gaucher's disease, and dysbarism.

There are very few reports describing this complication in patients receiving corticosteroids for pulmonary diseases.[120,121] Usually these patients had been receiving corticosteroids at high doses for many years, and it is extremely rare in the first three months of therapy.

The precise mechanism of avascular osteonecrosis is unknown, but it is generally felt that interruption of the blood supply for one reason or another is the most likely primary event, with fat embolization to the subchondral arterioles and localized bone cell death being the most widely-accepted theory.[22]

Prevention is the best treatment. Clearly, corticosteroids should be avoided in patients with conditions that predispose them to this complication, if at all possible. Nevertheless, in instances where the respiratory disease is progressive, severe and/or life threatening, (e.g. status asthmaticus or idiopathic pulmonary fibrosis) a trial of corticosteroid therapy should not be withheld for fear of this uncommon side-effect. A single daily dose appears to be less detrimental than divided daily doses, and the lower the dose, the less likely the complication.

Once the patient has established disease no satisfactory management regimen exists. Conservative treatments include: (1) Reduction or discontinuation of the corticosteroid therapy. This will not have an effect on the established lesion, but will likely lessen the risk of osteonecrosis at other sites; (2) Avoidance of weight-bearing may help prevent progression in weight-bearing joints (i.e. hip, knee); (3) Pain relief can occasionally be obtained by the application of heat and mild antiinflammatory analgesics (e.g., aspirin, indomethacin, ibuprofen); (4) In advanced cases with collapse of the femoral head, conventional total hip arthroplasty should be performed.

Ocular Side Effects

Posterior subcapsular cataracts. Posterior subcapsular cataracts are the most common ocular side effect of daily or alternate-day corticosteroid therapy.[123] The prevalence of cataracts ranges from 2.4 percent to 38 percent and is related to dose and duration of therapy with suggestive evidence that children are affected more frequently than adults, at lower dosages and with shorter periods of therapy. The earlier the appearance of cataract changes the higher the risk of developing extensive cataracts with subsequent visual impairment.

The corticosteroid-induced cataract can usually be distinguished from senile or diabetic cataracts in that it is frequently bilateral; the lesion usually occupies the polar region of the posterior cortex just within the lens capsule; and may extend forward into the cortex in an irregular manner but its borders are usually sharply defined.[124]

Management of this complication requires early identification and reduction of the dose of corticosteroid or conversion to alternate-day therapy. Patients who are receiving corticosteroids should have an ophthalmologic examination at each visit and slit-lamp examination every 6–12 months.

If used for airway disease, inhaled corticosteroids may delay the progression of the cataracts and allow control of the disorder. If the dose cannot be reduced and the cataracts progress, then removal of the lens is the only alternative. Fortunately, this is not frequently necessary.

Increased intraocular pressure.[124,125] Corticosteroid-induced increases in intraocular pressure complicate topical therapy more frequently than systemic therapy. It also develops in Cushing's syndrome. Susceptibility to the development of raised intraocular pressure seems to be inherited although the exact mode of inheritance is unclear. Similarly, the mechanism of the increased intraocular pressure is unknown.

Clinical signs of increased intraocular pressure, (i.e. cupping of the optic disc and visual field defects) may not be found in these patients so that measurement of the intraocular pressure is frequently required to make the diagnosis.

Interestingly, diabetics with corticosteroid-induced increases in intraocular pressure tend not to have diabetic retinopathy. It is postulated that the increase in pressure prevents the leak of blood from the retinal capillaries.

Other ocular side effects. Swelling of the eyelids, ptosis, and chemosis are findings associated with the "moon faces" resulting from systemic corticosteroids. Exophthalmos occurs in Cushing's disease, but is a very rare complication of long-term corticosteroid therapy. Extraocular muscle myopathy may complicate systemic therapy. Subconjunctival and retinal hemorrhages in patients with purpura and easy bruisability have been reported. Minor refractive changes are known to occur as a result of corticosteroid therapy; the exact mechanism is unknown.[125]

Psychiatric Disturbances[126,127]

Cushing's syndrome and high-dose corticosteroid therapy may be complicated by almost any form of psychological disturbance. Euphoria is most common but slight mood changes ranging from insomnia, increased appetite, nervousness, irritability, anxiety, and hyperkinesis to psychotic episodes (including manic-depressive or paranoid states and acute toxic psychoses) have been reported occasionally. It is difficult to predict which patient will develop these psychological reactions to corticosteroid therapy. Although there is very little support, a previously widely-held view was that serious psychological disturbances are more closely related to the patient's baseline personality structure than to the actual dose of the hormone prescribed. Interestingly, patients may become psychologically dependent on corticosteroids with surreptitious abuse of the drug.

Management, especially of severe depression, requires the gradual withdrawal of corticosteroid therapy. Occasionally antidepressant therapy is required. Untoward psychological reaction to a previous course of corticosteroids is not an absolute contraindication to a second course of treatment. Similarly, previous uneventful treatment does not preclude untoward psychological reactions during subsequent courses of therapy.

Intracranial Hypertension[128-130]

Benign intracranial hypertension ("pseudotumor cerebri") is a rare complication of prolonged corticosteroid therapy[131] whose mechanism is not certain. It occurs most commonly in children or young women. The most widely-held explanation is decreased cerebrospinal fluid (CSF) absorption. Most cases have occurred following a reduction in corticosteroid dosage or a change in preparation. The main features of benign intracranial hypertension are moderate to severe (general, episodic) throbbing morning headache, dizziness, irritability, vomiting, disturbance of visual acuity (e.g. blurring, obscurations, diplopia, blindness), tinnitus, and sixth cranial nerve palsy. The cerebrospinal fluid is normal except for increased pressure (above 200 mm H$_2$O). Management requires increasing the corticosteroid dose until symptoms are controlled. Repeated lumbar punctures (every 2 days to every week) and surgical shunting may be required, the latter when medical treatment fails or in case of rapidly failing vision.[132] Acetazolamide, a carbonic anhydrase inhibitor that reduces CSF production, has been recommended but the results are conflicting.

Increased Susceptibility to Infection[133,134]

Corticosteroids alter host defenses, and high doses for prolonged periods may be associated with increased susceptibility to infection. The key factor that determines the role of corticosteroid therapy in promoting infection is the underlying disease for which the corticosteroids are used. Often the primary disease lowers host resistance to infection even in the absence of corticosteroid therapy. Furthermore, other drugs taken concurrently may contribute to lowered host resistance. It has been suggested that the risk of infection may be greatest in those patients receiving very high doses of corticosteroid therapy, but this may simply reflect the fact that high risk patients receive the most intensive therapy. Low doses of corticosteroid therapy do not seem to increase the risk of infection even in diseases associated with a high incidence of secondary infection.

Bacterial infections. Most secondary infections occurring in "corticosteroid treated patients" are caused by bacteria. They include pneumonia, endocarditis, bacteremia, pyelonephritis, peritonitis, liver abscess, osteomyelitis, and septicemia.

Reactivation of Tuberculosis.[135] Corticosteroid therapy depresses cell-mediated immune responses and inhibits the cutaneous reaction to tuberculin, and has been considered a risk factor for reactivation of tuberculosis. Cutaneous anergy can develop within 2 weeks of starting prednisone. Although the true risk of corticosteroid-induced reactivation of tuberculosis is unknown, available studies suggest that it is quite low.[80,122,136,137] Routine prophylactic isoniazid therapy is not indicated when patients with a positive PPD are started on corticosteroids. Serial chest roentgenograms, may be indicated in order to identify reactivation in patients with previous disease.

Fungal infections. Candida is by far the most prevalent pathogen, about 30 percent of all systemic infection with this organism occurring in the setting of corticosteroid therapy. Diabetics and patients receiving intravenous hyperalimentation or antibiotic therapy are particularly susceptible. Corticosteroid therapy has also been associated with at least 50 percent of pulmonary or disseminated aspergillosis cases, the majority of such cases having occurred in association with cytotoxic chemotherapy for malignant diseases. An increased incidence of nocardiosis, mucormycosis, cryptococcosis, and pneumocystis carinii has also been reported in patients receiving corticosteroid therapy.

Viral infection. There is limited evidence that corticosteroids increase the incidence or severity of viral infections, although varicella-herpes zoster, herpes simplex, and cytomegalovirus infections do appear to be enhanced by corticosteroid therapy. Such infections are more likely in patients with underlying hematologic, connective tissue or reticuloendothelial system diseases, and only rarely occur in asthmatic patients treated with corticosteroids.

Parasitic infection. Patients with malaria, amebiasis, or strongyloidiasis have been reported to have increased complications on corticosteroid therapy.

Cutaneous Disturbances

There are multiple cutaneous manifestations of prolonged systemic corticosteroid therapy including: thinning of the skin, acneform eruptions, hirsutism, striae, purpura, and impaired wound healing. Atrophic skin is thought to occur as a result of corticosteroid-induced alterations in fibroblast biosynthesis of collagen and atrophy of collagen bundles and fibers. Hirsutism occurs in 3-13 percent of patients depending on the duration of corticosteroid administration. Acneform skin lesions are not well understood, but occur less often than hirsutism and tend to differ somewhat from acne vulgaris. Striae occur primarily on the back and lower abdomen. Purpuric lesions resemble those of senile purpura and occur on the extensor surface of the forearms, hands, as well as the neck and face. The mechanism is not clear, but probably results from tearing of poorly supported cutaneous vessels by shearing injuries.[138] Minor trauma may result in major skin damage in patients receiving corticosteroids.[139]

Uncommonly, hyperhidrosis, telangiectasia, hyperpigmentation, rolled hair in association with keratosis pilaris, bullous herpetiform lesions, acanthosis nigricans, nodular panniculitis, and hemorrhagic longitudinal linear tearing and necrosis have been reported in association with prolonged corticosteroid therapy.

Renal and Metabolic Disturbances

Although the kidney itself is relatively spared of severe corticosteroid side effects, the chronic administration of pharmacologic doses of corticosteroids does result in increases in glomerular infiltration rate, fluid delivery into the distal tubule, increased hydrogen, potassium and calcium excretion, as well as a decrease in sodium excretion.[140] Animal studies suggest that the chronic administration of potent corticosteroids results in increased endogenous acid production and stimulates renal tubular hydrogen ion secretion and ammonia production. The net effect on systemic acid base status is determined by the dose administered.[141]

Corticosteroids

Salt and water retention occur primarily in response to the mineralocorticoid activity of corticosteroids. When high doses are used, salt and water retention leads to edema, hypertension, and even left ventricular dysfunction. The edema is best treated by prevention, (i.e., dietary restriction of sodium intake at the onset of corticosteroid therapy). If it persists, the patient should be switched to a corticosteroid preparation less likely to produce sodium retention (see Table 2). Obviously, caution is required if large doses of corticosteroids are to be given to patients with cardiovascular or renal disease, where even mild degrees of fluid retention may be hazardous.

Potassium loss is usually slight with small doses of corticosteroids and is easily replaced by dietary potassium, but supplemental potassium may be required when large doses of corticosteroids are given. Severe hypokalemia is rare, but may cause asthenia, paralysis or arrhythmias, if undetected. Hypokalemic alkalosis may be produced by prolonged high doses of corticosteroids. The incidence of hypokalemia is related to the mineralocorticoid activity of the particular corticosteroid preparation. Potassium-wasting diuretics must be taken with caution in association with corticosteroid therapy. It should be noted that the renal sodium-retention and potassium-wasting actions of corticosteroids are independent of each other and that enhancement of potassium excretion is more consistent than the retention of sodium.

Corticosteroids cause a decrease in intestinal absorption of calcium and an increase in its urinary clearance, which is probably due to both enhanced glomerular filtration and diminished tubular reabsorption. The overall effects of this change in calcium metabolism are discussed in the section on osteoporosis. Corticosteroids have been used to treat selected conditions associated with hypercalcemia, namely hypervitaminosis D, sarcoidosis, and certain malignant states such as multiple myeloma, leukemia, lymphoma, and carcinoma of the breast. Unfortunately, patients with hypercalcemia due to primary hyperparathyroidism or a malignancy generally do not respond to corticosteroids.

Glomerular lesions have been detected in some patients with the nephrotic syndrome treated with corticosteroids.[109] However, the significance of these lesions is unclear. An increased urinary leukocyte count often associated with microscopic hematuria has been reported in patients on long-term therapy. It does not appear to be associated with renal infection.[142]

It has been claimed that corticosteroid therapy may be associated with a greater incidence of amyloid renal disease, although the validity of this observation has been challenged. Glycosuria has been noted in 3–10 percent of patients on corticosteroid therapy and is discussed in the section on diabetes mellitus.[109]

The relationship between corticosteroids and antidiuretic hormone (ADH) remains to be completely elucidated. Some data suggest that corticosteroids inhibit ADH release, while others have failed to show such a corticosteroid–ADH relationship.[109]

Growth Retardation

When genetic and socio-economic factors are taken into account, there is little doubt that asthmatic children tend to be short in stature irrespective of their treatment.[143] It appears that the growth stunting effect depends on the severity of the symptoms and the age at which the asthma developed, with increased effects, if it developed very early in life. Both chronic anorexia and chronic hypoxia appear to be factors responsible for this poor growth.[144] Unfortunately, corticosteroids in pharmacologic doses appear to exaggerate this growth retardation in asthmatic children.

Growth-stunting is apparent in children who had regular daily corticosteroids and correlates with the duration and dosage. Alternate-day corticosteroid therapy can reduce the growth retardation although this is not universal.[143,145] It has been demonstrated that catch-up growth can occur with use of less than 15 mg prednisone every other day, while high dose therapy (greater than 20 mg every other day) causes further growth suppression in asthmatic children during treatment with alternate-day corticosteroid.[146]

In patients with corticosteroid induced growth retardation, the bone age is delayed proportionately with the age and height.[144] Long term treatment with inhaled corticosteroids does not appear to retard growth or skeletal maturation in children.[147] It appears that the dwarfism results from corticosteroid-induced antagonism of the effects of human growth hormone at the peripheral tissue level.[148,149] Inhibition of sulfate incorporation into cartilage and of the generation of somatomedin A appear to be most important in growth suppression. Unfortunately, administration of human growth hormone fails to accelerate the growth of children with corticosteroid-induced suppression despite its effectiveness in some children with other forms of dwarfism.[148] If the corticosteroid dose is reduced below the threshold level that causes growth suppression or is discontinued completely, a catch-up growth phase occurs in many children.[145,150,151] Unfortunately, this catch-up growth may be incomplete and may result in a permanently short stature.[143,152]

Diabetes Mellitus

Prolonged corticosteroid therapy may unmask latent diabetes mellitus or aggravate preexisting disease,[153] presumably because corticosteroids induce peripheral resistance to insulin, while promoting gluconeogenesis. This adverse reaction does not appear to be related to the dose given,[108] but, hyperglycemia has rarely been reported with alternate-day corticosteroid therapy.[154] Glycosuria is a common finding in patients on corticosteroid therapy appearing in 3–10 percent of patients.[109] Although the incidence of acute pancreatitis appears to be higher in corticosteroid treated patients, it does not appear that this is the mechanism of the hyperglycemia and corticosteroid-induced diabetes found in this group.

In most cases the diabetes disappears soon after the corticosteroid is withdrawn. Acidosis, ketosis, and severe increases in blood glucose level occur, but are uncommon. The presence of frank diabetes mellitus or the demonstration of impaired glucose tolerance, although not precluding the use of corticosteroids, should temper the physician's decision to institute this form of therapy. Rarely, patients with corticosteroid-induced diabetes may require continued insulin therapy even after stopping the corticosteroids. The vast majority of patients can be managed by dietary restriction or the use of oral hypoglycemic agents. Glucose in the urine or serum should be measured as this may become evident within a few days of starting therapy. Onset of symptoms averages 26 days from the initiation of corticosteroid treatment in children, and therefore, is not the most reliable way to follow such patients.[154,155] Supplementation with high chromium brewer's yeast (a rich source of glucose tolerance factor) has been shown to improve glucose tolerance and lower serum lipids in diabetics as well as healthy controls, but it is not known if this will help decrease the incidence of corticosteroid-induced hyperglycemia or diabetes.[156]

Reproductive System

Fertility. The effect of corticosteroid therapy on human fertility is unknown. In contrast to endogenous Cushing's disease, women of child bearing age given corticosteroid therapy do not appear to have a significant increase in menstrual abnormalities or infertility.[109] In Cushing's disease, oligomenorrhea and infertility occur in as many as 70–90 percent of such patients. Prednisone has been used for the induction of ovulation and treatment of female infertility, when it is suspected that the etiology of the infertility is a mild abnormal elevation of the adrenal androgen level.[157] Therapy is discontinued after the confirmation of conception.

Male libido can be increased, decreased, or unchanged in patients given larger doses of corticosteroid therapy. No consistent changes in testicular size or function, spermatogenesis, or Leydig cell morphology has been reported following large doses of corticosteroids. Although there are variable changes in the sperm count, no profound effects on fertility have been reported.

Pregnancy. There is conflicting data as to whether the use of prednisone during pregnancy results in increased maternal or fetal complications.[158] Pregnant asthmatic patients treated with corticosteroids have not been shown to have increased complications.[159] Consequently, it has been recommended that if corticosteroid therapy is required during pregnancy, the patient should be treated as one would in the nongravid state. Obviously one should be extremely cautious in using these agents in patients with preeclampsia, fluid retention, or other complications of pregnancy.

Maternal corticosteroid therapy does not appear to result in fetal adrenal insufficiency. This may be because the human placenta converts cortisol to cortisone, which does not inhibit the HPA axis. Although the marked hyperestrogenemia during pregnancy greatly increases plasma transcortin (and hence the binding of cortisol), this does not result in a larger dose-requirement for corticosteroids in pregnant women.

Interestingly prenatal administration of betamethasone reduces the incidence and severity of the respiratory distress syndrome and neonatal mortality in infants delivered between 26 and 34 weeks of gestation,[160,161] without complications such as infection and growth derangement. However, hypoglycemia did occur more often in the infants from betamethasone-treated mothers than in the controls. The long term effects of this therapy on the fetus are unknown.

Side Effects of Corticosteroid Aerosols

At the recommended dosage, corticosteroid aerosols are free of systemic side effects.[23] The most common side effects of corticosteroid aerosols are dysphonia, which can affect up to 50 percent of patients treated with beclomethasone dipropionate,[162] and colonization of the oropharynx with Candida. The dysphonia improves with voice rest and does not appear to result in chronic sequelae. Oropharyngeal colonization with Candida is relatively common in patients receiving corticosteroid aerosol, particularly those receiving concomitant broad-spectrum antibiotics, although it causes symptoms in only about 5 percent of patients. Oropharyngeal candidiasis is not associated with tracheobronchial colonization and responds well to nystatin.

Some simple measures can decrease the frequency of these undesirable complications of corticosteroid aerosol.[162] Correct inhalational technique is extremely important to ensure minimal deposition of the drug in the oral cavity and pharynx. In addition, the use of a spacer will reduce the frequency of oropharyngeal candidiasis in addition to increasing the drug's antiasthmatic potency.[163] Rinsing out the oral cavity with tap water after each aerosol inhalation can decrease the frequency of oropharyngeal complications, and thus should be taught to all patients starting on corticosteroid aerosol. Finally, deliberate avoidance of voice stress such as frequent hawking or shouting may reduce the problem of dysphonia.

Adrenal suppression can result from inhaled beclomethasone dipropionate, but only when high doses (e.g. 800–1600 mg per day) are utilized. If inhaled beclomethasone is used with alternate-day prednisone, the HPA suppressive effects are additive. One needs to be aware that when a patient is switched from chronic oral corticosteroids to the aerosol, signs of adrenal insufficiency may develop. Consequently, during periods of stress, these patients should be covered with stress doses of systemic corticosteroids.

Corticosteroids

Side Effects of Inappropriately Rapid Withdrawal

Hypothalamic–Pituitary–Adrenal Suppression

Suppression of normal hypothalamic–pituitary–adrenal (HPA) function is a unique and feared consequence of prolonged corticosteroid therapy. The shortest duration or the smallest dose that will result in HPA suppression is unknown, since the response varies from patient to patient. However, HPA suppression can develop rapidly; pituitary ACTH release falls within minutes to hours and there is anatomic evidence of HPA suppression within 5–10 days after the institution of a daily regimen of 15–20 mg of prednisone or its equivalent. Fortunately, the clinical significance of these changes appear minor unless the patient undergoes major stress such as surgery, trauma, infection, or severe emotional disturbance. Clinically apparent impairment of HPA function has been demonstrated in patients who receive 20 mg to 30 mg/day of prednisone for 5–13 days.[164] However, prolonged therapy with replacement doses of corticosteroids, (approximately 5 mg of prednisone or its equivalent) do not cause HPA suppression as long as it is given as a single dose early each day.[165] It is important to remember that the HPA axis is more susceptible to corticosteroid inhibition if the corticosteroids are given during the evening hours. Furthermore, alternate-day corticosteroid regimens, and use of short acting preparations, are likely to maintain an intact hypothalamic–pituitary–adrenal function.

The symptoms and signs of corticosteroid-induced adrenal insufficiency are very similar to those associated with Addisonian crisis. The most common manifestations are easy fatigability, lassitude, weakness, depression, postural hypotension (occasionally shock), hemoconcentration and marked symptoms in the face of what appears to be a minor illness. Hyperkalemia, hyponatremia, increased BUN, and Addisonian pigmentation are rarely present due to absence of mineralocorticoid-insufficiency and marked elevation of ACTH. Diagnosis of HPA suppression rests on demonstration of the clinical syndrome, absence of recurrent disease with symptoms that mimic HPA suppression, rigorous laboratory examination to identify HPA insufficiency, and the relief of clinical syndrome by replacement of corticosteroids.

After prolonged treatment with large doses of corticosteroids (greater than 30 mg of prednisone or equivalent per day) one should determine whether or not HPA axis suppression is present before discontinuing the drug, or during periods of severe stress such as general anesthesia or severe infection which may result in severe hypotension. If adrenal insufficiency is not suspected, the hypertension can become intractable and may result in death. Interestingly, it appears that the hypothalamic-pituitary axis recovers first (within 5–9 months), and the adrenal cortical recovery lags behind (between 9–12 months), so that the time taken for the HPA system axis to fully recover and react appropriately to stress is 12–16 months following corticosteroid withdrawal.[142,166] The administration of

ACTH during treatment with corticosteroid therapy does not minimize the HPA suppression.

If HPA suppression is suspected, the adequacy of adrenocortical function should be assessed by the ACTH stimulation test.[167] A positive response correlates well with the ability of the patient to tolerate general anesthesia and surgery.[168] It should be remembered that corticosteroids administered by a variety of routes can induce HPA suppression, i.e. oral, intravenous, intramuscular, cutaneous (especially with occlusive dressings), rectal, aerosol inhalation, topical eye instillation, etc.[109]

Corticosteroid Withdrawal Syndrome[169]

Psychologic or physical dependence on corticosteroids presumably is a result of the euphoria and the sense of well-being associated with corticosteroid therapy. Importantly, many of these symptoms can occur with normal levels of plasma glucocorticoid and in patients with normal responsiveness of HPA system.[170,171] Furthermore, many patients who feel fine while withdrawing from corticosteroids may have a strong emotional reluctance to further dose reduction because previous attempts at withdrawal had resulted in unpleasant relapses of their underlying disease. The corticosteroid withdrawal syndrome is characterized by anorexia, nausea, emesis, lethargy, headache, fever, desquamation of the skin of the face and extremities, arthralgia, myalgia, stiffness, joint pain, and limping. Interestingly, pseudorheumatism occurs more commonly in patients with pulmonary tuberculosis and asthma (i.e., patients who should ordinarily not have these symptoms). Obviously, the diagnosis is extremely difficult in patients with underlying active arthritis. Since most patients with corticosteroid withdrawal syndrome usually suffer from concomitant HPA suppression, appropriate tests to define HPA function should be performed.

The signs and symptoms of the corticosteroid withdrawal syndrome are alleviated by pharmacologic, but not replacement or physiologic doses of corticosteroids. Interestingly, the majority of cases occur when corticosteroids are withdrawn rapidly.

DRUG INTERACTIONS[172]

The metabolism of corticosteroids may be altered by certain disease states or by interactions with other drugs (Table 5-7). As discussed earlier, corticosteroid metabolism is decreased in patients with severe liver diseases. Patients with thyroid diseases can also have altered corticosteroid metabolism. Hyperthyroidism accelerates corticosteroid metabolism so that higher than the usual replacement dose may be required to treat adrenal insufficiency, whereas hypothyroidism slows corticosteroid metabolism and Cushing's syndrome may develop on relatively low doses of corticosteroids.

Table 5-7
Alterations in Corticosteroid Metabolism

	Pathophysiologic states	Drugs
Increased steroid metabolism	hyperthyroidism	phenytoin phenobarbital ephedrine rifampin
Decreased steroid metabolism	hypothyroidism liver disease	troleandomycin erythromycin

Drugs Which Affect Corticosteroid Action

Most of the drugs that affect corticosteroid action do so by altering the hepatic metabolism of corticosteroids.[172]

Macrolide Antibiotics[173,174]

Troleandomycin (TAO), a macrolide antibiotic structurally similar to erythromycin, was introduced in 1957 for the treatment of gram-positive infections, was noted to produce dramatic clinical improvement in certain asthmatics, which could not be attributed to its antibiotic property. TAO has been shown to improve pulmonary function in some corticosteroid-dependent asthmatics,[175,176] and allowed many patients to be managed on a much reduced dose of methylprednisolone, often on an alternate day basis. TAO and erythromycin, another macrolide antibiotic, reduce theophylline clearance,[177,178] but erythromycin is associated with a lesser " 'corticosteroid sparing' effect."[179]

Mechanism of Action

The corticosteroid-sparing property of TAO appears to be specific for methylprednisolone[175,180] and is due to its effect on corticosteroid metabolism. TAO significantly decreases methylprednisolone elimination and prolongs plasma half-life of methylprednisolone from 2.5 to 4.6 hours.[181] This effect of TAO on methylprednisolone elimination appears to persist for at least one month after TAO is started. Clinical experience suggests that adding TAO is not simply equivalent to increasing the dose of methylprednisolone.[175]

A trial of TAO is indicated in patients with severe chronic asthma who remain symptomatic despite theophylline, β-adrenergic agents and chronic corticosteroid therapy. Before TAO is prescribed the corticosteroid should be changed to an equivalent dose of methylprednisolone for at least one week.[176] Since the major toxicity of TAO is on the liver, hepatic function should be assessed prior to the initiation of TAO treatment and weekly thereafter, and in the setting of active liver disease, TAO therapy is probably contraindicated. After stabilization with methylprednisolone, TAO is started at 250 mg q.i.d. (or 14 mg/kg/day) for the first week, then reduced to 250 mg t.i.d. the second week, 250 mg b.i.d. the third week and finally 250 mg every morning beginning in the fourth week.

As explained in Chapter 2, theophylline dosage should be reduced concomitantly. If the patient is receiving more than 32 mg/day of methylprednisolone, the corticosteroid dosage should also be reduced by 25 percent with the initiation of TAO. If there is no improvement in symptoms or spirometry after two weeks, TAO may be discontinued and the original dose of corticosteroid reinstituted. If there is clinical improvement, the daily dose of methylprednisolone should be tapered by 4 mg per week. When a dose of 4–8 mg/day is reached, the patient should be switched to an alternate day regimen giving three times the daily dose in the morning every other day. Once the patient is stable on alternate day methylprednisolone, TAO can also be switched to 250 mg every other day given on the same day as methylprednisolone.

Side Effects

Side effects seen with TAO therapy include transient increase in corticosteroid-induced side effects such as cushingoid features, fluid retention, osteoporosis, and cataracts. Transient gastrointestinal upsets with nausea and abdominal cramps may be reduced when the serum theophylline levels are monitored carefully. Less common side effects include rash and aspirin intolerance.[175,176] However, the side effects of TAO are primarily hepatic.[182] Evidence of mild hepatocellular damage (elevated SGOT and SGPT) occur in 24 to 50 percent of patients.[175,176,182] Overt jaundice or hepatitis is uncommon (less than 4 percent of cases). Most changes occur after 3 to 4 weeks of therapy. The liver function tests return to normal when the drug is stopped and, occasionally, spontaneously with reduction in the dosage. Chronic therapy with 250 mg of TAO daily is rarely associated with abnormalities in liver function tests.

As noted earlier, TAO and erythromycin can also cause a significant elevation of serum theophylline levels,[178] and a reduction of 25–50 percent of baseline theophylline dose is advisable on initiation of TAO. Frequent serum theophylline levels are needed for proper theophylline dosage as the TAO dose is altered. Similarly, when erythromycin is given to asthmatics treated with methylprednisolone, one needs to consider the interaction of erythromycin with both theophylline and methylprednisone.

Rifampin

Rifampin, an antituberculous antibiotic, can increase cortisol metabolism due to the induction of hepatic microsomal enzymes.[183] When rifampin is initiated in patients on chronic corticosteroid therapy, the dose of the corticosteroids may need to be increased by as much as two fold.[172]

Anticonvulsants

The anticonvulsants, diphenylhydantoin and phenobarbital, are powerful inducers of hepatic microsomal enzymes important in drug metabolism. Diphen-

Corticosteroids

ylhydantoin[184] and phenobarbitate[185] increase the metabolic clearance of prednisolone; the magnitude of the effect on corticosteroid clearance appears to be proportional to the initial half-life of the corticosteroid. Thus, corticosteroids with the longest half-life, such as dexamethasone, are affected more than those with the shortest half-life, such as hydrocortisone. Therefore, it has been suggested that the corticosteroid dose should be doubled when either diphenylhydantoin or phenobarbital is initiated.

Sympathomimetic agents

Ephedrine, a component of several over-the-counter antiasthma medications including Bronkaid® (Winthrop Consumer Products, New York, New York 10016) and Primatene® (Whitehall Laboratories, New York, New York 10017) tablets, has been reported to increase the plasma clearance of dexamethasone.[186] This could potentially cause a decrease in corticosteroid action, leading to exacerbation of asthma. This effect of ephedrine was attributed to a combination of increased liver blood flow and induction of hepatic microsomal enzymes. Whether β-adrenergic agonists other than ephedrine affect corticosteroid metabolism is unknown.

Effects of Corticosteroids on Other Drugs

One of the most important effects of corticosteroids in airway disease is prevention or reversal of tachyphylaxis to β-adrenergic agonists. Corticosteroids do not appear to alter either the metabolism or bioavailability of other drugs commonly used in the treatment of respiratory diseases.[187]

Corticosteroids do affect the metabolism or action of several other drugs including salicylates, anticholinesterase drugs, and pancuronium.[172] Corticosteroids increase the metabolism of salicylates and lead to suboptimal serum salicylate levels, so that corticosteroid withdrawal in a patient also receiving salicylates should prompt a reduction in the salicylate dose as well. In patients with myasthenia gravis, corticosteroids can block the therapeutic effects of anticholinesterase drugs, and thus, lead to increased weakness. Hydrocortisone, prednisolone, and methylprednisolone are the preparations most likely to interfere with the action of anticholinesterase drugs, whereas dexamethasone is said not to exhibit this property. In the presence of hydrocortisone and prednisolone, the duration of neuromuscular blockade by pancuronium is decreased. Again the mechanism of this interaction is unclear, but may be due to direct competition at the myoneural junction.

Finally, although corticosteroids may not interact with certain drugs directly, the powerful metabolic effects of corticosteroids may lead to interference with the therapeutic action of some drugs. Drugs in this category include insulin and diuretics. Because corticosteroid therapy can aggravate hyperglycemia and fluid and salt retention, the dosages of these drugs must be regulated with care when corticosteroids are added to the therapeutic regimen.

REFERENCES

1. Axelrod L: Glucocorticoid therapy. Medicine 55:39-65, 1976
2. Thompson EB, Lippman ME: Mechanism of action of glucocorticoids. Metabolism 23:159-202, 1974
3. Parrillo JE, Fauci AS: Mechanisms of glucocorticoid action on immune processes. Ann Rev Pharmacol Toxicol 19:179-201, 1979
4. Fauci AS, Dale DC, Balow JE: Glucocorticosteroid therapy: Mechanisms of action and clinical consideration. Ann Intern Med 84:304-315, 1976
5. Bovornkitti S, Kangsdal P, Sathirapat P, et al: Reversion and reconversion rate of tuberculin skin reactions in correlation with the use of prednisone. Dis Chest 38:51-55, 1960
6. Balow JE, Rosenthal AS: Glucocorticoid suppression of macrophage migration inhibitory factor. J Exp Med 137:1031-1041, 1973
7. Shoenfeld Y, Gurewich Y, Gallant LA, et al: Prednisone-induced leukocytosis. Am J Med 71:773-778, 1981
8. Casey FB, Ciosek CP: Lipid mediators: An overview. Adv in Inf Res 7:13-15, 1984
9. Lewis RA: Leukotrienes and other lipid mediators of asthma. Chest 87:5S-10S, 1985
10. Spector SL: The use of corticosteroids in the treatment of asthma. Chest 87:73S-79S, 1985
11. Blackwell GJ, Carnuccio R, DiRosa M, et al: Macrocortin: A polypeptide causing the anti-phospholipase effect of glucocorticoids. Nature 287:147-149, 1980
12. Hirada F: Roles of lipomodulin: A phospholipase inhibitory protein in immunoregulation. Adv in Inflamm Res 7:71-77, 1984
13. Holgate ST, Baldwin CJ, Tattersfield AE: Beta-adrenergic agonist resistance in normal human airways. Lancet 2:375-377, 1977
14. Cutroneo KR, Rokowski R, Counts DF: Glucocorticoids and collagen synthesis: Comparison of *in vivo* and cell culture studies. Collagen Rel Res 1:557-568, 1981
15. Cole RB: Drug treatment of respiratory diseases. New York, Churchill-Livingstone, Inc., 1981, pp 220-252
16. Melby JC: Systemic corticosteroid therapy: Pharmacology and endocrinologic considerations. Ann Intern Med 81:505-512, 1974
17. Myles AB, Daly JR: Corticosteroids and ACTH Treatments. London, Edward Arnold, LTD, 1974, pp 183-204
18. Powell LW, Axelsen Z: Corticosteroids in liver disease: Studies on the biological conversion of prednisone to prednisolone and plasma protein binding. Gut 13:690-696, 1972
19. Harter JG: Corticosteroids: Their physiologic use in allergic disease. NY State J Med 66:827-834, 1966
20. Nugent CA, Ward J, MacDiarmid WD, et al: Glucocorticoid toxicity: Single contrasted with divided daily doses of prednisolone. J Chron Dis 18:323-332, 1965
21. Rabhan NB: Pituitary-adrenal suppression and Cushing's Syndrome after intermittent dexamethasone therapy. Ann Intern Med 69:1141-1148, 1968

22. Tse CST, Bernstein IL: Corticosteroid aerosols in the treatment of asthma. Pharmacotherapy 4:334–342, 1984
23. Williams MH: Beclomethasone dipropionate. Ann Intern Med 95:464–467, 1981
24. Shim C, Stover DE, Williams MH, Jr: Response to corticosteroids in chronic bronchitis. J Allergy Clin Immunol 62:363–367, 1978
25. Byyny RL: Withdrawal from glucocorticoid therapy. N Engl J Med 295:30–32, 1976
26. Christy NP: Corticosteroid withdrawal. In Bayless TM, Brian MC, Cherniack RM (eds): Current Therapy in Internal Medicine 1984–1985. Philadelphia, B.C. Decker Inc., 1984, pp 535–545
27. Christy NP: Principles of systemic corticosteroid therapy in nonendocrine disease, in Bayless TM, Brain MC, Cherniack RM (eds): Current Therapy in Internal Medicine 1984–1985. Philadelphia, B.C. Decker Inc., 1984, pp 524–535
28. Morris HG: Pharmacology of corticosteroids in asthma, in Middleton E, Jr, Ellis EF (eds) Allergy: Principles and Practice. St. Louis, C.V. Mosby Co, St. Louis, 1983, pp 593–611
29. Barach AL, Bickerman HA, Beck GJ: Clinical and physiological studies on the use of metacortandracin in respiratory disease. Dis Chest 27:515–527, 1955
30. Controlled trial of effects of cortisone acetate in status asthmaticus: Report to the Medical Research Council. Lancet 2:803–806, 1956
31. Hench PS, Kendall EC, Slocumb CH, et al: The effect of a hormone of the adrenal cortex and of pituitary adrenocorticotropic hormone on rheumatoid arthritis. Proc Staff Meetings Mayo Clinic 24:181–197, 1949
32. Ricketti AJ, Greenberger PA, Mintzer RA, et al: Allergic bronchopulmonary aspergillosis. Arch Intern Med 143:1553–1557, 1983
33. Basich JE, Gravis TS, Baz MN, et al: Allergic bronchopulmonary aspergillosis in corticosteroid-dependent asthmatics. J Allergy Clin Immunol 68:98–102, 1981
34. Safirstein BH, D'Souza MF, Simon G, et al: Five year follow-up of allergic bronchopulmonary aspergillosis. Am Rev Respir Dis 108:450–459, 1973
35. Wang JLF, Patterson R, Roberts M, et al: The management of allergic bronchopulmonary aspergillosis. Am Rev Respir Dis 120:87–92, 1979
36. Sahn SA: Corticosteroids in chronic bronchitis and pulmonary emphysema. Chest 73:389–396, 1978
37. Stokes TC, Shaylor JM, O'Reilly JF, et al: Assessment of steroid responsiveness in patients with chronic airflow obstruction. Lancet 2:345–348, 1982
38. Rudd R: Corticosteroids in chronic bronchitis. Br Med J 1:1553–1554, 1984
39. Harding SM, Freedman S: A comparison of oral and inhaled steroids in patients with chronic airways obstruction: Features determining response. Thorax 33:214–218, 1978
40. Blair GP, Light RW: Treatment of chronic obstructive pulmonary disease with corticosteroids: Comparison of daily vs alternate-day therapy. Chest 86:524–528, 1984
41. Mendella LA, Manfreda J, Warren CPW, et al: Steroid response in stable chronic obstructive pulmonary disease. Ann Intern Med 96:17–21, 1982
42. Albert RK, Martin TR, Lewis SW: Controlled clinical trial of methylprednisolone in patients with chronic bronchitis and acute respiratory insufficiency. Ann Intern Med 92:753–758, 1980

43. Meltzer EO: The current outlook on chronic allergic rhinitis. J Respir Dis 6:100-123, 1985
44. Applebaum ML, Hunninghake GW: Collagen-vascular lung disorders. In Cherniack RM (ed) Current Therapy of Respiratory Disease 1984-1985, Philadelphia, BC Decker, Inc., 1984 pp 187-192
45. Schwarz MI, King TE Jr: Lung involvement in the collagen vascular diseases. In Mitchell RS, Petty TL (eds), Synopsis of Clinical Pulmonary Disease. St. Louis, CV Mosby Co., 1982, pp 296-306
46. Yount WJ, Utsinger PD, Puritz EM, et al: Corticosteroid therapy of the collagen vascular disorders. Med Clinic of North Am 57:1343-1355, 1973
47. Decker JL, Steinberg AD, Reinersten JL, et al: Systemic lupus erythematosus: evolving concepts. Ann Intern Med 91:587-604, 1979
48. Wasner CK, Fried JF: Treatment decisions in systemic lupus erythematosus. Arthrit Rheumat 23:283-286, 1980
49. Fauci AS: Corticosteroids in autoimmune disease. Hosp Pract 18:99-114, 1983
50. Carette S, Klippel JH, Decker JL, et al: Controlled studies of oral immunosuppressive drugs in lupus nephritis. A long-term follow-up. Ann Intern Med 99:1-8, 1983
51. Rossi GA, Bitterman PB, Rennard SI, et al: Evidence for chronic inflammation as a component of the interstitial lung disease associated with progressive systemic sclerosis. Am Rev Respir Dis 131:612-617, 1985
52. Metzer AL, Bohan A, Goldberg LS, et al: Polymyositis and dermatomyositis: Combined methotrexate and corticosteroid therapy. Ann Intern Med 81:182-189, 1979
53. Bohan A, Peter JB, Bowman RL, et al: A computer-assisted analysis of 153 patients with polymyositis and dermatomyositis. Medicine 56:255-286, 1977
54. Salmeron G, Greenberg SD, Lidsky MD: Polymyositis and diffuse interstitial lung disease. A review of the pulmonary histopathologic findings. Arch Intern Med 141:1005-1010, 1981
55. Songcharoen S, Raju SF, Pennebaker JB: Interstitial lung disease in polymyositis and dermatomyositis. J Rheumatol 7:353-360, 1980
56. Fauci AS, Haynes BF, Katz P, et al: Wegener's granulomatosis: Prospective clinical and therapeutic experience with 85 patients for 21 years. Ann Intern Med 98:76-85, 1983
57. Fauci AS, Wolff SM: Wegener's granulomatosis: Studies in eighteen patients and a review of the literature. Medicine 52:535-558, 1973
58. Israel HL, Patchefsky AS, Saldona MJ: Wegener's granulomatosis, lymphomatoid granulomatosis and benign lymphocytic angiitis and granulomatosis of lung. Recognition and treatment. Ann Intern Med 87:691-699, 1977
59. Harrison HL, Linshaw MA, Lindsley CB, et al: Bolus corticosteroids and cyclophosphamide for initial treatment of Wegener's granulomatosis. JAMA 244:1599-1600, 1980
60. Dee PM, Arora NS, Innes DJ, Jr: The pulmonary manifestations of lymphomatoid granulomatosis. Radiology 143:613-618, 1982
61. Sordillo PP, Epremian B, Koziner B, et al: Lymphomatoid granulomatosis. An analysis of clinical and immunologic characteristics. Cancer 49:2070-2076, 1982
62. Fauci AS, Haynes BF, Costa J, et al: Lymphomatoid granulomatosis. Prospective clinical and therapeutic experience over 10 years. N Engl J Med 306:68-74, 1982

63. Koss MN, Robinson RG, Hochholzer L: Bronchocentric granulomatosis. Human Path 12:632–638, 1981
64. Clee MD, Lamb D, Clark RA: Bronchocentric granulomatosis: A review and thoughts on pathogenesis. Br J Dis Chest 77:227–234, 1983
65. Katzenstein AL, Liebon AA, Friedman PJ: State of the art: bronchocentric granulomatosis, mucoid impaction, and hypersensitivity reactions to fungi. Am Rev Respir Dis 11:497–548, 1975
66. Robinson RG, Wehunt WD, Tsou E, et al: Bronchocentric granulomatosis: roentgenographic manifestations. Am Rev Respir Dis 125:751–756, 1982
67. Mankare S: Influence of corticosteroid treatment on the course of farmer's lung. Eur J Respir Dis 64:283–293, 1983
68. Reynolds HY: Hypersensitivity pneumonitis. Clinics in Chest Med 3:503–519, 1982
69. Schlueter DP: Infiltrative lung disease hypersensitivity pneumonitis. J Allergy Clin Immunol 70:50–55, 1982
70. Stankus RP, Salvaggio JE: Hypersensitivity pneumonitis. Clinics in Chest Med 4:55–62, 1983
71. Leitch AG: Pulmonary eosinophilia. Basic of RD 7:1–6, 1979
72. Reich JM, Johnson RE: Course and prognosis of sarcoidosis in a nonreferral setting. Analysis of 86 patients observed for 10 years. Am J Med 78:61–67, 1985
73. DeRemee RA: The present status of treatment of pulmonary sarcoidosis: A house divided. Chest 71:388–393, 1977
74. Harkleroad LE, Young RL, Savage PJ, et al: Pulmonary sarcoidosis. Long-term follow-up of the effects of steroid therapy. Chest 82:84–87, 1982
75. Crystal RG, Bitterman PB, Rennard SI, et al: Interstitial lung disease of unknown cause. N Engl J Med 310:154–166, 235–244, 1984
76. Schwarz MI, King TE Jr: Idiopathic pulmonary fibrosis, in Cherniack RM (ed) Current Therapy of Respiratory Disease 1984–1985. Philadelphia, B.C. Decker, Inc., 1984 pp 178–182
77. Turner-Warwick M: Approaches to therapy. Semin in Respir Med 6:92–102, 1984
78. Friedman PJ, Liebow AA, Sokoloff J: Eosinophilic granuloma of lung: Clinical aspects of primary pulmonary histiocytosis in the adult. Medicine 60:385–396, 1981
79. Basset F, Corrin B, Spencer H, et al: Pulmonary histiocytosis X. Am Rev Respir Dis 118:811–820, 1978
80. Hawley PC, Whitcomb ME: Bronchiolitis fibrosa obliterans in adults. Arch Intern Med 141:1324–1327, 1981
81. Seggev JS, Mason UG, III, Worthen S, et al: Bronchiolitis obliterans. Report of three cases with detailed physiologic studies. Chest 83:169–174, 1983
82. Epler GR, Colby TV: The spectrum of bronchiolitis obliterans. Chest 83:161–162, 1983
83. Davison AG, Heard BE, McAllister WAC, et al: Cryptogenic organizing pneumonitis. Q J Med 52:382–394, 1983
84. Epler GR, Colby TV, McLoud TC, et al: Bronchiolitis obliterans organizing pneumonia. N Engl J Med 312:152–158, 1985
85. Petty TL, Fowler AA 3d: Another look at ARDS. Chest 82:98–104, 1982
86. Nicholson DP: Glucocorticoids in the treatment of shock and the adult respiratory distress syndrome. Clin Chest Med 67:121–131, 1982

87. Brigham KL, Bowers RE, McKeen CR: Methylprednisolone prevention of increased lung vascular permeability following endotoxemia in sheep. J Clin Invest 67:1103–1110, 1981
88. Shumer W: Steroids in the treatment of clinical septic shock. Ann Surg 184:333–341, 1976
89. Sibbald WJ, Anderson RR, Reid B, et al: Alveolo-capillary permeability in human septic ARDS. Chest 79:133–141, 1981
90. Sprung CL, Caralis PV, Marcial EH, et al: The effect of high-dose corticosteroids in patients with septic shock: A prospective, controlled study. N Engl J Med 311:1137–1143, 1984
91. Bynum LJ, Pierce AK: Pulmonary aspiration of gastric contents. Am Rev Respir Dis 114:1129–1136, 1976
92. Wynne JW, Modell JH: Respiratory aspiration of stomach contents. Ann Intern Med 87:466–474, 1977
93. Wolfe JE, Bone RC, Ruth WE: Effects of corticosteroids in the treatment of patients with gastric aspiration. Am J Med 63:719–722, 1977
94. Moylan JA, Evenson MA: Diagnosis and treatment of fat embolism. Ann Rev Med 28:85–90, 1977
95. Ashbaugh DG, Petty TL: The use of corticosteroids in the treatment of respiratory failure associated with massive fat embolism. Surg Gynecol Obstet 123:493–500, 1966
96. Alho A, Saikku K, Eerola P, et al: Corticosteroids in patients with a high risk of fat embolism syndrome. Surg Gynecol Obstet 147:358–361, 1978
97. Schonfeld SA, Ploysongsang Y, DiLisio R, et al: Fat embolism prophylaxis with corticosteroids. Ann Int Med 99:438–443, 1983
98. Murray HW, Tauzon CU, Kirmani N, et al: The adult respiratory distress syndrome associated with miliary tuberculosis. Chest 73:37–43, 1978
99. Meyers BR: Tuberculous meningitis. Med Clin North Am 66:755–762, 1982
100. Hockaday JM, Smith HMV: Corticosteroids as an adjuvant to the chemotherapy of tuberculous meningitis. Tubercle 47:75–91, 1966
101. O'Toole RD, Thornton GF, Mukherjee MK, et al: Dexamethasone in tuberculous meningitis. Ann Intern Med 70:39–48, 1969
102. Rooney JJ, Crocco JA, Lyons HA: Tuberculous pericarditis. Ann Intern Med 72:73–78, 1970
103. Singh MM, Bhargava AN, Jain KP: Tuberculous peritonitis. N Engl J Med 281:1091–1094, 1969
104. Borhanmanesh F, Hekmat K, Vaezzadeh K, et al: Tuberculous peritonitis. Ann Intern Med 76:567–572, 1972
105. Lakshminarayan S: Inhalation injury of the lungs, in Sahn SA (ed): Pulmonary emergencies. New York, Churchill Livingstone, 1982, pp 375–386
106. Horvath EP, doPico GA, Barbee RA, et al: Nitrogen dioxide-induced pulmonary disease. J Occup Med 20:103–109, 1978
107. Gross NJ: Pulmonary effects of radiation therapy. Ann Intern Med 86:81–92, 1977
108. The Boston Collaborative Drug Surveillance Program: Acute adverse reactions to prednisone in relation to dosage. Clinical Pharmaco and Therapeutics 13:694–698, 1972

109. David DS, Grieco MH, Cushman P Jr: Adrenal glucocorticoids after twenty years. A review of their clinically relevant consequences. J Chron Dis 22:637-711, 1970
110. Askari A, Vignos PJ, Jr, Moskowitz RW: Steroid myopathy in connective tissue disease. Am J Med 61:485-492, 1976
111. Mandel S: Steroid myopathy. Postgrad Med 72:207-215, 1982
112. Khaleeli AA, Edwards RHT, Gohil K, et al: Corticosteroid myopathy: A clinical and pathological study. Clinical Endocrinology 18:155-166, 1983
113. Guyatt GH, Webber CE, Mewa AA, et al: Determining causation-A case study: Adrenocorticosteroids and osteoporosis. J Chron Dis 37:343-352, 1984
114. Baylink DJ: Glucocorticoid-induced osteoporosis. N Engl J Med 309:306-308, 1983
115. Adinoff AD, Hollister JR: Steroid-induced fractures and bone loss in patients with asthma. N Engl J Med 309:265-268, 1983
116. Smith DM, Johnston CC Jr, Yu PL: *In vivo* measurement of bone mass: Its use in demineralized states such as osteoporosis. JAMA 219:325-329, 1972
117. Heimann WG, Freiberger RH: Avascular necrosis of the femoral and humeral heads after high-dosage corticosteroid therapy. N Engl J Med 263:672-675, 1960
118. Williams PL, Corbett M: Avascular necrosis of bone complicating corticosteroid replacement therapy. Annals of the Rheumatic Diseases 42:276-279, 1983
119. Madell SH, Freeman LM: Avascular necrosis of bone in Cushing's syndrome. Radiology 83:1068-1077, 1964
120. Richards JM, Santiago SM, Klaustermeyer WB: Aseptic necrosis of the femoral head in corticosteroid-treated pulmonary disease. Arch Intern Med 140:1473-1475, 1980
121. Smyllie HC, Connolly CK: Incidence of serious complications of corticosteroid therapy in respiratory disease. Thorax 23:571-581, 1968
122. Fisher DE: The role of fat embolism in the etiology of corticosteroid-induced avascular necrosis: Clinical and experimental results. Clin Orthop 130:68-80, 1978
123. Lubkin VL: Steroid cataract-a review and conclusion. J Asthma Res 14:55-59, 1977
124. David DS, Berkowitz JS: Ocular effects of topical and systemic corticosteroids. Lancet 2:149-151, 1969
125. Crews SJ: Adverse reactions to corticosteroid therapy in the eye. Proc Roy Soc Med 58:533-535, 1965
126. Cordess C, Folstein M, Drachman D: Psychiatric effects of alternate-day steroid therapy. Brit J Psychiat 138:504-506, 1981
127. Glaser GH: Psychotic reactions induced by corticotrophin (ACTH) and cortisone. Psychosmat Med 15:280-291, 1953
128. Editorial: Intracranial hypertension and steroids. Lancet 2:1052-1053, 1964
129. Greer M: Benign intracranial hypertension. II. Following corticosteroid therapy. Neurology 13:439-441, 1963
130. Vyas CK, Talwar KK, Bhatnagar V, et al: Steroid-induced benign intracranial hypertension. Postgrad Med J 57:181-182, 1981
131. Walker AE, Adamkiewicz JJ: Pseudotumor cerebri associated with prolonged corticosteroid therapy. JAMA 188:779-784, 1964

132. Ahlskog JE, O'Neill BP: Pseudotumor cerebri. Ann Intern Med 97:249-256, 1982
133. Beisel WR, Rapoport MI: Inter-relations between adrenocortical functions and infectious illness. N Engl J Med 280:541-546, 596-604, 1969
134. Grieco MH: The role of corticosteroid therapy in infection. Hosp Prac 19:131-135, 139-143, 1984
135. Editorial: Tuberculosis in corticosteroid-treated asthmatics. Brit Med J 2:266-267, 1976
136. Mayfield RB: Tuberculosis occurring in association with corticosteroid treatment. Tubercle (Lond) 43:55-60, 1962
137. Haanaes OC, Bergmann A: Tuberculosis emerging in patients treated with corticosteroids. Eur J Resp Dis 64:294-297, 1983
138. Gottlieb NL, Penneys NS: Spontaneous skin tearing during systemic corticosteroid treatment. JAMA 243:1260-1261, 1980
139. David DJ: Skin trauma in patients receiving systemic corticosteroid therapy. Brit Med J 2:614-161, 1972
140. Baylis C, Brenner BM: Mechanism of the glucocorticoid-induced increase in glomerular filtration rate. Am J Physiol 234:166-170, 1978
141. Hulter HN, Licht JH, Bonner EL Jr, et al: Effects of glucocorticoid steroids on renal and systemic acid-base metabolism. Am J Physiol 239:30-43, 1980
142. Charpin J, Arnaud A, Boutin C, et al: Long-term corticosteroid therapy and its effects on the kidney. Acta Allerg 24:49-56, 1969
143. Chang KC, Miklich DR, Barwise G, et al: Linear growth of chronic asthmatic children: The effects of the disease and various forms of steroid therapy. Clinical Allergy 12:369-378, 1982
144. Murray AB, Fraser BM, Hardwick DF, et al: Chronic asthma and growth failure in children. Lancet 2:197-198, 1976
145. Morris HA: Growth and skeletal maturation in asthmatic children: Effect of corticosteroid treatment. Pediatr Res 9:579-583, 1975
146. Reimer LG, Morris HG, Ellis EF: Growth of asthmatic children during treatment with alternate-day steroids. J Allergy Clin Immunol 55:224-231, 1975
147. Graff-Lonnevig V, Kraepelien S: Long-term treatment with beclomethasone dipropionate aerosol in asthmatic children, with special reference to growth. Allergy 34:57-61, 1979
148. Morris HG, Jorgensen JR, Elrick H, et al: Metabolic effects of human growth hormone in corticosteroid-treated children. J Clin Invest 47:436-451, 1968
149. Root AW, Bongiovanni AM, Eberlein WR: Studies of the secretion and metabolic effects of human growth hormone in children with glucocorticoid-induced growth retardation. J Pediatr 75:826-832, 1969
150. Blodgett FM, Burgin L, Iezzoni D, et al: Effects of prolonged cortisone therapy on the statural growth, skeletal maturation and metabolic status of children. N Engl J Med 254:636-641, 1956
151. Loeb JN: Corticosteroids and growth. N Engl J Med 295:547-552, 1976
152. Prader A: Catch-up growth. Postgrad Med J 54:S133-146, 1978
153. Miller SEP, Neilson J McE: Clinical features of the diabetic syndrome appearing after steroid therapy. Postgrad Med J 40:660-669, 1964
154. Lohr KM: Precipitation of hyperosmolar nonketotic diabetes on alternate-day corticosteroid therapy (letter). JAMA 252:A628, 1984

155. Perlman K, Ehrlich RM: Steroid diabetes in childhood. Am J Dis Child 136:64-68, 1982
156. McCarty MF: "Nutritional insurance" supplementation and corticosteroid toxicity. Medical Hypotheses 9:145-156, 1982
157. Reinisch JM, Simon NG, Karow WG, et al: Prenatal exposure to prednisone in humans and animals retards intrauterine growth. Science 202:436-438, 1978
158. Worrell DW, Taylor R: Outcome for the fetus of mothers receiving prednisolone during pregnancy. Lancet 1:117-118, 1968
159. Schatz M, Patterson R, Zeitz S, et al: Corticosteroid therapy for the pregnant asthmatic patient. JAMA 233:804-807, 1975
160. Ballard RA, Ballard PL, Granberg JP, et al: Prenatal administration of betamethasone for prevention of respiratory distress syndrome. J Pediatr 94:97-101, 1979
161. Papageorgiou AN, Desgranges MF, Masson M, et al: The antenatal use of betamethasone in the prevention of respiratory distress syndrome: A controlled double-blind study. Pediatrics 63:73-79, 1979
162. Toogood JH, Jennings B, Greenway RW, Chuang L: Candidiasis and dysphonia complicating beclomethasone treatment of asthma. J Allergy Clin Immunol 65:145-153, 1980
163. Toogood JH, Baskerville J, Jennings B, et al: Use of spacers to facilitate inhaled corticosteroid treatment of asthma. Am Rev Respir Dis 129:723-729, 1984
164. Christy NP, Wallace EZ, Jailer JW: Comparative effects of prednisone and of cortisone in suppressing the response of the adrenal cortex to exogenous adrenal corticotropin. J Clin Endocrinol Metab 16:1059-1073, 1956
165. Danowski TS, Bonessi JV, Sabeh G, et al: Probabilities of pituitary-adrenal responsiveness after steroid therapy. Ann Intern Med 61:11-26, 1964
166. Livanou T, Ferriman D, James VHT: Recovery of hypothalamo-pituitary-adrenal function after corticosteroid therapy. Lancet 2:856-859, 1967
167. Kehlet H, Blichert-Toft M, Lindholm J, et al: Short ACTH test in assessing hypothalamic-pituitary-adrenocortical function. Br Med J 1:249-251, 1976
168. Kehlet H, Binder C: Value of an ACTH test in assessing hypothalamic-pituitary-adrenocortical function in glucocorticoid-treated patients. Br Med J 2:147-149, 1973
169. Amatruda TT, Hurst MM, D'Esopu ND: Certain endocrine and metabolic facets of the steroid withdrawal syndrome. J Clin Endocrinol Metab 25:1207-1217, 1965
170. Amatruda TT Jr., Hollingsworth DR, E'Esopu ND, et al: A study of the mechanism of the steroid withdrawal syndrome. Evidence for integrity of the hypothalamic-pituitary-adrenal system. J Clin Endocrinol Metab 20:339-354, 1960
171. Morgan HC, Boulnois J, Burns-Cox C: Addiction to prednisone. Brit Med J 2:93-94, 1973
172. Jubiz W, Meikle AW: Alterations of glucocorticoid actions by other drugs and disease states. Drugs 18:113-121, 1979
173. Brenner M: Macrolide antibiotics, in Bukstein DA, Strunk RC (eds): Manual of Clinical Problems in Asthma Allergy and Related Disorders. Boston, Little, Brown and Co., 1984, pp 177-187
174. Itkin IH, Menzel ML: The use of macrolide antibiotic substances in the treatment of asthma. J Allergy 45:146-162, 1970

175. Spector SL, Katz FH, Farr RS: Troleandomycin: Effectiveness in steroid-dependent asthma and bronchitis. J Allergy Clin Immunol 54:367-379, 1974
176. Zeiger RS, Schatz M, Sperling W, et al: Efficacy of troleandomycin in outpatients with severe, corticosteroid-dependent asthma. J Allergy Clin Immunol 66:438-446, 1980
177. LaForce CF, Miller MF, Chai H: Effect of erythromycin on theophylline clearance in asthmatic children. J Pediatrics 99:153-156, 1981
178. Weinberger M, Hudgel D, Spector S, et al: Inhibition of theophylline clearance by troleandomycin. J Allergy Clin Immunol 59:228-231, 1977
179. LaForce CF, Szefler SJ, Miller MF, et al: Inhibition of methylprednisolone elimination in the presence of erythromycin therapy. J Allergy Clin Immunol 72:34-39, 1983
180. Szefler SJ, Ellis EF, Brenner M, et al: Steroid-specific and anticonvulsant interaction aspects of troleandomycin-steroid therapy. J Allergy Clin Immunol 69:455-462, 1982
181. Szefler SJ, Rose JQ, Ellis EF, et al: The effect of troleandomycin on methylprednisolone elimination. J Allergy Clin Immunol 66:447-451, 1980
182. Ticktin HE, Zimmerman HJ: Hepatic dysfunction and jaundice in patients receiving triacetyloleandomycin. N Engl J Med 267:964-968, 1962
183. Edwards OMK, Courtenay-Evans RJ, Galley JM, et al: Changes in cortisol metabolism following rifampin therapy. Lancet 2:549-551, 1974
184. Petereit LB, Meikle AW: Effectiveness of prednisolone during phenytoin therapy. Clin Pharmacol Ther 22:912-916, 1977
185. Brooks SM, Werk EE Jr, Ackerman SJ, et al: Adverse effect of phenobarbital on corticosteroid metabolism in patients with bronchial asthma. N Eng J Med 286:1125-1128, 1972
186. Brooks SM, Sholiton LJ, Werk EE Jr, et al: The effects of ephedrine and theophylline on dexamethasone metabolism in bronchial asthma. J Clin Pharm 17:308-318, 1977
187. Leavengood DC, Bunker-Soler AL, Nelson HS: The effect of corticosteroids on theophylline metabolism. Ann Allergy 50:249-251, 1983

Leslie C. Watters

6

Cytotoxic Drugs For Nonneoplastic Disorders of the Respiratory System

"For extreme illnesses, extreme treatments are most fitting"
Hippocrates; Aphorisms I,6.

Cytotoxic therapy has been used with gradually increasing frequency over the last 15 years for nonneoplastic disorders affecting the respiratory system. The use of cytotoxic drugs (including cyclophosphamide, azathioprine, and chlorambucil), however, is relatively uncommon in the day-to-day practice of pulmonary medicine, especially when compared to such classes of drugs as theophyllines or corticosteroids. The disorders for which cytotoxic therapy is useful are generally chronic, progressively disabling processes, often characterized by a disordering of immunoregulatory mechanisms. Despite the progressive, potentially fatal natural history of many of these disorders, there has been a justifiable reluctance among chest physicians to initiate cytotoxic therapy, because of the multiple, serious (and sometimes fatal) potential side effects. For most of the entities listed in Table 6-1 (with the notable exceptions of Wegener's granulomatosis, lymphomatoid granulomatosis, and Goodpasture's syndrome), cytotoxic agents serve as second-line drugs, used only after the failure of corticosteroids, and/or after the induction of intolerable toxic side effects by corticosteroid therapy. With a few exceptions, the use of cytotoxic drugs for nonneoplastic respiratory ailments has not been prospectively evaluated. Thus, because of the anecdotal nature of many of the reports, firm recommendations of the most efficacious cytotoxic drug for a given illness cannot be made.

Because of their more common usage, cyclophosphamide and azathioprine

DRUGS FOR THE RESPIRATORY SYSTEM
ISBN 0-8089-1818-4

Copyright © 1986 by Grune & Stratton, Inc.
All rights of reproduction in any form reserved.

Table 6-1
Diseases Affecting the Respiratory Tract for
Which Cytotoxic Drugs Have Been Used

A. Vasculitides
   1. Wegener's granulomatosis
   2. Lymphomatoid granulomatosis
   3. Churg-Strauss syndrome
   4. Benign lymphocytic angiitis and granulomatosis
   5. Behcet's syndrome
   6. Polyarteritis nodosa
   7. Rheumatoid pulmonary arteritis
B. Interstitial Lung Diseases
   1. Idiopathic pulmonary fibrosis
   2. Lymphocytic interstitial pneumonitis
   3. Plasma cell interstitial pneumonitis
   4. Connective tissue diseases
      a. rheumatoid disease
      b. systemic lupus erythematosus
      c. polymyositis/dermatomyositis
      d. progressive systemic sclerosis
      e. mixed connective tissue disease
   5. Sarcoidosis
C. Diffuse Alveolar Disease
   1. Goodpasture's syndrome
   2. Idiopathic pulmonary hemosiderosis
D. Neurological Disease
   1. Myasthenia gravis
   2. Multiple sclerosis
E. Miscellaneous
   1. Angio-immunoblastic lymphadenopathy
   2. Relapsing polychondritis (tracheal collapse)
   3. Asthma

will be emphasized, with a briefer description of the less-frequently employed drug, chlorambucil. The use of these cytotoxic agents for the therapy of neoplastic disease of the thorax is beyond the scope of this chapter.

MECHANISM OF ACTION

Cyclophosphamide

Cyclophosphamide (CYT) is a nitrogen mustard alkylating agent that interferes with DNA replication and with the transcription of RNA.[1] Its effects are cell cycle nonspecific, (i.e., it reacts with DNA during any phase of the cell cycle.[2]) The theoretical benefit of CYT in immunologically-mediated pulmonary disease is exerted via a reduction in the number and activity of immune effector cells in the target organ by suppressing the production of such cells in the bone marrow and by suppressing their function in the peripheral blood and tissues.

CYT causes neutropenia via marrow depression, an effect that may be important in the therapy of some processes dependent upon the neutrophil in their pathogenesis. More work has been done in investigation of the effect of CYT on lymphocyte number and function. The number of T and B cells are reduced in response to CYT therapy for Wegener's granulomatosis.[3,4] A decreased antibody response to a number of antigens was shown to be due to depletion of B cells from lymphoid follicles.[5] In addition to a depletion effect, CYT also suppresses the differentiation of B cells in murine lupus.[6] Although CYT-induced suppression of humoral immunity is dose-dependent, it is not directly related to the peripheral leukocyte count.[7] CYT appears to be a more potent inhibitor of antibody synthesis than either azathioprine or chlorambucil.[8]

CYT may have varying effects on T-lymphocyte populations, depending on the disease entity and the dose of the drug. The usual effect of chronic CYT therapy is an inhibition of delayed hypersensitivity.[7] It has, however, also been shown to actually potentiate delayed hypersensitivity reactions to some antigens by decreasing the modulating effect of T-suppressor cells.[5] In addition, CYT may activate or potentiate natural killer T-lymphocyte function.[9] The effect of CYT on both humoral and cell-mediated immunity is likely dependent on dose and individualized host-response. For example, augmentation of both cell-mediated and humoral immunity was shown in a small group of patients with advanced cancer after administration of one relatively low-dose of CYT,[10] presumably via ablation of the modulatory effect of T-suppressor cells. One might speculate as to the possibility that such an augmentation of immune responses might play a role in the development of CYT-induced interstitial lung disease, which usually occurs in patients with an underlying lymphoproliferative process.

CYT is well-absorbed when given orally. There is negligible binding to plasma proteins.[11] It is distributed throughout the body, including transplacentally and into breast milk. CYT, in its original form is converted to its active metabolites in the liver, and both CYT and these active metabolites are excreted into the urine.[1] Because enzymes in the hepatic pathway for CYT are inducible and shared by other drugs, the plasma half-life (and thus the degree of effect) of CYT may be altered by other drugs (see Drug Interactions).[7] Seven to 14 days are usually required for daily oral CYT to exert any clinically-relevant effect. Although rate of metabolism and toxicity of CYT relate better to body surface area than to weight, the doses are traditionally calculated per Kg body weight.[7]

Azathioprine

Azathioprine (AZA) is a purine analog, used chiefly as an immunosuppressive agent (unlike CYT, which is chiefly used as an anti-neoplastic drug). The exact mechanisms of AZA-induced immunosuppression are incompletely understood, but it is clear that there is a consistent reduction in T-lymphocyte function, accompanied by variable changes in antibody production.[1] AZA reduces the number of monocytes available for migration into sites of inflammation by reducing marrow promonocytes, leading to a reduction in peripheral blood monocytes, and ultimately a decrease in tissue macrophages.[12] AZA therapy also results in a reduction in circulating granulocytes. Although the subcellular mechanisms of these effects are unknown, there are several possibilities,[1] the most likely of which is that AZA arrests the cell cycle of promonocytes late in the DNA synthesis phase or in the post-synthesis (G_2) phase, and mitosis does not occur.[12] When given in lower concentrations, AZA may result in enhancement of immunoglobulin synthesis due to selective inactivation of suppressor T-cells. Higher drug concentrations lead to suppression of helper T-cell function, as well as suppression of B cell differentiation.[13]

AZA is well-absorbed enterally, and is metabolized to 6-mercaptopurine. It is dialyzable even though it is approximately 30 percent bound to plasma proteins. AZA and its metabolites are excreted in the urine.[1] The interval between institution of daily oral AZA and any clinical evidence of therapeutic response is usually two to four weeks.[12]

Chlorambucil

Chlorambucil (CHL), like cyclophosphamide, is a nitrogen mustard alkylating agent. It interferes with DNA replication and transcription of RNA, resulting in disruption of nucleic acid function. CHL is the slowest-acting and least toxic of the nitrogen mustard derivatives.[1] It is well-absorbed from the gastrointestinal tract, bound to plasma and tissue proteins and distributed throughout the body. It is metabolized in the liver to active metabolites, which are excreted in the urine.[1]

The mechanism by which CHL exerts its therapeutic effect in granulomatous diseases such as sarcoidosis is unknown. Speculation has centered on a chlorambucil-induced reduction in mononuclear cells available for granuloma formation via a decrease in marrow production of monocytes and also via a decrease in lymphocyte-derived monocyte chemotactic factor.

INDICATIONS AND DOSAGES

Vasculitides

Wegener's Granulomatosis

This disorder is characterized by a granulomatous vasculitis of the upper and lower respiratory tracts with or without glomerulonephritis and disseminated vasculitis of small systemic arteries and veins.[14] Before corticosteroid and chemotherapeutic modalities became available, patients almost invariably died within months of diagnosis, usually from renal failure, respiratory failure, or superimposed infection. Wegener's is the entity for which CYT has achieved its most favorable therapeutic response. There has been some controversy about total acceptance of the most common treatment regimen, CYT plus prednisone, because no randomized trials comparing this regimen to other potentially less toxic regimens have been carried out.[15] Most investigators, however, have been reluctant to embark upon such a trial because mortality rates have so markedly improved compared to pre-CYT therapy rates.[16,17] In addition, while there have not been randomized, prospective trials, data have been reported that suggest that CYT may exert a more beneficial effect than AZA in the initial therapy of Wegener's. In one report, 10 of 11 patients with Wegener's, initially begun on AZA, had progressive organ dysfunction on therapy. All 10 of these patients enjoyed a complete remission when switched to CYT.[17] A single case was reported in which a patient with Wegener's underwent a successful kidney transplant, and was maintained on chronic AZA therapy. After four years, the manifestations of Wegener's recurred with the patient still on AZA. When CYT was substituted for AZA, a complete remission was induced.[18]

A complete remission rate of 93 percent has been reported in patients treated at the National Institute of Health with a treatment regimen consisting of prednisone and CYT.[17] (A complete remission is well-defined and consists of the following: (1) pulmonary infiltrates must be cleared or only be manifest by stable residual scarring; (2) renal function must be stable/improved with no active renal sediment; (3) systemic inflammatory disease, as manifest by serositis and fever, must resolve; (4) erythrocyte sedimentation rate must be normal, or if slightly elevated, attributable to smoldering sinus infection). Such complete remissions had a mean duration of 48 months.[17] There was about a 30 percent rate of relapse after CYT was withdrawn (usually a year after achievement of complete remission). Fortunately, most of these patients achieved a second complete remission when retreated with prednisone and CYT.[17] Similarly high rates of complete remission have also been reported by other investigators in response to a similar regimen.[19] Improved patient survival has resulted in complications not previously seen; some of these late complications, such as sub-glottic stenosis, have responded to re-institution of CYT therapy.[20]

The NIH treatment regimen for Wegener's consists of CYT–2 mg/kg/day in one oral dose, plus prednisone–1 mg/kg/day for 2–4 weeks. This is followed by a reduction in prednisone to 60 mg orally every other day, with maintenance of the original CYT dose. The prednisone is gradually tapered to zero over a 6 to 12 month period.[17] If the course of the disease prior to diagnosis has been indolent, some authors recommend CYT alone (in the same dose) without corticosteroids.[21] If the course has been fulminant prior to diagnosis, the CYT dose may be started at 4–5 mg/kg/day, using the leukocyte count to adjust dosage. If the patient is so ill as to make oral administration difficult, CYT may be given intravenously. In fulminant disease, corticosteroid dose would also be higher initially, e.g. 2 mg/kg/day of prednisone, or an equivalent parenteral dose.[17]

CYT should be continued for 12 months after induction of a complete remission, and then tapered in 25 mg decrements every 2–3 months until completely withdrawn, or until the patient has a relapse involving a major organ system. An increase in sinus symptoms should not be considered as a "flare-up" sufficient to justify increasing or reinstituting CYT therapy because the most common cause of such an exacerbation in Wegener's patients is infection (especially *Staphlylococcus aureus*). Such exacerbations should be treated with drainage and antibiotics, not with an increase in CYT.[17] Persistent joint symptoms may respond to non-steroidal anti-inflammatory agents, not necessitating an increase in CYT. By avoiding the resumption of CYT for sinus or joint symptoms after the initial remission, some of CYT's potentially devastating side effects may be avoided.

The complete blood count (CBC) of patients on CYT should be checked every 2–3 days at the start of therapy, and then every 1–2 weeks. The total leukocyte count should not be allowed to drop below 3000–3500/mm^3 and the total neutrophil count should be at least 1000–1500/mm^3. Occasionally, patients may not respond to the standard regimen, and more intensive therapy may be required, in which case the leukocyte counts should be even more closely monitored. For example, a patient has been reported with severe necrotic purpuric skin lesions (with lung and kidney disease as well), who did not respond to the routine regimen, but who did respond to CYT-500 mg intravenously once a week plus 60 mg/day prednisone.[22]

Although most physicians treat Wegener's with corticosteroids and CYT, the disease has also responded to AZA therapy.[17,23-25] AZA is clearly the drug of choice in patients with Wegener's who have had a complete remission on CYT/prednisone therapy, but who later develop cystitis as a toxic side effect of CYT. When such patients have been switched from CYT to AZA, complete remission has been maintained in almost 90 percent.[17] The dose of AZA given for Wegener's is 2–3 mg/kg/day, usually 150–250 mg per day.

CHL was one of the earliest successful cytotoxic treatments for Wegener's granulomatosis,[26] although it has now been supplanted by either CYT/prednisone or AZA/prednisone. It was previously recommended as the initial therapy for Wegener's because of its relative lack of toxicity.[27] However, since CYT is more likely to induce a complete remission, it has become uncommon for CHL to be used for Wegener's.

Lymphomatoid Granulomatosis

This is an uncommon disorder characterized by infiltration of the lung and other organs (especially skin, kidney, CNS) with atypical lymphocytoid and plasmacytoid cells along with angiocentric, angio-invasive necrotizing granulomatous inflammation.[28,29] The diagnosis is usually made by open lung biopsy. The prognosis of lymphomatoid granulomatosis has been very poor, with a mortality rate of greater than 60 percent within two years of onset,[30] despite therapy. However, in one series, over half of the patients who received CYT achieved complete remission. Among the remainder, the mortality was high, death commonly being associated with a transformation from lymphomatoid granulomatosis to frank lymphoma.[31] Most of the patients who developed lymphoma and subsequently died had not had treatment for lymphomatoid granulomatosis for an "adequate" period of time, so that early recognition of this entity and treatment with CYT and prednisone may alter ultimate outcome. The dose of CYT for lymphomatoid granulomatosis is the same as that for Wegener's, with concomitant prednisone also recommended.[29,31,32]

Churg-Strauss Syndrome

The Churg-Strauss syndrome (allergic angiitis and granulomatosis) is a disorder characterized by systemic vasculitis, asthma, and eosinophilia.[33] The diagnosis may be made by biopsy of skin, kidney, or lung, showing necrotizing vasculitis, tissue inflammation with eosinophils, and extra-vascular granulomata,[34] although some authors feel the diagnosis may be made on clinical grounds.[33] Such a diagnosis might be made in a patient with a history of allergic rhinitis and asthma for several years, who develops blood/tissue eosinophilia, and later, systemic vasculitis involving at least two extra-pulmonary organs.

Although the majority of patients will respond to corticosteroids, some also require the addition of cytotoxic therapy, including CYT,[29,35] AZA,[36,37] and CHL.[38] One course of action would be to use CYT early in the severely ill patient who fails to respond to corticosteroids, and to use AZA for maintenance therapy in refractory disease.[33] Such a treatment plan is subjective, however, and based on no systematic data evaluating the effects of cytotoxic drugs in this disease. If CYT were used in a patient deteriorating despite corticosteroids, the dose would be the same as for Wegener's, (i.e., 2 mg/kg/day).

Benign Lymphocytic Angiitis and Granulomatosis

Benign lymphocytic angiitis and granulomatosis (BLAG) is a disease entity characterized by cellular infiltrates composed of lymphocytes, plasma cells and histiocytes, usually confined to the lungs (uncommonly involving skin). The patient may be asymptomatic (with abnormal routine chest x-rays showing multiple nodular infiltrates) or may present with cough and fever.

The prognosis is good with CHL therapy, although some patients later develop lymphomatoid granulomatosis, usually after several years.[30,39] In fact, some authorities regard BLAG as the favorable end of a spectrum that progresses through lymphomatoid granulomatosis to frank lymphoma. After CHL is begun, a response should be evident within a few weeks.

Behcet's Syndrome

This is a systemic vasculitis characterized by oral/genital ulcers, iritis, phlebitis, meningo-encephalitis, venous thrombo-embolism and, uncommonly, pulmonary vasculitis or pulmonary aneurysm.[40] Other associated (but uncommon) problems of interest are superior vena cava thrombosis, hemoptysis, and pulmonary infiltrates.[41]

The pulmonary abnormalities may respond to CYT, although the dosage schedule is not standardized. CHL has been shown to be effective therapy for the uveitis and meningo-encephalitis[42] of Behcet's, but has not been evaluated specifically for the pulmonary vascular abnormalities. The dose of CHL given for Behcet's is 0.1 mg/kg/day, given once daily.[42]

Polyarteritis Nodosa

There is controversy about whether or not there is a difference between polyarteritis nodosa involving the lung and the Churg-Strauss syndrome. In a report that differentiated between the two, a lack of peripheral blood eosinophils in polyarteritis seems to have been the differentiating point,[43] but for practical purposes, there is probably no utility in trying to differentiate polyarteritis nodosa with lung involvement from the Churg-Strauss syndrome.[40] Thus, the same guidelines for use of CYT in Churg-Strauss would apply to "polyarteritis nodosa of the lung."

Rheumatoid Pulmonary Vasculitis

Pulmonary arteritis may be a feature of rheumatoid arthritis, but it is uncommon and may not be associated with interstitial lung disease.[44] The patient may present only after chronic rheumatoid pulmonary vasculitis has led to pulmonary hypertension and cor pulmonale.[45] Because of the poor results with corticosteroid therapy, one might consider treatment with a cytotoxic agent such as CYT, but experience with CYT for this indication has been limited.

Interstitial Lung Diseases

Idiopathic Pulmonary Fibrosis (IPF)

Idiopathic pulmonary fibrosis (cryptogenic fibrosis alveolitis) is an interstitial lung disease of unknown etiology, characterized by both cellular infiltration (composed of lymphocytes, plasma cells, macrophages, eosinophils, and neutrophils) and fibrosis involving the alveolar walls, interstitium, and small airways, associated with proliferation of type II alveolar epithelial cells.

The treatment of choice is systemic corticosteroid therapy, but when patients deteriorate despite therapy, or when corticosteroids are contraindicated, CYT or AZA may be used.[46-51] Although data have not been reported on different dosages of CYT for IPF, the usual dose is the same as that for Wegener's, (i.e., 2 mg/kg/day orally.) Follow-up of leukocyte counts has been outlined previously. Although anecdotal reports have described a beneficial response to CYT when given as the initial therapeutic regimen, the results of randomized, prospective trials using CYT from the time of diagnosis have not been published. There has been no systematic evaluation of the relative efficacy of CYT and AZA in idiopathic pulmonary fibrosis (IPF). AZA was used in addition to prednisone in one study of IPF in a dose of 3 mg/kg/day.[52] Although all patients also received corticosteroids, the data suggest that further improvement may be obtained from the addition of AZA. Another study reported better results with AZA plus prednisolone than with prednisolone alone.[53] However, definition of the proper places of both AZA and CYT in the chronic therapy of IPF awaits the results of long-term, prospective, randomized trials.

Lymphocytic Interstitial Pneumonitis (LIP)

This is an entity characterized by interstitial cellular infiltration by lymphocytes, plasma cells, and immunoblasts. LIP may exist alone, but is often associated with other diseases, (e.g., Sjørgren's syndrome, systemic lupus, myasthenia gravis, pernicious anemia, and chronic active hepatitis).[54] The initial treatment of LIP is corticosteroids,[55] although the concomitant use of CYT has been reported, with a favorable outcome.[56]

Plasma Cell Interstitial Pneumonitis (PIP)

This entity is usually considered to be a variant of LIP, which is characterized by interstitial infiltration by plasma cells, as well as lymphocytes. Improvement has been reported in response to the combination of corticosteroids and CYT,[57] although the dosage was unclear.

Connective Tissue Disorders

Cytotoxic agents have also been used for interstitial lung disease (ILD) associated with connective tissue diseases, including rheumatoid disease, systemic lupus erythematosus, polymyositis/dermatomyositis, progressive systemic sclerosis, and mixed connective tissue disease. Such therapy is usually reserved for patients with progressive involvement, unresponsive to corticosteroid therapy.

Rheumatoid Disease

Cyclophosphamide has been used for rheumatoid arthritis, (RA)[7,58] although its effect on the interstitial lung disease of RA has not been evaluated. For example, the combination of CYT and methylprednisolone has been shown to be effective in treating a group of rheumatoid patients with systemic vasculitis.[59] Although 38 percent of these patients had pulmonary involvement, we do not know if the pulmonary manifestations improved with this regimen. It has been reported that treatment with AZA led to improvement in pulmonary function (despite further deterioration of joint disease) in a patient with rheumatoid interstitial lung disease.[60] When AZA is empirically given for rheumatoid arthritis, the dose varies from 1.0 mg/kg/day to 2.5 mg/kg/day, with an "adequate" therapeutic trial being at least 12 weeks.[1]

Systemic Lupus Erythematosis

Systemic lupus erythematosis may be associated with an acute or subacute noninfectious pneumonitis, which may progress to a chronic interstitial lung disease. Pleuropulmonary involvement is probably more common in SLE than in any other connective disease,[44] and may be manifest as pleural effusion, atelectasis, acute pneumonitis, chronic interstitial lung disease, uremic pneumonitis, and diaphragmatic dysfunction with volume loss. In an autopsy series, the incidence of parenchymal disease was 18 percent.[61] Unfortunately, infiltrates in patients with SLE are very often due to infection, which must be carefully ruled out before aggressive immunosuppressive/cytotoxic therapy is begun.

Most patients with acute lupus pneumonitis respond to corticosteroid therapy, but some improve only after the addition of AZA. The usual dose of AZA is 2.5 mg/kg/day.[62,63] Many patients have recurrent episodes of lupus pneumonitis. Occasionally chronic interstitial lung disease develops, and is usually treated with corticosteroids.[64] The utility of cytotoxic therapy in the subset of these patients who do not respond to corticosteroids has not been evaluated, although AZA has been used in order to allow a reduction in corticosteroid dose in patients with lupus ILD.[65]

Polymyositis/Dermatomyositis

The most common type of lung disease associated with polymyositis/dermatomyositis (PM/DM) is interstitial lung disease, which occurs in approximately five percent of patients.

About one half of patients with interstitial lung disease associated with PM/DM will respond to corticosteroids alone.[66-68] In the remainder, if the ILD appears to be progressive, a trial of CYT is justified. It should be pointed out that interstitial infiltrates in this disease may be due to recurrent aspiration; and thus would be unlikely to respond to CYT.

Progressive Systemic Sclerosis

Progressive systemic sclerosis (scleroderma) is a disorder that leads to severe lung parenchymal fibrosis, with concomitant thickening of the pleura, and frequent pulmonary hypertension. In patients with the CREST syndrome (calcinosis, Raynaud's phenomenon, eosophageal dysfunction, sclerodactyly, and telangiectasia), the pulmonary hypertension may be severe, even without significant fibrotic parenchymal disease. Cytotoxic therapy has not been shown to be beneficial in pulmonary scleroderma.

Mixed Connective Tissue Disease

Mixed connective tissue disease (MCTD) has features which overlap with those of SLE, polymyositis, and scleroderma. While an early report of lung disease associated with MCTD suggested that it is usually steroid-responsive,[69] there appears to be a subset of patients who have progressive disease in whom early treatment with CHL (in a dose up to 8 mg/kg/day), in addition to corticosteroids, may be advisable.[70]

Sarcoidosis

Sarcoidosis is a multisystem chronic granulomatous disorder in which the lung is the most frequent organ involved.[71] Usually, these lesions respond at least partially to corticosteroid therapy. CHL has been given to patients with severe, progressive disease, unresponsive to prednisone,[72] or to patients with contraindications to high-dose corticosteroids.[73] In spite of such a preselection of the sickest patients, there have been favorable responses in a significant percentage of patients.[72,73] If a response is to be gained from CHL therapy, it is usually apparent within two to three months. The dose of CHL for sarcoidosis is initially 4–6 mg/day orally once a day, and may be increased by a 2 mg/day every 2–3 weeks to a maximum of 10–12 mg/day if the leukocyte and platelet counts remain adequate. Complete blood counts with platelet counts should be monitored weekly until stable, keeping the WBC above 3500 and the platelet count 100,000.[70]

Alveolar Hemorrhage

Goodpasture's Syndrome

This disorder includes pulmonary hemorrhage, glomerulonephritis, and circulating antiglomerular basement membrane antibody.[74] The current therapy of Goodpasture's syndrome consists of prednisone, CYT, and plasmapheresis.[75-80] The dose of CYT is 2 mg/kg/day, as in Wegener's, and the duration of therapy is at least as long as plasmapheresis continues, (i.e., until clear-cut clinical improvement, with a reduction in anti-GBM.)[80] CYT is usually continued for several months after the disappearance of anti-GBM.

Idiopathic Pulmonary Hemosiderosis (IPH)

This is a disorder characterized by intermittent diffuse intrapulmonary hemorrhage with hemoptysis, cough, iron deficiency anemia, and widespread alveolar infiltrates. The usual therapy consists of oxygen and blood transfusions as needed, along with systemic corticosteroids. AZA has also been reported to be of benefit in prevention of recurrences of hemoptysis[81] and in amelioration of ongoing lung infiltrates.[82] In both of these reports, the dose of AZA was not specified in mg/kg, but ranged from 50 to 100 mg/day. CYT has also been used for patients with IPH.[83]

Neurological Disease

Neurologic diseases such as myasthenia gravis and multiple sclerosis may affect the respiratory system by impairment of ventilatory muscles or by impairment of the coordinated pharyngeal/laryngeal muscle functions which normally protect the airway from aspiration. AZA has been reported to be of some benefit in myasthenia gravis.[2,83,84] One report, which studied myasthenic patients who had already undergone thymectomy and prednisone therapy, cited a 47 percent incidence of improvement solely attributable to AZA.[84] The time required to perceive benefit may be long, with an initial response after 4–10 months of therapy and peak improvement after 14 months. In this study, there was also 100 percent relapse with one year of cessation of AZA.[84] The dosage of AZA for myasthenia was begun at 50 mg/day orally, with weekly increments of 50 mg, until a dose of 2–3 mg/kg/day was attained, or until toxic side effects became apparent.[84] Although cytotoxic therapy theoretically might be beneficial in multiple sclerosis via an effect on T-lymphocytes,[85] no practical value has been demonstrated in patients.[83,86]

Miscellaneous Disorders

Angio-immunoblastic Lymphadenopathy (AIL)

This is a systemic disease characterized by fever, lymphadenopathy, hepatosplenomegaly, rash, hypergammaglobulinemia, Coomb's-positive hemolytic anemia, and pulmonary infiltrates (less than 15 percent of patients).[87] The pattern of pulmonary histopathology is not distinctive enough to render a definitive diagnosis from lung biopsy,[88] and the diagnosis is usually obtained from lymph node biopsy.

Although it has been suggested that corticosteroids alone may be as effective as combinations including immunosuppressives,[89] CYT has often been included in the therapeutic regimen for these patients.[88,90] Unfortunately, the prognosis is bleak. For example, although three of seven patients treated with prednisone and CYT obtained a remission, only one patient survived for two years.[90] The administration of CYT for AIL is different from the other entities discussed in this chapter. For example, it has been given in a single dose of 1200–2000 mg IV (along with vincristine IV and continuous oral prednisone) at three-week intervals.[85]

Relapsing Polychondritis

This condition may involve the trachea and require tracheostomy. Although systemic corticosteroids are the treatment of choice, AZA has been used to lower the steroid dosage.[91]

Asthma

Cytotoxic drugs have been used in the past for the therapy of chronic, severe asthma,[92,93] although such use is now only of historical interest.

SPECIAL CONSIDERATIONS

Cyclophosphamide

Conventionally, immunosuppressive therapy is not begun immediately after an operative procedure such as an open lung biopsy unless the patient's situation is deteriorating, because of concerns of impairment of wound healing. This concern may or may not be clinically important, although the only data come from animal studies. At doses comparable to those used for non-malignant respiratory illnesses (2 mg/kg/day), no decrease in wound tensile strength was shown in mice given CYT compared to controls,[94] although abnormalities in wound tensile strength have been shown in animals after administration of other cytotoxic drugs.[95]

Therapy with CYT and the other cytotoxic agents requires close monitoring for the potentially severe side effects. During early induction therapy, a check of the white count may be justified as often as every second day.[17] The complete blood count (including platelet count) should be checked once a week for 1–3 months, then once every two to three weeks (assuming a stable dose and stable blood count) for the duration of therapy.[1] A peripheral white count of at least 3000–3500/mm^3 should be maintained. It is very important for patients on CYT to be adequately hydrated, in order to minimize bladder complications so the physician must emphasize adequate fluid intake and frequent voiding. CYT should be avoided in pregnancy because of its potential teratogenicity, and because of its possible prolonged effect even after cessation, contraception should ideally be continued for at least four months after the discontinuation of CYT. In mothers on CYT, breast feeding is not advised because the drug is excreted into the milk. Another potentially relevant concern about the use of CYT is the fact that the tablets contain tartrazine, which may lead to significant bronchospasm in susceptible individuals.[1]

Azathioprine

Like CYT, AZA therapy requires frequent monitoring of the peripheral WBC. In addition, because of potential for hepatic damage, baseline liver enzymes are necessary. AZA should also be avoided in pregnancy.

Chlorambucil

Hematologic abnormalities are the major side effects; thus one must monitor the CBC twice a week during the first 3-6 weeks, then once a week for 3 months, then every 4 weeks if stable.[1]

SIDE EFFECTS

Cyclophosphamide

While the frequency of significant side effects of chronic low-dose CYT therapy is not extremely high, these side effects may be very severe, and both physician and patient should be well aware of them before embarking on a course of therapy including CYT. The most common toxic side effects are marrow depression with its attendant immunosuppression, skin test anergy, bladder hemorrhage, nonspecific gastrointestinal distress, alopecia (usually reversible after removal of the drug), and gonadal dysfunction.[2] Less frequent, but obviously important, side effects include malignancy (most frequently leukemia, lymphoproliferative neoplasia, and urinary tract neoplasia), drug-induced interstitial lung disease, thrombocytopenia, and liver enzyme abnormalities. Uncommon side effects include the syndrome of inappropriate anti-diuretic hormone secretion and myocarditis.[2,96]

Marrow Depression/Immunosuppression

CYT therapy usually results in a degree of leukopenia, affecting both granulocytes and lymphocytes. Avoidance of most infectious complications of CYT therapy can be achieved if the leukocyte count is maintained above 3000-3500, and a neutrophil count above 1000-1500/m,m^3. Using such guidelines, investigators at the NIH following Wegener's patients on long-term CYT have avoided a significant incidence of opportunistic bacterial and fungal infection, but have noted a significantly increased susceptibility to cutaneous herpes zoster.[17,97] Other investigators have also reported a notable lack of infectious complications in patients undergoing long-term CYT therapy.[19] There has been an occasional case report, however, so that the possibility of opportunistic infection in these patients should not be overlooked. The mechanisms by which chronic CYT therapy could theoretically result in an increased susceptibility are three-fold.

Obviously leukopenia (including both neutropenia and monocytopenia) could increase such susceptibility. In addition, qualitative defects in cellular function[66] could contribute. An additional possibility, only shown in experimental animals to date, is that CYT may cause ciliary stasis, decreasing the clearance of pathogens from the lung and increasing susceptibility to superimposed infection.[98]

Urinary Tract Abnormalities–(Nonmalignant)

Hemorrhagic cystitis was first reported in 1959,[99] and the reported incidence has varied widely from less than 5 percent to greater than 35 percent of patients. The clinical manifestations include dysuria, frequency, urgency, and gross or microscopic hematuria.[96] The onset may be within days of institution of the drug or even several weeks after the drug has been withdrawn. Cystoscopy during the episode may show mucosal hyperemia, telangiectasia, or mucosal ulceration/necrosis.[96] Urinary cytology during an acute episode shows cellular atypia.[100] Acute hemorrhagic cystitis usually resolves with discontinuation of the drug and hydration of the patient, although microscopic hematuria may continue for months.[96] Occasionally, the bleeding may be massive and life-threatening, requiring surgical intervention. In a recent review of the complications of chronic CYT treatment in Wegener's patients, hemorrhagic cystitis was fairly frequent, with 34 percent of the patients showing some degree of cystitis (usually mild).[17] These authors recommend early cystoscopy. Long-term therapy with CYT may also result in bladder fibrosis with vesico-ureteral reflux, seen at autopsy in 25 percent of patients who underwent chronic CYT therapy.[101] Half of these patients had been asymptomatic.[101]

Malignancy

Approximately ¾ of the malignancies associated with chronic CYT therapy have belonged to the broad groups of leukemia, lymphoma, or urinary tract neoplasia.[102] Acute nonlymphoblastic leukemias (acute myeloblastic leukemia and acute myelomonocytic leukemia) are the most common forms of leukemias complicating long-term therapy with CYT.[103,104] It has been suggested that clinically-important marrow toxicity may precede the development of overt leukemia, and that such patients should be watched more closely.[105] Diffuse histiocytic lymphoma has been reported after long-term CYT therapy for Wegener's granulomatosis,[106] systemic lupus erythematosus,[107] Sjogren's syndrome,[108] and sarcoidosis.[109]

Urinary tract neoplasia represents the largest group of solid nonlymphoproliferative malignancies secondary to CYT therapy. Renal immunoblastic sarcoma,[110] as well as carcinoma of the renal pelvis,[111] have been reported following chronic CYT therapy for nonmalignant disease. Transitional cell carcinoma of the ureter has also been reported in a patient on CYT for interstitial lung disease.[112] More common than renal or ureteral neoplasia has been carcinoma of the bladder, presumably developing at sites of chronic cystitis and fibrosis. It has been suggested that patients on chronic CYT therapy have their urine cytology routinely monitored,[113] although there may be cellular atypia in the absence of malignancy.[100]

Other malignancies reported to have complicated long-term CYT therapy include squamous cell carcinoma of the stomach,[114] squamous cell carcinoma of the skin,[115] and sarcoma.[116]

Gonadal Dysfunction

Premenopausal women placed on long-term CYT almost invariably develop oligomenorrhea or amenorrhea, which may be irreversible.[17] Ovarian biopsy has shown this to be associated with a severe loss of ovarian follicles.[117] This loss of follicles, however, may be markedly attenuated by simultaneously administering birth control pills to premenopausal women for the duration of therapy with CYT,[117] a practice that has begun for Wegener's patients treated at the NIH.[17]

Significant impotence and loss of libido have been reported in male Wegener's patients on chonic CYT, along with decreased serum testosterone levels and oligospermia.[17]

Pneumonitis

Unfortunately, one of the potential side effects of CYT therapy may be pneumonitis, which could be especially devastating if CYT were originally given for a respiratory illness. The histologic features of CYT-induced pneumonitis include intraalveolar exudate, interstitial edema and round cell infiltrate, interstitial fibrosis, proliferation of atypical alveolar lining cells and occasional hyaline membrane.[118] CYT-induced pneumonitis usually has occurred after a cumulative dose of 40–250 grams, but has been reported after a total dose of only 5 grams.[118] It may be possible for CYT-induced pneumonitis to begin even after CYT has been stopped.[119] The mechanism by which CYT induces interstitial pneumonitis is unknown, although is has been suggested that there is an interaction between CYT and lymphoproliferative tissue, since a striking majority of cases of CYT-induced pneumonitis have occurred when CYT was given for a lymphoproliferative disorder.[66,120,121] Thus, this may not be of clinical importance when given, for example, to patients with steroid-resistant, progressive IPF. Therapy for CYT-induced pneumonitis consists of withdrawal of the drug. The addition of corticosteroids is of uncertain utility, but they are usually given.

Alopecia

Hair loss is usually insignificant when CYT is given in a dose of 2 mg/kg/day. If alopecia does become a significant problem, it is usually completely reversible after cessation of CYT.[17]

Azathioprine

The major toxic side effects of AZA are marrow depression (including leukopenia, anemia, and thrombocytopenia), gastrointestinal distress (including nausea, vomiting, diarrhea, and anorexia), mucus membrane ulceration, fever, alopecia, Raynaud's phenomenon, and biliary stasis. Uncommon side effects include esophagitis, pancreatitis, and interstitial pneumonitis/pulmonary edema.[1]

Marrow Depression

This is the chief toxic effect of AZA, and usually results in modest leukopenia and thrombocytopenia,[46] although there have been a few cases of acute idiosyncratic aplastic anemia.[2] The leukopenia and thrombocytopenia are generally dose-related.

Gastrointestinal Disturbances

These side effects may be conveniently divided into those with and without biliary stasis and its accompanying liver enzyme abnormalities. Liver dysfunction may be severe, dominated by biliary stasis, with marked elevations of serum alkaline phosphatase, and may progress to hepatic failure if AZA is not stopped. It is typically reversible after withdrawal of the drug.[1,2] The current theory of the pathogenesis of AZA-induced liver disease is that AZA acts as an idiosyncratic hepatotoxin resulting in a combination of cholestasis and hepatocellular injury.[122]

Other gastrointestinal side effects include nausea, vomiting, and anorexia, which may be minimized by giving the drug in a split dose after meals.[1] This nonspecific nausea is usually noted in the first two weeks of therapy.[2] If the nausea persists, one should keep in mind the possibility of drug-induced pancreatitis, which although uncommon, may be severe.[1] The diarrhea is occasionally intractable and has forced the cessation of AZA.[52]

Infections

When the white blood count is monitored routinely, infectious complications in patients on chronic AZA therapy appear to be relatively uncommon, although they have been reported.[52,123]

Lung Disease

Although AZA-induced interstitial lung disease was once thought to be rare,[124,125] it is unfortunately being recognized more frequently, especially in renal transplant patients.[126,127] AZA-induced ILD usually results in diffuse interstitial infiltrates, with no cavities, pleural effusions, or focal lesions. It has become manifest after a total AZA dose ranging from 2.9 grams to 28.6 grams. The infiltrates may resolve spontaneously after withdrawl of AZA, but unfortunately may continue to progress after drug cessation. The drug-induced histopathologic lesion appears to be related to prognosis. In a recent report of five patients whose lung tissue showed varying degrees of fibrosis and reorganization of distal airspaces, only one of five improved after cessation of AZA, whereas two of two patients with histopathologic evidence of diffuse alveolar damage improved after removal of the drug.[126] In three of these seven patients, atypical epithelial cells were seen in cytology specimens at the time of onset of x-ray abnormalities, suggesting that monitoring sputum cytology may be useful in following patients on such potentially pneumotoxic drugs.[126] The typical cell seen in such cytology specimens would theoretically have its origin as an epithelial cell lining a reorganized distal airspace. They are crescent-shaped, with granular, nonpigmented cytoplasm, atypical nuclei with prominent nucleoli and no inclusion bodies.[126] Besides serial follow-up of sputum cytology or bronchial washings for cellular atypia, it has also been suggested that gallium scanning may detect early drug-induced lung disease.[128]

Chlorambucil

Marrow Depression

Marrow depression is the most common side effect of CHL. While thrombocytopenia and anemia may result, leukopenia is the usual manifestation of this marrow depression.[1] With prolonged therapy, irreversible marrow damage has been reported.[1]

Gastro-Intestinal Effects

Relatively mild gastrointestinal side effects occur, including nausea, vomiting, abdominal discomfort, anorexia, and diarrhea.[1]

Infection

When given for treatment of sarcoidosis, systemic herpes infection may be a severe, potentially fatal side effect.[129] Other side effects noted in sarcoidosis patients given CHL include a maculopapular skin rash and herpes zoster, which may be focal or diffuse.[73]

Interstitial Pulmonary Fibrosis

Interstitial pulmonary fibrosis, while uncommon, has been reported.[130]

Malignancy

The development of acute leukemia and occasional solid tumors have appeared to result from chronic CHL therapy. This may be due to chromosome damage, which has been measured by sister chromatid exchanges in peripheral blood lymphocytes from patients with Behcet's disease on chronic CHL. The chromosomal damage was related to both daily dose and duration of therapy.[131]

Miscellaneous Side Effects

Uncommon side effects of CHL include seizures, hepatotoxicity, fever, peripheral neuropathy, cystitis, hyperuricemia, and oral ulceration.[1]

DRUG INTERACTIONS

Cyclophosphamide

Barbiturates and other drugs that induce liver microsomal enzymes may theoretically increase the toxicity of CYT because of increased conversion of CYT to its active metabolites.[11] This may not be clinically significant because the higher peak drug levels in patients on barbiturates are balanced by a more rapid decline in plasma alkylating metabolite level.[11] Concomitant allopurinol therapy is associated with an increased frequency (not severity) of marrow depression by an unknown mechanism,[132] although it may be due to an allopurinol-induced prolongation of CYT half-life.[11]

Corticosteroids may inhibit liver microsomal enzymes. Thus, if the steroid dose is abruptly decreased in a patient on CYT, there may be an excessive CYT effect due to the decrease in inhibition of microsomal enzymes, resulting in a higher peak of the active metabolites of CYT.[133] This assertion has been disputed, however,[134] and it is uncertain if this is clinically significant.

Azathioprine

AZA is metabolized to 6-mercaptopurine (6-MP), which is then metabolized to inactive 6-thiouric acid (6-TU) by xanthine oxidase.[1] Allopurinol inhibits xanthine oxidase, thereby impairing conversion of 6-MP to 6-TU. The resulting high level of 6-MP results in increased bone marrow toxicity. Thus, in patients on allopurinol, the dose of AZA should be decreased to about one fourth the usual dose.[135]

REFERENCES

1. McEvoy GK, ed., Drug information '84. American hospital formulary service. American Society of Hospital Pharmacists, Bethesda. pp 234–242 and 226–228, 1984
2. AMA Drug Evaluations, Fourth Edition, American Medical Association, Chicago, p 1123–1129, 1980
3. Kornblut AD, Wolff SM, Defries HO, et al: Wegener's granulomatosis. Laryngoscope 90:1453–1465, 1980
4. Wolff SM, Fauci AS, Horn RG, et al: Wegener's granulomatosis. Ann Int Med 81:513–525, 1974

5. Turk JL, Parker D. Effect of cyclophosphamide on immunlogical control mechanisms. Immunological Rev 65:99-113
6. Shiraki M, Fujiwara M, Tomura S: Long term administration of cyclophosphamide in MRL/1 mice. The effects on the development of immunological abnormalities and lupus nephritis. Clin Exp Immunol 55:333-339, 1984
7. Gershwin ME, Goetzl EJ, Steinberg AD: Cyclophosphamide: Use in practice. Ann Int Med 80:531-540, 1974
8. Dietrich FM: Inhibition of antibody formation to sheep erythrocytes by various tumor-inhibiting chemicals. Int Arch Allergy 29:313-328, 1966
9. Sharma B, Vaziri ND: Augmentation of human natural killer cell activity by cyclophosphamide *in vitro*. Cancer Res 44:3258-3261, 1984
10. Berd D, Maguire HC Jr., Mastrangelo MJ: Potentiation of human cell-mediated and humoral immunity by low-dose cyclophosphamide. Cancer Res 44:5439-5443, 1984
11. Bagley CM Jr, Bostick FW, DeVita VT Jr: Clinical pharmacology of cyclophosphamide. Cancer Res 33:226-233, 1973
12. van Furth R, Gassmann AE, Diesselhoff-Den Dulk MMC: The effect of azathioprine on the cell cycle of promonocytes and the production of monocytes in the bone marrow. J Exp Med 141:531-546, 1975
13. Gorski A, Korczak-Kowalska G, Nowaczyk M, et al: The effect of azathioprine on terminal differentiation of human B lymphocytes. Immunopharmacology 6:259-266, 1983
14. Fahey JL, Leonard E, Churg J, et al: Wegener's granulomatosis. Am J Med 17:168-179, 1954
15. Steinberg AD: Assessing treatments with cyclophosphamide. Ant Int Med 98:1026-1027, 1983
16. Walton EW: Giant cells granuloma of the respiratory tract (Wegener's granulomatosis). Br Med J 2:265-270, 1958
17. Fauci AS, Haynes BF, Katz P, et al: Wegener's granulomatosis: Prospective clinical and therapeutic experience with 85 patients for 21 years. Ann Int Med 98:76-85, 1983
18. Steinman TI, Jaffe BF, Monaco AP, et al: Recurrence of Wegener's granulomatosis after kidney transplantation. Am J Med 68:458-460, 1980
19. Reza MJ, Dornfeld L, Goldberg LS, et al: Wegener's granulomatosis. Long-term follow-up of patients treated with cyclophosphamide. Arthr Rheum 18:501-506, 1975
20. Flye MW, Mundinger GH, Fauci AS: Diagnostic and therapeutic aspects of the surgical approach to Wegener's granulomatosis. J Thor CV Surg 77:331-337, 1979
21. De Remee RA: Wegener's granulomatosis, in: Cherniack RM, (ed), Current Therapy of Respiratory Disease. 1984-1985. BC Decker Inc. Philadelphia and CV Mosby Co., St. Louis, pp 219-221, 1984
22. Nishioka K, Katayama J, Katayama I, et al: Wegener's granulomatosis: Successful treatment with high-dose cyclophosphamide. Dermatologica 164:142-147, 1982
23. Coutu RE, Klein M, Lessell S, et al: Limited form of Wegener granulomatosis. Eye involvement as a major sign. JAMA 233:868-871, 1975
24. Kaplan SR, Calabresi P: Drug therapy. Immunosuppressive agents (part 2). N Engl J Med 289:1234-1238, 1973

25. Bouroncle BA, Smith EJ, Cuppage FE: Treatment of Wegener's granulomatosis with imuran. Am J Med 42:314–318, 1967
26. McIlvanie SK: Wegener's granulomatosis. Successful treatment with chlorambucil. JAMA 197:90–92, 1966
27. Israel HL, Patchefsky AS: Treatment of Wegener's granulomatosis of the lung. Am J Med 58:671–673, 1967
28. Liebow AA, Carrington CRB, Friedman PJ: Lymphomatoid granulomatosis. Hum Pathol 3:457–458, 1972
29. Fauci AS: Granulomatous vasculitides–distinct but related. Ann Int Med 87:782–783, 1977
30. Israel HL, Patchefsky AS, Saldana MJ: Wegener's granulomatosis, lymphomatoid granulomatosis, and benign lymphocyte angiitis and granulomatosis of the lung. Ann Int Med 87:691–699, 1977
31. Fauci AS, Haynes BF, Costa J, et al: Lymphomatoid granulomatosis: Prospective clinical and therapeutic experience over 10 years. N Eng J Med 306:68–74, 1982
32. Fauci AS, Katz P, Haynes BF, et al: Cyclophosphamide therapy of severe systemic necrotizing vasculitides. N Eng J Med 301:235–238, 1979
33. Lanham JG, Elkon KN, Pusey CD, et al: Systemic vasculitis with asthma and eosinophilia: A clinical approach to the Churg-Strauss Syndrome. Medicine 63:65–81, 1984
34. Churg J, Strauss L: Allergic granulomatosis, allergic angiitis and periarteritis nodosa. Am J Pathol 27:277–301, 1951
35. Chumbley LC, Harrison EG, DeRemee RA: Allergic granulomatosis and angiitis (Churg-Strauss syndrome) Mayo Clin Proc 52:477–484, 1977
36. Degesys GE, Mintzer RA, Vrla RF: Allergic granulomatosis: Churg-Strauss syndrome. Am J Roent 135:1281–1282, 1980
37. Cooper BJ, Bacal E, Patterson R: Allergic angiitis and granulomatosis. Prolonged remission induced by combined prednisone-azathioprine therapy. Arch Int Med 138:367–371, 1978
38. Case records of the Massachusetts General Hospital Case 46–1980. N Eng J Med 303:1218–1225, 1980
39. Saldana MJ, Patchefsky AS, Israel HI, et al: Pulmonary angiitis and granulomatosis. The relationship between histological features, organ involvement, and response to treatment. Hum Pathol 8:391–409, 1977
40. Dreisin RB: Pulmonary vasculitis. Clin Chest Med 3:607–618, 1982
41. Cadman EC, Lundberg WB, Mitchell MS: Pulmonary manifestations in Behcet syndrome. Arch Int Med 136:944–947, 1976
42. O'Duffy JD, Robertson DM, Goldstein NP: Chlorambucil in the treatment of uveitis and meningoencephalitis of Behcet's disease. Am J Med 76:75–84, 1984
43. Cohen RD, Conn DL, Ilstrup DM: Clinical features, prognosis and response to treatment in polyarteritis. Mayo Clin Proc 55:146–155, 1980
44. Hunninghake GW, Fauci AS: Pulmonary involvement in the collagen vascular diseases. Am Rev Respir Dis 119:471–503, 1979
45. Shiel WC, Jr., Prete PE: Pleuropulmonary manifestations of rheumatoid arthritis. Semin Arthr Rheum 12:235–243, 1984
46. Brown CH, Turner-Warwick M: The treatment of cryptogenic fibrosing alveolitis with immunosuppressant drugs. Q J Med 158:289–306, 1971

47. Rudd RM, Haslam PL, Turner-Warwick M: Cryptogenic fibrosing alveolitis. Am Rev Respir Dis 124:1-8, 1981
48. Haslam PL, Turton CWG, Lukoszek A, et al: Bronchoalveolar lavage fluid cell counts in cryptogenic fibrosing alveolitis and their relation to therapy. Thorax 35:328-339, 1980
49. Weese WC, Levine BW, Kazemi H: Interstitial lung disease resistant to corticosteroid therapy. Chest 67:57-60, 1975
50. Meuret G, Fueter R, Gloor F: Early stage of fulminant idiopathic pulmonary fibrosis cured by intense combination therapy using cyclophosphamide, vincristine, and prednisone. Respiration 36:228-233, 1978
51. Turner-Warwick M: Interstitial lung disease. Approaches to therapy. Semin Resp Med 6:92-102, 1984
52. Winterbauer RH, Hammar SP, Hallman KO, et al: Diffuse interstitial pneumonitis. Clinicopathologic correlations in 20 patients treated with prednisone/azathioprine. Am J Med 65:661-672, 1978
53. Costabel U, Matthys H: Different therapies and factors influencing response to therapy in idiopathic diffuse fibrosing alveolitis. Respiration 42:141-149, 1981
54. Vath RR, Alexander CB, Fulmer JD: The lymphocytic infiltrative lung diseases. Clin Chest Med 3:619-634, 1982
55. Strimlan CV, Rosenow EC III, Weiland LH, et al: Lymphocytic interstitial pneumonitis Review of 13 cases. Ann Int Med 88:616-621, 1978
56. Case records of the Massachussets General Hospital Case 38-1977: N Eng J Med 297:652-660, 1977
57. Essig LJ, Timms ES, Hancock DE, et al: Plasma cell interstitial pneumonia and macroglobulinemia: A response to corticosteroid and cyclophosphamide therapy. Am J Med 56:398-405, 1974
58. Cooperating clinics committee of the American Rheumatism Association: A controlled trial of cyclophosphamide in rheumatoid arthritis. N Eng J Med 283:883-889, 1970
59. Scott DGI, Bacon PA: Intravenous cyclophosphamide plus methylprednisolone in treatment of systemic rheumatoid vasculitis. Am J Med 76:377-384, 1984
60. Cohen JM, Miller A, Spiera H: Interstitial pneumonitis complicating rheumatoid arthritis. Sustained remission with azathioprine therapy. Chest 72:521-524, 1977
61. Haupt HM, Moore GW, Hutchins GM: The lung in systemic lupus erythematosus. Analysis of the pathologic changes in 120 patients. Am J Med 71:791-798, 1981
62. Matthay RA, Hudson LD, Petty TL: Acute lupus pneumonitis: Response to azathioprine therapy. Chest 63:117-120, 1973
63. Matthay RA, Schwarz MI, Petty TL, et al: Pulmonary manifestations of systemic lupus erythematosus: Review of twelve cases of acute lupus pneumonitis. Medicine 54:397-409, 1975
64. Eisenberg H: The interstitial lung diseases associated with the collagen-vascular disorders. Clin Chest Med 3:565-578, 1982
65. McDonald CF, Fraser KJ, Barter CE, et al: Severe thoracic systemic lupus erythematosus. Aust NZ J Med 14:239-243, 1984
66. Dickey BF, Myers AR: Pulmonary disease in polymyositis/dermatomyositis. Semin Arth Rheum 14:60-76, 1984
67. Plowman PM, Stableforth DE: Dermatomyositis with fibrosing alveolitis: Response to treatment with cyclophosphamide. Proc R Soc Med 70:738-740, 1977

68. Schwarz MI, Matthay RA, Sahn SA, et al: Interstitial lung disease in polymyositis and dermatomyositis: Analysis of six cases and review of the literature. Medicine 55:89–104, 1976
69. Harmon C, Wolfe F, Lillard S, et al: Pulmonary involvement in mixed connective tissue disease (MCTD). Arthritis and Rheumatism 19:801, 1976. (Abstract)
70. Wiener-Kronish JP, Solinger AM, Warnock ML, et al: Severe pulmonary involvement in mixed connective tissue disease. Am Rev Respir Dis 124:499–503, 1981
71. Mayock RL, Bertrand P, Morrison CE, et al: Manifestations of sarcoidosis. Am J Med 35:67–89, 1963
72. Israel HL, Fouts DW, Beggs RA: A controlled trial of prednisone treatment of sarcoidosis. Am Rev Respir Dis 107:609–614, 1973
73. Kataria YP: Chlorambucil in sarcoidosis. Chest 78:36–43, 1980
74. Briggs WA, Johnson JP, Teichman S, et al: Antiglomerular basement membrane antibody-mediated glomerulonephritis and Goodpasture's syndrome. Medicine 58:348–361, 1979
75. Teichman S, Briggs WA, Knieser MR, et al: Goodpasture's syndrome: Two cases with contrasting early course and management. Am Rev Respir Dis 113:223–232, 1976
76. Fitzcharles MA, Benatar SR: Goodpasture's syndrome. Case report of a survivor. S Afr Med J 53:63–66, 1978
77. Finch RA, Rutsky EA, McGowan E, et al: Treatment of Goodpasture's syndrome with immunosuppression and plasmapheresis. South Med J 72:1288–1290, 1979
78. Rossen RD, Duffy J, McCredie KB, et al: Treatment of Goodpasture's syndrome with cyclophosphamide, prednisone and plasma exchange transfusions. Clin Exp Immunol 24:218–222, 1976
79. Lockwood CM, Boulton-Jones JM, Lowenthal RM, et al: Recovery from Goodpasture's syndrome after immunosuppressive treatment and plasmapheresis. Br Med J 2(5965):252–254, 1975
80. Erickson SB, Kurtz SB, Donadio JV Jr, et al: Use of combined plasmapheresis and immunosuppression in the treatment of Goodpasture's syndrome. Mayo Clin Proc 54:714–720, 1979
81. Byrd RB, Gracey DR: Immunosuppressive treatment of idiopathic pulmonary hemosiderosis. JAMA 226:458–459, 1973
82. Yeager H, Powell D, Weinberg RM, et al: Idiopathic pulmonary hemosiderosis. Arch Int Med 136:1145–1149, 1976
83. Gerber NL, Steinberg AD: Clinical use of immunosuppressive drugs: Part II. Drugs II: 90–112, 1976
84. Witte AS, Cornblath DR, Parry GJ, et al: Azathioprine in the treatment of myasthenia gravis. Ann Neurol 15:602–605, 1984
85. Brinkman CJJ, Nillesen WM, Hommes OR: The effect of cyclophosphamide on T lymphocytes and T lymphocyte subsets in patients with chronic progressive multiple sclerosis. Acta Neurol Scand 69:90–96, 1984
86. Dau P, Peterson R: Transformation of lymphocytes from patients with multiple sclerosis. Arch Neurol 23:32–40, 1970
87. Frizzera G, Moran EM, Rappaport H: Angio-immunoblastic lymphadenopathy: Prognosis and clinical course. Am J Med 59:803–818, 1975
88. Bradly SL, Dines DE, Banks PM, et al: The lung in immunoblastic lymphadenopathy. Chest 80:312–318, 1981

89. Nathwani BN, Rappaport H, Moran EM, et al: Malignant lymphoma arising in angio immunoblastic lymphadenopathy. Cancer 41:578-606, 1978
90. Cullen MH, Stansfield AG, Oliver RTD, et al: Angioimmunoblastic lymphadenopathy: Report of 10 cases and review of the literature. Q J Med 48:151-177, 1979
91. Waller ES, Raebel MA: Relapsing polychondritis in a Latin American man. Am J Hosp Pharm 36:806-810, 1979
92. Waldbott GL: Nitrogen mustard in the treatment of bronchial asthma. Ann Allergy 10:428-432, 1952
93. Cohen EP, Petty TL, Szentivanyi A, et al: Clinical and pathologic observations in fatal bronchial asthma. Report of a case treated with the immunosuppressive drug, azathioprine. Ann Int Med 62:103-109, 1965
94. Desprez JD, Kiehn CL: The effects of cytoxan (cyclophosphamide) on wound healing. Plast Reconstr Surg 26:301-308, 1960
95. Bland KI, Palin WE, von Fraunhofer JA, et al: Experimental and clinical observations of the effects of cytotoxic chemotherapeutic drugs on wound healing. Ann Surg 199:782-790, 1984
96. Schein PS, Winokur SH: Immunosuppressive and cytotoxic chemotherapy: Long-term complications. Ann Int Med 82:84-95, 1975
97. Cupps TR, Silverman GJ, Fauci AS: Herpes zoster in patients with treated Wegener's granulomatosis. A possible role for cyclophosphamide. Am J Med 69:881-885, 1980
98. Rowatt JD, Hill JO, Lundgren DL: Respiratory infection with cyclophosphamide-treated mice with pseudomonas aeruginosa. Exp Lung Res 5:305-316, 1983
99. Coggins PR, Ravdin RG, Eisman SM: Clinical pharmacology and preliminary evaluation of cytoxan. Cancer Chemother Rep 3:9-11, 1959
100. Forni AM, Koss LG, Geller W: Cytologic study of the effect of cyclophosphamide on the epithelium of urinary bladder in man. Cancer 17:1348-1355, 1964
101. Johnson WW, Meadows DC: Urinary bladder fibrosis and telangiectasia associated with long-term cyclophosphamide therapy. N Engl J Med 284:290-294, 1971
102. Puri HC, Campbell RA: Cyclophosphamide and malignancy. Lancet 1:1306, 1977
103. Chang J, Geary CG: Therapy-linked leukemia. Lancet 1:97, 1977
104. Grunwald HW, Rosner F: Acute leukemia and immunosuppressive drug use. Arch Int Med 139:461-466, 1979
105. Wheeler GE: Cyclophosphamide-associated leukemia in Wegener's granulomatosis. Ann Int Med 94:361-362, 1981
106. Ambrus JL Jr., Fauci AS: Diffuse histiocytic lymphoma in a patient treated with cyclophosphamide for Wegener's granulomatosis. Am J Med 76:745-747, 1984
107. Louie S, Daoust PR, Schwartz RS: Immunodeficiency and the pathogenesis of non-Hodgkins lymphoma. Semin Oncol 7:267-284, 1980
108. Kassan SS, Thomas TL, Moutsopoulos HM, et al: Increased risk of lymphoma in sicca syndrome. Ann Int Med 89:888-892, 1978
109. Brinker H, Wilbek E: The incidence of malignant tumors in patients with respiratory sarcoidosis. Br J Cancer 29:247-251, 1974
110. Sant GR, Ucci AA, Meares EM: Renal immunoblastic sarcoma complicating immunosuppressive therapy for Wegener's granulomatosis. Urology 21:632-634, 1983

111. McDougal WS, Cramer SF, Miller R: Invasive carcinoma of the renal pelvis following cycolphosphamide therapy for non-malignant disease. Cancer 48:691-695, 1981
112. Schiff HI, Finkel M, Schapira HE: Traditional cell carcinoma of the ureter associated with cyclophosphamide therapy for benign disease. J Urol 128:1023-1024, 1982
113. Chasko SB, Keuhnelian JG, Gutowski WT III, et al: Spindle cell cancer of bladder during cyclophosphamide therapy for Wegener's granulomatosis. Am J Surg Pathol 4:191-196, 1980
114. McLoughlin GA, Cave-Bigley DJ, Tagore V, et al: Cyclophosphamide and pure squamous cell carcinoma of the stomach. Br Med J 280:524-525, 1980
115. Louie S, Schwartz RS: Immunodeficiency and the pathogenesis of lymphoma and leukemia. Semin Hematol 15:117-138, 1978
116. Marks JS, Scholtz CL: Sarcoma complicating therapy with cyclophosphamide. Postgrad Med J 53:48-49, 1977
117. Chapman RM, Sutcliffe SB: Protection of ovarian function by oral contraceptives in women receiving chemotherapy for Hodgkin's disease. Blood 58:849-851, 1981
118. Spector JI, Zimbler H, Ross JS: Early-onset cyclophosphamide-induced interstitial pneumonitis. JAMA 242:2852-2854, 1979
119. Patel AR, Shah PC, Rhee HL, et al: Cyclophosphamide therapy and interstitial pulmonary fibrosis. Cancer 38:1542-1549, 1976
120. Alvarado CS, Boat TF, Newman AJ: Late-onset pulmonary fibrosis and chest deformity in two children treated with cyclophosphamide. J Pediatrics 92:443-446, 1978
121. Spector JI, Zimbler H: Cyclophosphamide pneumonitis (letter) N Eng J Med 307:251, 1982
122. DePinho RA, Goldberg CS, Lefkowitch JH: Azathioprine and the liver. Evidence favoring idiosyncratic, mixed cholestatic-hepatocellular injury in humans. Gastroenterology 86:162-165, 1984
123. So SY, Chau PY, Leung YK, et al: Successful treatment of melioidosis caused by a multiresistant strain in an immunocompromised host with third generation cephalosporins. Am Rev Respir Dis 127:650-654, 1983
124. Rubin G, Baume P, Vandenberg R: Azathioprine and acute restrictive lung disease. Austr NZ J Med 3:272-274, 1972
125. Weisenburger DD: Interstitial pneumonitis associated with azathioprine therapy. Am J Clin Pathol 69:181-185, 1978
126. Bedrossian CWM, Sussman J, Conklin RH, et al: Azathioprine-associated interstitial pneumonitis. Am J Clin Pathol 82:148-154, 1984
127. Carmichael DJS, Hamilton DV, Evans DB, et al: Interstitial pneumonitis secondary to azathioprine in a renal transplant patient. Thorax 38:951-952, 1983
128. Krowka MJ, Breuer RI, Kehoe TJ: Azathioprine-associated pulmonary dysfunction Chest 83:696-698, 1983
129. Sahgal SM, Sharma OP: Fatal herpes simplex infection during chlorambucil therapy for sarcoidosis. J Royal Soc Med 77:144-146, 1984
130. Cole SR, Myers TJ, Klatsky AU: Pulmonary disease with chlorambucil therapy. Cancer 41:455-459, 1978

131. Palmer RG, Dore CJ, Denman AM: Chlorambucil-induced chromosome damage to human lymphocytes is dose-dependent and cumulative. Lancet 1:246–249, 1984
132. Boston Collaberative Drug Surveillance Program: Allopurinol and cytotoxic drugs. Interaction in relation to bone marrow depression. JAMA 227:1036–1040, 1974
133. Kaplan SR, Calabresi P: Immunosuppressive agents. N Eng J Med 289:952–955, 1973
134. Faber OK, Mouridsen HT: Cyclophosphamide activation and corticosteroids (letter). N Eng J Med 291:211, 1974
135. Hansten PD: Drug interactions, 4th ed, Lea and Febiger, Philadelphia, p 183, 1979

Gary R. Cott

7

Drug Therapy in the Management of Cough

Cough is only one of several physiological mechanisms that clears the airways of secretions and foreign materials. The rarity of cough in the healthy individual indicates the efficiency of other clearance mechanisms, particularly the cellular mechanisms of the macrophage and mucociliary system. When these cellular mechanisms fail or are overwhelmed, however, coughing can become a particularly rapid and efficient means of facilitating respiratory clearance.

At some point in many conditions, cough is no longer just a normal physiologic response and becomes a symptom of the underlying illness or even a pathologic mechanism by itself. A patient may seek medical attention solely for a cough that is annoying because of its frequency or persistence. In other cases, a patient may suffer one or more of the secondary complications of a vigorous and persistent cough. Therapeutic intervention may also be required in a patient who manifests an ineffective cough and retains secretions. Each of these patients is likely to require a different form of drug therapy for treatment of his cough.

MECHANISMS OF COUGH

Before discussing drug therapy of cough, a brief review of the mechanisms and physiology of cough is in order. The cough reflex can be described in terms of a classic reflex arc involving a receptor, afferent pathway, central cough center, efferent pathway, and motor response.[1,2] Stimulation of any one of a number of pulmonary or extrapulmonary receptors may initiate a cough reflex,[3] but the primary receptors involved appear to be the irritant receptors of the airways.[2] These receptors are located predominantly in the larynx, trachea, and bronchi and are sensitive to both mechanical and chemical stimuli. Of note is the associated bronchoconstriction that can occur with stimulation of these irritant receptors,[2] and the possible converse situation, where bronchoconstriction may initiate the cough reflex in some cases.[4] The afferent pathway (usually traveling through the vagus, glossopharyngeal, or trigeminal nerve) terminates in the "cough center." This center is probably located in the medullary and pontine area of the hindbrain and is closely linked with the respiratory center.[4] It also appears to be under cortical influence and as such may be voluntarily initiated, modified, or suppressed. The efferent pathway (vagus, phrenic, and spinal motor nerves) innervates respiratory and airway muscles. The action of these muscles on a normal lung "bellows" is responsible for the mechanical phases of an effective cough. These phases are: (1) an inspiratory phase, (2) a compressive phase in which the glottis is closed, and (3) an expiratory blast phase.[1] A mechanically effective cough is capable of developing intraalveolar pressures of 100 mm Hg or more and expiratory flows of 12 liters/sec or more.[1]

Cough can be produced or markedly altered by any disease process that impacts upon any component of the reflex arc.[1,3,5] Examples of disorders that can stimulate irritant receptors or afferent pathways and produce coughing are listed in Table 7-1. Disorders affecting the efferent limb of the reflex arc generally

Table 7-1
Examples of Disorders That Cause Coughing

Pulmonary	
Inhaled irritants:	tobacco smoke, noxious gases, chemical vapors, dusts, foreign bodies
Neoplasms:	benign or malignant, primary or metastatic
Inflammation:	acute or chronic bronchitis, bronchiolitis, bronchiectasis, pneumonitis
Allergy:	asthma, systemic allergic reactions
Others:	pulmonary emboli, congestive heart failure, retained respiratory secretions, airway compression (e.g. by adenopathy, enlarged heart, aneurysms, esophageal cysts or tumors)
Extrapulmonary	
Upper respiratory tract:	rhinitis, sinusitis, pharyngitis, laryngitis, tracheitis, improper phonation, elongated uvula, postnasal drip
Thoracic:	pleural, diaphragmatic, or pericardial inflammation/irritation
Others:	gastric distention, disorders of the external auditory canal or tympanic membrane
Central	
Psychogenic	

Drug Therapy in the Management of Cough 167

result in a mechanically altered or ineffective cough (i.e., one which is not effective in clearing secretions from the tracheo-bronchial tree) (Table 7-2). In addition, an ineffective cough may, by nature of the retention of respiratory secretions, stimulate irritant receptors and thus be a mechanism for perpetuating cough.[6]

INDICATIONS FOR TREATMENT

Three forms of therapy may be chosen for the patient with a cough: specific treatment, symptomatic (or nonspecific) treatment, or no treatment.[7] No treatment is usually indicated for the patient with an acute, selflimited illness causing a nonproblematic cough. In other patients specific and/or symptomatic therapy will be indicated based upon the causitive underlying etiology, and the pathologic potential of the cough. In general, specific therapy is directed towards the etiology and symptomatic therapy is directed towards preventing pathologic or secondary complications of cough.

A key in successful management is to determine, if possible, the precise etiology of, and thus specific therapy for the cough.[8,9] Irwin, et al[8] found a 97 percent success rate for specific therapy alone in the treatment of chronic persistent cough in 49 adults, the majority of whom had asthma, postnasal drip, or both. Thus, specific drug therapy may be definitive in eliminating the cause of

Table 7-2
Examples of Disorders That Cause an Ineffective Cough

Pulmonary	
Decreased receptor sensitivity:	adaptation, topical anethesia, endotracheal tube, chronic inflammation or irritation
Abnormal airways:	chronic obstructive pulmonary disease, asthma, endobronchial lesions or foreign bodies, airway compression, airway collapse (e.g., secondary to tracheo- and/or bronchomalacia)
Abnormal secretions:	cystic fibrosis, dehydration, asthma
Neuromuscular	
Drugs:	cholinesterase inhibitors, curare-like drugs
Others:	spinal cord injuries, myasthenia, amyotrophic lateral sclerosis, weakness (e.g., secondary to cachexia or inanition)
Central	
Central depression:	head injury, systemic illness, drugs, hyperthermia, age
Voluntary:	secondary to pain

cough in many patients. Likewise, the patient with an ineffective cough may be significantly aided by specific therapy directed at the disorder responsible for decreasing the effectiveness of his cough. Further discussion of specific drug therapy for each of the disorders listed in Tables 7-1 and 7-2 is beyond the scope of this chapter. The reader is referred to Chapters 1–4 for discussion of drugs used in treating asthma, a common cause of cough.

Symptomatic treatment of cough is indicated either when no specific cause for the cough can be determined or when the cough is "abnormal." An abnormal cough performs no useful function and has pathologic potential for causing secondary complications (Table 7-3). These complications are generally the result of either the mechanical phases of cough or the pooling of secretions in the case of an ineffective cough.[1,3] Under these conditions, symptomatic therapy is indicated using medications from one or more of three pharmacological categories: antitussive, expectorant or mucolytic. The fact that "cough/cold" medications are the fifth most commonly prescribed category of drugs demonstrates the frequency with which physicians utilize drug therapy to treat the cough.[10] The enormous number of prescription and over-the-counter cough preparations available offers a bewildering array of medications from which to choose. An understanding of the clinical pharmacology of these drugs is essential in choosing the appropriate therapy for a given patient.

ANTITUSSIVE THERAPY

One should not use symptomatic antitussive therapy with the goal of eliminating cough. Elimination is the goal of specific therapy directed at the underly-

Table 7-3
Complications of Cough

Secondary to Mechanical Phase	
Pulmonary:	pneumothorax, pneumomediastinum, local airway or laryngeal trauma, (?) pulmonary emphysema, (?) reflex bronchoconstriction
Musculoskeletal:	strained or torn muscles or cartilage, rib fractures
Central:	tussive syncope
Cardiovascular:	transient bradycardia, transient A-V block, venous rupture (e.g., subconjunctival, nasal or anal vein)
Others:	hernias, vaginal prolapse, urinary incontinence, wound dehiscence, insomnia, vomiting, headache
Secondary to an Ineffective Cough	
Pulmonary:	retained respiratory secretions, airway obstruction, atelectasis, infection, respiratory failure

ing disorder whose pathophysiology is responsible for causing the cough. Since most disorders causing cough are associated with excess material in the airway, the cough is an essential physiologic response necessary for maintaining respiratory clearance. Therefore, the ideal antitussive drug would reduce the frequency of excessive and potentially pathologic coughing, but not jeopardize respiratory function by inhibiting the cough necessary to maintain patent airways. The ideal drug does not exist.

Two problems arise in considering the clinical pharmacologic properties of antitussive drugs. First, the precise mechanism of action for many of these drugs is not completely understood. Theoretically, it would be possible for antitussive drugs to reduce the frequency of cough by inhibiting the reflex arc anywhere along its path. In practice, however, most antitussives either act peripherally at the site of irritant receptors or centrally at the cough center. Second, the efficacy of many of the marketed antitussives is uncertain. Investigators have induced coughing in animals or healthy human volunteers, or have used patients with coughs due to a variety of causes in the evaluation of antitussives. The mechanisms producing cough and thus the response to an antitussive may be different for each of these subjects. In addition, a variety of techniques have been used to gather data including subjective scoring, patient diaries, cough counting, and physiologic measurements. As a result, comparing antitussive studies can be difficult and the findings can often be inconsistent or even conflicting.[11] Therefore, we will discuss only those agents for which clinical efficacy has been proven and/or are in common use.

Peripherally Acting Antitussives

Agents in this category suppress cough by reducing local irritation within the respiratory tract. They mediate their effect on peripheral irritant receptors by either a direct anesthetic action or an indirect soothing effect created by altering respiratory tract fluid.

Anesthetics

Local anesthetics including benzocaine, benzyl alcohol, phenol, and phenol containing salts can be found as ingredients in many over-the-counter cough lozenges.[12] At the concentrations found in most lozenges, these anesthetics may ameliorate pharyngeal irritation and the cough associated with stimulation of pharyngeal irritant receptors. However, they probably have little efficacy in the treatment of cough caused by disorders of the lower respiratory tract.

Lidocaine. The topical application of local anesthetics (e.g., tetracaine, cocaine, and lidocaine) to the upper respiratory tract and major airways has been very effective in limiting the cough associated with bronchoscopy and related procedures. Inhaled anesthetic therapy in the symptomatic treatment of cough has not been well studied, but inhaled lidocaine (400 mg) has been anecdotally demonstrated to suppress chronic cough for periods of one to six weeks.[13-15] However, several cautions regarding the use of inhaled lidocaine at these doses should be emphasized: (1) The risk of aspiration may persist for hours after a single treatment; (2) Any sensitivity to topical anesthetics should preclude its use; (3) Following inhalation treatment with lidocaine, an increase in airways resistance was noted by Howard et al[13] in all patients studied; (4) Finally, there is a risk of systemic toxic effects including arrhythmias and seizures; particularly in patients in whom hepatic and/or cardiac disease results in decreased lidocaine metabolism. Thus, inhaled lidocaine is not generally recommended in the symptomatic treatment of cough. Nevertheless, it should be considered in a limited number of patients with known pulmonary pathology who have a chronic disabling cough that is unresponsive to conventional specific and symptomatic therapy.

Benzonatate. Benzonatate is chemically related to tetracaine and has local anesthetic action when applied topically. It is, however, as an orally administered agent that benzonatate has gained acceptance as an effective antitussive. Animal studies have demonstrated anesthesia of a number of peripheral receptors including the pulmonary stretch receptors following parenteral administration of the drug.[16] Benzonatate may have a central antitussive effect as well, but it is this peripheral action that is felt to be predominantly responsible for the drug's antitussive effect. Although not well controlled, a number of clinical studies in patients with a variety of disorders have shown moderate to excellent symptomatic relief of cough.[16] Benzonatate does not depress respiration at recommended doses and may, in asthmatic patients, result in an increase in vital capacity and a decrease in the sense of dyspnea.[17] The drug is generally well tolerated, but adverse side effects may include rash, constipation, nasal congestion, slight vertigo, headache, nausea, drowsiness, hypersensitivity reactions, and a vague "chilly" sensation.[18] The usual recommended dosage for adults and children over 10 years of age is 100 mg orally three times daily; if necessary up to 600 mg/day.[19] For children under 10 years of age, 8 mg/kg daily in three to six divided doses is recommended.[19]

Demulcents

Demulcents are agents often containing local sialogogues that may have a soothing effect by coating an irritated pharyngeal mucosa and preventing mucosal drying. These agents may be used as vehicles for other antitussive agents or be marketed as over-the-counter syrups or lozenges containing honey, acacia, glycerin, wild cherry, or licorice. In addition, many traditional home remedies fall in this category. An example is the popular "sugar and honey with whiskey or rum in a glass of hot water with lemon juice."[20] There is no objective data to indicate that demulcents have a significant antitussive effect, but they are by and large harmless and may result in the subjective improvement of pharyngeal symptoms.

Expectorants

Expectorants are agents that augment respiratory tract secretions in such a way as to promote their expulsion from respiratory passages. The mechanisms of action and efficacy of individual expectorants are discussed in more detail in a later section. Many expectorants are touted to have an indirect antitussive effect as well,[16] but there is little objective evidence to support this contention. Kuhn et al,[21] found that 96 percent of young adults with acute respiratory disease receiving guaifenesin reported a decrease in sputum thickness compared to 54 percent of the patients receiving the syrup vehicle only, but there were no significant differences in objective cough counts between the two groups. Similar results were obtained in a study of cough induced in healthy volunteers, but guaifenesin may have enhanced the antitussive activity of a combination cough medicine.[22] Therefore, until objective data is available to indicate otherwise, we would suggest that the decision to use an expectorant be based solely on the merits of the drug as an expectorant and not on a potential antitussive effect.

Centrally Acting Antitussives

Centrally acting antitussive agents suppress cough by raising the threshold necessary to stimulate the central cough center. In addition, the sedative or hypnotic effect of many of these drugs may help the patient adapt by making him less aware of his cough even though its severity or frequency has not changed.[23] In general, these drugs can be classified into two groups: the narcotic and nonnarcotic antitussives.

Narcotics

Among the opium alkaloids are the phenanthrenes (e.g., morphine and codeine). These opioids and their derivatives possess a number of pharmacologic properties that make them clinically useful as analgesics, antitussives, sedatives, antidiarrheal agents, and adjunctive therapy in certain forms of cardiogenic pulmonary edema.[24] It is their many undesirable effects, however, that limit their usefulness in clinical practice. Among these adverse effects are physical and psychological addiction, nausea and vomiting, biliary colic, ureteral spasm, constipation, bronchospasm, and respiratory depression.[24]

Some of these adverse effects may be of particular concern when considering antitussive therapy for patients with various pulmonary disorders. The opioids can cause the release of histamines which, along with other mediators, has been postulated to cause the bronchospasm reported in animals and some patients receiving large parenteral doses of narcotics.[24,25] This effect, however, is rarely seen with the doses used for oral antitussive therapy in man. Narcotics can also impair mucociliary clearance by inhibiting bronchial mucous gland secretion and ciliary activity.[23,25] When compared to a number of other morphine derivatives, codeine appeared to have the least ciliary inhibitory activity per antitussive dose.[25] Finally, all the opioids are capable of depressing the central respiratory centers and decreasing the central respiratory response to changes in CO_2.[24] The respiratory depressant effects of narcotics and other CNS depressants (including sleep) appear to be additive.[26] Equal analgesic doses of different opioids appear to cause the same degree of respiratory depression.[26] However, at equal antitussive doses (which are substantially less than those needed to produce analgesia) codeine has only ¼ the respiratory depressant effect of morphine.[23]

Codeine

Codeine remains one of the most popular prescription antitussive drugs and is the standard for evaluating the potency of other cough suppressants.[25,27] Its effectiveness as an antitussive has been demonstrated in a variety of animal and human subject studies.[25,28,29] The optimum single oral dose for effective antitussive therapy and minimal side effects ranges from 10 to 30 mg.[25,28,29]

Although all of the narcotics are probably effective cough suppressants, codeine has several advantages over other narcotics. In contrast to morphine and most other narcotics, codeine is well absorbed and has a high oral potency; ⅔ that of a parenterally administered dose.[24] In addition, the dependency and abuse liability of codeine are less than with most other narcotics, particularly heroin and morphine.[24,30] This relatively small addictive potential may stem from the fact that an equal antitussive dose of codeine has less of a psychic and euphoric effect than morphine.[25] Finally, as previously discussed, codeine causes less respiratory depression and mucocilliary clearance inhibition than most other narcotics. Despite its relative safety, codeine has the potential to produce any or all of the above adverse effects in some high-risk patients or when it is improperly prescribed.

Adverse side effects are infrequent with the usual oral doses of codeine administered for cough. However, nausea, vomiting, constipation with repeated doses, dizziness, sedation, palpitation, pruritis and, rarely, excessive perspiration and agitation have been reported.[19] In addition, codeine may potentiate the effects of other opiate agonists, general anesthetics, tranquilizers, sedatives and hypnotics, tricyclic antidepressants, monoamine oxidase inhibitors, alcohol, and other CNS depressants.[19]

When used as an antitussive, the usual dosage of codeine, codeine phosphate, codeine sulfate or codeine resin for adults and children 12 years of age or older is 10–20 mg orally every 4–6 hours, not to exceed 120 mg/day.[18,19] Lesser dosages are indicated in poor-risk patients, in the very young or very old and in patients receiving other CNS depressants. The usual dosage for children 6–11 years of age is 5–10 mg orally every 4–6 hours, not to exceed 60 mg/day; for children 2–5 years, 2.5–5 mg every 4–6 hours not to exceed 30 mg/day is recommended.[18,19] For further information concerning the use of codeine antitussives in children the reader is referred to the American Academy of Pediatrics Committee on Drugs recommendations for the use of codeine cough syrups in pediatrics.[31]

Hydrocodone

Hydrocodone, a hydrogenated ketone derivative of codeine found in a number of proprietary cough medications, has a narcotic antitussive effect similar to that of codeine. On a milligram basis, hydrocodone may be a more effective antitussive agent but has a greater dependency liability than codeine.[19,25] Other than possibly causing less constipation, hydrocodone has adverse reactions and side effects similar to codeine.[18,19] Thus, hydrocodone offers no clear advantage over codeine. The usual adult antitussive dose of hydrocodone bitartrate or hydrocodone resin is 5–10 mg orally every 4–6 hours.[19] Children may receive 0.6 mg/kg daily administered in 3–4 divided doses.[19]

Other Narcotics

Other derivatives of morphine and codeine have significant antitussive properties and some, including hydromorphone and pholcodine (not available in the United States), are marketed as cough suppressants. Many of these agents (with the possible exception of pholcodine), however, have a higher addictive potential than codeine and offer no particular therapeutic advantage over codeine for most coughs. The antitussive properties of these narcotics are reviewed elsewhere.[20,25,27]

Nonnarcotics

Dextromethorphan. Dextromethorphan is probably the best known and most well studied of the nonnarcotic antitussives. It is the dextro-isomer of the narcotic analgesic levorphanol, but unlike the latter, dextromethorphan appears to have no significant analgesic or addictive effect.[24,25] The drug's effectiveness as a cough suppressant has been documented in a number of clinical studies.[25,29,32] As with codeine, a dose dependent antitussive effect has been noted and comparable effectiveness has been observed for these drugs.[29,32]

Adverse effects with dextromethorphan at therapeutic doses are uncommon. Ciliary activity is not inhibited at dose levels below 5 mg/kg in animals, but whether or not dextromethorphan has a "drying effect" on respiratory mucosa is still uncertain.[23] If present, this drying effect is probably not of clinical significance. Nausea, dizziness, and slight drowsiness are occasional side effects and the drug is contraindicated in patients receiving monoamine oxidase inhibitors.[19] CNS depression has been noted clinically only in accidental poisonings.[23]

The recommended dosage of dextromethorphan hydrobromide for adults and children 12 years of age or older is 10–20 mg orally every four hours or 30 mg every six–eight hours, not to exceed 120 mg/day.[18,19] For children 6–11 years of age the usual dosage is 5–10 mg orally every 4 hours or 15 mg every 6–8 hours, not to exceed 60 mg/day; for children 2–6 years, 2.5–5 mg every 4 hours or 7.5 mg every 6–8 hours not to exceed 30 mg/day is recommended.[18,19]

Noscapine. Noscapine is a naturally occurring benzylisoquinoline opium alkaloid that is nonaddicting.[23,24] In animals noscapine has been shown to produce antispasmodic papaverine-like effects including coronary vasodilation and bronchodilation.[25] In man, however, at therapeutic doses the drug appears to have little effect on smooth muscle and no significant central respiratory or analgesic effect.[23,25] Clinical studies have demonstrated a significant antitussive effect that is comparable to codeine.[23] It may also have expectorant properties, but its effect on bronchial secretions is still somewhat controversial.[23,25] Only occasional adverse side effects such as slight drowsiness, mild nausea, acute allergic vasomotor rhinitis, and conjunctivitis have been reported.[19] Although the usual adult dosage of noscapine is 15–30 mg orally every 4–6 hours not to exceed 120 mg/day; single doses as high as 60 mg have been given safely for the control of paroxysmal coughing.[19,23] Children from 2–12 years of age may receive 7.5–15 mg every 3–4 hours, not to exceed 60 mg/day.[19]

Caramiphen. Caramiphen edisylate is a phenylcyclopentylakylamine that is chemically unrelated to the opioids and has exhibited both central antitussive and atropine-like pharmacological properties. Clinical studies with caramiphen have not always been objective or well-controlled, but in general the antitussive effect of caramiphen appears to be somewhat variable and is probably less than that of codeine.[23,25] Adverse side effects are few but include slight nausea, dizziness, and occasional drowsiness. Because of its weak anticholinergic properties, caramiphen should be used with caution in patients with glaucoma or urinary retention. Its effect on bronchial reactivity, respiratory secretions, and mucocilliary clearance has not been well-established. The usual dosage for adults and children over 12 years of age is 10–20 mg orally 3–4 times daily. The dosage of sustained release combination medications will vary.

Carbetapentane. Carbetapentane citrate and tannate are from the same chemical and pharmacologic class of drugs as caramiphen. Carbetapentane also has mild atropine-like properties and local anesthetic effects as well. Animal studies have suggested that it has greater antitussive activity than an equivalent dose of codeine, and that it has a quicker onset and longer duration of action.[33] These observations have not been confirmed in humans. Although an antitussive effect has been demonstrated in man, further well-controlled, objective studies are needed to establish the clinical usefulness of this drug.[23,25] Known adverse side effects and precautions for carbetapentane are similar to those of caramiphen. The usual dosages are not well established and, as carbetapentane is found in combination cold and cough preparations, dosages should be individualized as per the prescribing information for each proprietary product.

Diphenhydramine. Diphenhydramine, other antihistamines, and a number of other antihistaminic-like drugs including the phenothiazine promethazine have been reported to have antitussive properties.[25] Again, too few well-controlled, objective clinical studies have been conducted to fully establish the clinical usefulness of these drugs. Diphenhydramine has been shown to have a significant but variable response in reducing experimentally induced coughs[23] and chronic coughs related to bronchitis.[34] Animal studies suggest diphenhydramine is less effective than codeine.[35] The mechanism of action of these drugs is not completely understood. Although a central effect has been suggested by animal studies, it is also possible that a sedative action, peripheral action, or specific action (e.g., in patients with allergic rhinitis and/or postnasal drip) may play a role in the therapeutic response of individual patients. The adverse side effects of these drugs can include a drying effect on respiratory secretions and mucosa, drowsiness, and occasional CNS excitation. Because of their anticholinergic effects, these drugs should be used cautiously in patients with glaucoma, urinary retention, and impaired pulmonary function. Concommittant therapy with other anticholinergic drugs, CNS depressants, or CNS stimulants is also cautioned. The recommended antitussive doses for diphenhydramine hydrochloride are 25 mg orally every four hours not to exceed 100 mg/day for adults, 12.5 mg every four hours not to exceed 50 mg/day for children age 6–12 years, and 6.25 mg every four hours not to exceed 25 mg/day for children age 2–5 years.[18]

EXPECTORANT THERAPY

As listed in Table 7-2, there are a variety of disorders that can result in an ineffective cough. In most instances specific therapy directed at these disorders will improve the effectiveness of a patient's cough. In some cases, however, particularly when chronic illnesses or disorders lead to protracted periods of ineffective coughing, symptomatic therapy may be warranted to help avoid the complications of an ineffective cough.

Symptomatic therapies that promote the clearance of respiratory secretions from the lung are referred to as mucokinetics by Ziment.[36] Theoretically, mucokinetics could act on any number of factors including sputum, the mucociliary system, the airways, or the cough reflex mechanism. In practice, however, symptomatic drug therapy for an ineffective cough utilizes mucokinetic drugs in an attempt to alter respiratory secretions in order to ease or facilitate their removal. Mucolytic drugs, which will be considered later in this chapter, directly alter the physiochemical properties of respiratory tract mucus. Expectorants are defined as those mucokinetic drugs that appear to have their major effect by causing an augmentation of respiratory tract fluid.

A number of points are worth emphasizing before considering the effectiveness of mucokinetic drugs. As with antitussive drugs, difficulties may arise in comparing studies which have examined the effects of mucokinetics in different types of subjects (i.e., animal vs. human). A second problem concerns the relevance of the parameters measured.[37] Sputum characteristics such as volume, adhesiveness, consistency, and viscoelastic properties may be determined. How an alteration in one of these characteristics, particularly as measured *in vitro*, affects respiratory clearance and in turn the course of a specific pulmonary disorder is in many cases uncertain. Thus, if a mucokinetic drug alters the properties of respiratory secretions in what would appear to be a beneficial manner, the effect of this alteration on the patient's clinical status must be determined before a drug can truly be termed effective.

Expectorant drugs have traditionally been given in mild self-limiting diseases often with the primary aim of lessening cough in part by a demulcent action of respiratory secretions on inflamed airway epithelium. As discussed earlier, what little objective evidence is available suggests that expectorant drugs probably don't have a major independent antitussive effect. In addition, most expectorants at the doses recommended have not been documented to significantly increase the clearance of respiratory secretions or consistently improve a patient's clinical condition. The inevitable conclusion is that there are very few indications for the use of expectorant drugs.

Vagally Mediated Expectorants

Guaifenesin

Guaifenesin or glyceryl guaiacolate is the most commonly found expectorant in both prescription and nonprescription proprietary cough preparations.[38] Animal studies have shown that large doses of guaifenesin administered orally will produce an increase in respiratory tract fluid in autumn months.[39] It is postulated that gastric mucosal irritation by the drug produces reflex stimulation of the bronchial glands via the vagus nerve.[36] Similarly, subemetic doses of other gastric mucosal irritants including ipecacuanha can cause an increase in the output of respiratory tract fluid.[16] The possibility of direct bronchial gland stimulation by guaifenesin has been suggested as well.[40] Although the drug does enter the respiratory tract secretions, no significant mucolytic or other action on mucous has been demonstrated.[41]

Despite the fact that guaifenesin and other guaiacol derivatives like potassium guaiacol sulfonate have enjoyed widespread use as expectorants their clinical value is debatable.[42,43] Objective studies with chronic bronchitis have shown that guaifenesin at the usual adult dosages has no significant effect on sputum or its clearance when compared to a placebo.[41,44] A mucokinetic effect has been found in a few studies but the dosages required were well above the conventional adult dosage.[45,46] Thus, it would appear that at currently recommended doses, guaifenesin has little, if any, expectorant activity.

The adverse side effects of guaifenesin are few. Nausea and vomiting, and rarely drowsiness may occur at large doses. The drug has been reported to decrease platelet adhesiveness, but does not cause prolongations of bleeding time.[47] Finally, guaifenesin may produce a false-positive response for urinary 5-hydroxyindolacetic acid (5-HIAA) and vanillylmandelic acid (VMA).[18]

The usual dosage of guaifenesin for adults and children 12 years of age and older is 200–400 mg orally every four hours, not to exceed 2.4 g/day. For children age 6–11 years, 100–200 mg every four hours not to exceed 1.2 g/day; and for children age 2–5 years, 50–100 mg every four hours not to exceed 600 mg/day is recommended.[19]

Terpin Hydrate

Terpine hydrate is the most popular of a number of volatile oils including eucalyptus oil, lemon oil, and terpentine oil that have been touted to have expectorant properties. These drugs are believed to have their effect through indirect and direct mechanisms similar to those of the guaiacol derivatives. Like guaifenesin, however, the doses of terpin hydrate necessary to cause an increase in respiratory tract fluid are considerably higher and more poorly tolerated than conventional doses.[48] Adverse side effects with terpin hydrate are rare but include nausea and vomiting. In addition, the high alcohol content in terpin hydrate elixir may preclude its use in some patients. Thus, the dose of terpin hydrate usually given in most combination "cough medicines" is safe but insufficient to cause any mucokinetic effect, and probably serves mainly as a vehicle for other active drugs.

Ammonium Chloride

Although little data exists to support its clinical efficacy, ammonium chloride is found as an expectorant ingredient in a number of proprietary "cough medicines." Its mechanism of action is felt to be predominantly through the indirect vagal reflex, but it is doubtful that in conventional doses its irritant action on the gastric mucosa significantly contributes to any expectorant action.[48] Large doses of ammonium chloride may induce nausea, vomiting, and a metabolic acidosis.

Iodides

The iodides have been popular expectorants for many years. A number of mechanisms have been postulated as contributing to the action of iodides on respiratory secretions. Iodide appears to directly stimulate bronchial, nasal, and salivary gland secretion. There may also be an indirect stimulation through the gastropulmonary mucokinetic vagal reflex. However, animal studies suggest that the doses necessary to cause a significant increase in bronchial gland secretion are well above the recommended adult dosages.[39] A second mechanism may be through a mucolytic effect. The direct addition of iodide to sputum *in vitro* results in a rapid decrease in viscosity.[49] Since iodide is found in respiratory secretions shortly after administration, it is postulated that iodides may have a mucolytic effect *in vivo*. In addition, iodides potentiate the enzymatic activity of natural proteases in respiratory tract secretions and may thereby enhance the endogenous breakdown of viscous mucoproteins.[50] A final mechanism may be an increase in ciliary beating seen with iodides.[51]

Most of the clinical studies with iodides have been plagued by a lack of objectivity, poorly controlled experiments, and difficulties comparing and interpreting data. Subjective studies involving large numbers of asthmatic or chronic bronchitic adult patients suggest that iodides may be helpful in clearing secretions, but the incidence of undesirable side effects can be significant particularly at larger doses.[52,53] Falliers et al[54] in a controlled study of chronic severely ill asthmatic children reported a "significant improvement" of asthma in 18 percent while 36 percent showed no improvement. Of note in this study is that the incidence of toxicity was significant and that no meaningful correlation could be established between serum iodide levels and either sputum viscosity or response to therapy.

Adverse side effects can occur in up to 50 percent of patients and have warranted discontinuance of iodide expectorants in over 10 percent.[3] Among the hypersensitivity reactions ascribed to iodides are angioedema, serum sickness, urticaria, thrombotic thrombocytopenia purpura, and fatal periarteritis. Long-term side effects of iodides (iodism) are both time and dose dependent. Manifestations of iodism include a metallic taste, increased salivation, coryza, headache, acneiform eruptions, swelling and tenderness of the parotid and submaxillary glands, and gastric irritation.[19] Prolonged use of iodides may also suppress thyroid function and result in adenoma or goiter formation and occasionally myxedema. Thyrotoxicosis is a rare complication of iodide therapy in patients with preexisting goiter.

As a result of the relatively low therapeutic index for iodide expectorants the American Academy of Pediatrics Committee on Drugs has advised that iodides are contraindicated during pregnancy, breast feeding, and adolescence.[55] In addition, they recommend that "iodides should be used as expectorants only in patients with chronic disease who have a reproducible clear-cut amelioration which cannot be obtained with a less toxic agent." The recommended expectorant dosage of potassium iodide is 300–650 mg orally 3–4 times daily in adults or 60–250 mg orally four times daily in children,[19] while the recommended expectorant dosage of hydriodic acid solution (70 mg/5 ml) in adults is 5 ml orally with a glass of water 3–4 times daily.[19]

Iodinated glycerol is an organic iodide, which is more stable in storage and is claimed to cause less gastric irritation but also contains less iodide per dose. The usual adult dosage of iodinated glycerol is 60 mg orally with water four times daily, and children may receive up to one-half the adult dosage.[19]

Miscellaneous Expectorants

Bromhexine and Ambroxol

Bromhexine and its metabolite ambroxol are not available in the United States but are marketed in Europe as expectorants. Bromhexine is obtained from the alkaloid component vasicine of the Asian plant *Adhatoda vasica*. Animal studies have demonstrated that bromhexine will increase the volume and reduce the viscosity of respiratory tract secretions. The mechanisms involved appear to include: (1) a direct and indirect (vagally mediated) stimulation of tracheobronchial mucous secretion with possible associated structural changes in the serous cells,[56,57] (2) increased ciliary beating,[58] and (3) a mucolytic action as demonstrated by a fragmentation of sputum acid glycoprotein fibers.[59] Additional evidence has suggested that these agents may stimulate surfactant production and as such may have efficacy in the treatment of the neonatal respiratory distress syndrome.[60,61]

A number of investigators have examined the effects of bromhexine and ambroxol in patients with chronic bronchitis. Using radiolabeled clearance measurement techniques, these drugs did not consistently show significantly improved mucociliary clearance in the groups studied.[62,63] Well-controlled clinical trials with bromhexine have yielded conflicting results but may be summarized as follows: (1) subjective improvement in respiratory status is variable, may be seasonally and dose related, and does not always coincide with spirometric improvement,[64-66] (2) increases in sputum volume and decreases in viscosity may not be associated with spirometric improvement or subjective improvement in respiratory status,[67] and (3) when spirometric improvement is seen it may correlate with patients having a milder or more reversible obstruction.[67-69] Preliminary reports with ambroxol indicate that it may be somewhat more effective than bromhexine, but further studies are needed to define its true clinical usefulness.[70]

Bromhexine and ambroxol are relatively well tolerated but may cause epigastric discomfort and nausea. Caution should be used in administering these drugs to patients with peptic ulceration. In addition, transient rises in serum aminotransferases have been reported. Bromhexine doses usually range between 8-16 mg orally three times daily; while daily doses of ambroxol are generally between 45 and 60 mg daily.

OTHER THERAPIES

Fluids

The oral intake of water has long been recommended as important adjunctive therapy in helping to prevent the inspissation of secretions in disorders such as asthma and chronic bronchitis. Animal and patient studies, however, suggest that the oral administration of water has no effect on the volume or viscosity of respiratory tract fluid in the absence of severe dehydration.[71,72] Thus, maintaining adequate hydration in patients is important, but there is no evidence that excess hydration acts as an expectorant and it may be dangerous in the elderly.

The aerosolization of water vapor, with or without saline, by mist, steam, or ultrasonic nebulizer has been a popular home remedy for lessening "chest congestion." Aerosolized water therapy may have a demulcent effect and lessen the viscosity of secretions in the larger upper airways. However, most experimental evidence would suggest that regardless of which administration technique is used, insufficient amounts of water are delivered to the peripheral respiratory airways to affect respiratory secretions.[73-75] Parks et al[76] in a study with panting dogs has suggested that water nebulization may increase mucous transport by cough but not by the mucociliary system. The clinical value of mist tent and aerosol therapy is less clear. One group has reported a beneficial improvement in lung function in cystic fibrosis patients.[77,78] However, a number of other investigators examining a variety of pulmonary disorders including cystic fibrosis have failed to show a beneficial effect of aerosolized water therapy and in some cases the inhalation of may make lung function worse.[79] For example, the inhalation of either hypo- or hyperosmotic aerosols can cause bronchospasm in asthmatics[80] and the bacterial contamination of aerosolization equipment is relatively common.[79] It should be emphasized that these above mentioned studies are in reference to nonventilated and nontracheotomized patients. In patients requiring artificial airways or permanent tracheostomies the normal humidification chambers of the nose and sinuses are bypassed and control of inspired air temperature and humidity becomes more important.[72]

Detergents and Wetting Agents

In an attempt to improve the hydration of airway secretions, various detergents and wetting agents including tyloxapol, 2-ethylhexyl sulfonate, and propylene glycol have been added to inhalation agents.[36,72,75,81] Although some of these agents may improve the airway deposition of inhaled aerosols they appear to have little if any significant effect on patient sputum.[72,75,81] Likewise, a clinical trial in COPD patients failed to show symptomatic improvement or significant improvement in pulmonary function testing.[82]

MUCOLYTIC THERAPY

The clearance of respiratory secretions from the airways is a complex process that is dependent at least in part on the characteristics of respiratory tract mucus secretions.[75,83] The combined properties of mucus viscosity and elasticity

Drug Therapy in the Management of Cough

influence clearance by both the mucociliary and cough transport systems.[76,84] The principle determinant of mucus viscoelasticity appears to be mucus glycoprotein content, although other factors such as pH, DNA content, calcium and serum proteins may also be important.[85]

Mucolytics, as defined earlier, are mucokinetic drugs that directly alter the physiochemical properties of respiratory tract mucus in such a way as to reduce its viscosity. They are used as adjunctive therapy to remove mucus from the conducting airways when it is significantly obstructing airflow. Thus, to warrant the use of a mucolytic drug, a patient must demonstrate the presence of severe airflow limitation, abnormally viscous respiratory secretions, an ineffective cough, and, in most cases, a failure to respond to specific and more traditional symptomatic therapies. These conditions are most clearly defined in acute respiratory failure associated with mucus impaction. The efficacy of these drugs for long-term therapy in patients with chronic pulmonary disorders associated with abnormally viscous sputum is less clear. This stems in part from the uncertainty as to whether decreasing respiratory mucus viscosity will significantly affect the course of illness such as asthma, cystic fibrosis, and chronic bronchitis. For this reason objective, well-controlled clinical trials are needed to establish the true benefit of these drugs in chronic pulmonary disorders.

Acetylcysteine

Acetylcysteine is the N-acetyl derivative of L-cysteine and is probably the best known of the mucolytic drugs. Its mucolytic activity is conferred by a free sulfhydryl group that splits the disulfide bonds between mucus glycoprotein strands and thus produces a less viscous mucus. This activity has been shown *in vitro* to be sustained and dependent on both concentration of drug and pH (most effective between pH 5-8).[16] There is no evidence that acetylcysteine breaks down DNA or has any action on fibrin or blood clots.[86]

The direct administration of acetylcysteine by catheter or bronchoscope appears to produce an immediate local mucolytic action and may markedly increase the amount of respiratory secretions retrieved.[16,75] It is uncertain whether this effect is due entirely to the drug's mucolytic action or in part to its hypertonicity.[87] Perruchoud et al[88] using bronchoscopic lavage with acetylcysteine in an uncontrolled study, reported that atelectasis caused by mucus inpaction could either be completely or partially relieved in over 90 percent of their patients. The bronchoscopic administration of acetylcysteine has also been reported to relieve mucus plugging and impaction in patients with status asthmaticus who have failed to respond to more traditional forms of therapy.[89] This agent has also been used to locally remove mucus in tracheostomy care and in the preparation of patients for bronchograms and other bronchial studies.[16]

In general, the results appear to be less impressive when the drug is nebulized into the respiratory tract. Aerosolized acetylcysteine in both short term and longer duration (3–7 weeks) studies with chronic bronchitics decreased the measured viscosity of sputum when compared to controls.[90–93] Aerosolized acetylcysteine therapy in these studies, however, failed to produce an improvement in lung function as manifested by pulmonary function testing or an improvement in subjective clinical status. Likewise, a controlled study in asthmatic patients with abnormally viscid or inspissated sputum reported no significant changes in spirometric tests between acetylcysteine treated and control groups, despite significant sputum thinning in the experimental group.[94] Most studies of acetylcysteine inhalation therapy in cystic fibrosis report that inhalation therapy may reduce sputum viscosity, but fail to reproducibly demonstrate a beneficial clinical effect.[86,95,96] Thus, this form of therapy in cystic fibrosis remains controversial. Finally, one possible reason that acetylcysteine aerosolization has not been more successful in the management of these illnesses, is that aerosol deposition may largely be limited to those airways that are unobstructed and well ventilated.

Of note is that either the direct instillation or inhalation of acetylcysteine can produce bronchospasm in both asthmatic and nonasthmatic patients, and is occasionally associated with a temporary deterioration in gas exchange.[75] As a result the prophylactic or concommittant use of an inhaled β-agent bronchodilator is recommended.

Recently, several European investigators have examined the efficacy of oral acetylcysteine therapy at dosages of 200 mg b.i.d. or t.i.d. in disorders associated with viscous bronchial secretions. Several well controlled studies have been performed to assess the effects of oral acetylcysteine in patients with chronic bronchitis.[97–99] The results of these studies may be summarized as follows: (1) symptoms of cough severity, sputum consistency, and ease of expectoration significantly improved in the acetylcysteine treated patients,[97,99] (2) a quantitative increase in sputum volume and decrease in "thickness" (as determined by an increase in pourability) was found to correlate with acetylcysteine therapy,[97] (3) spirometric values showed a small but statistically significant improvement in one study,[97] but were either not available or incomplete in the other studies,[98,99] and (4) "acute exacerbations" were reduced for patients receiving acetylcysteine.[98,99] These studies are largely subjective in nature and further well-designed, objective studies are needed to fully define the nature and mechanism of the "beneficial effect" of oral acetylcysteine therapy in chronic bronchitis. Similar well controlled studies are needed in other chronic pulmonary disorders with associated viscous sputum production.

Adverse side effects are uncommon but include stomatitis, nausea, vomiting, drowsiness, clamminess, severe rhinorrhea, and rarely fever and chills. Systemic toxicity is uncommon because the drugs are rapidly metabolized to cysteine and acetate. The liquid preparation has a slightly disagreeable sulfurous odor and taste, which may contribute to the incidence of nausea. Irritation of oral and tracheal mucosa occasionally occurs with persistent use. As mentioned previously, cough and bronchospasm may develop in some patients and warrants the use of prophylactic or concommittent use of an inhaled β-bronchodilator. Acetylcysteine can also inhibit ciliary activity[100] and though no deleterious effect has been correlated with this inhibition, this fact remains a concern in the long term treatment of patients who already have impaired respiratory secretion clearance.

Acetylcysteine is a reducing agent and as such, is incompatible with oxidizing agents. The drug will react with rubber and some metals including iron and copper, but not with glass, plastic, aluminum, chromed metal, or stainless steel.[19] It is also reported to inhibit the antibacterial activity of some antibiotics and thus solutions of acetylcysteine should not include amphotericin B, erythromycin lactobionate, ampicillin, oxacillin, cloxacillin, or methicillin.[19,101] Acetylcysteine solutions are also incompatible with hydrogen peroxide, iodized oil, chymotrypsin, and trypsin.

For direct instillation, 1-2 ml of 10-20 percent solution may be instilled as often as every hour.[18,19] The usual inhalation dose is 1-10 ml of the 20 percent solution or 2-20 ml of the 10 percent nebulized every 2-6 hours.[18,19] Oxygen supplementation may be used. The 20 percent solution may be associated with more frequent episodes of bronchospasm and mucosal irritation. Ultrasonic nebulization is not recommended since it intensifies the irritating effect of the aerosol. Acetylcysteine solutions should not be placed directly into the chamber of heated (hot-pot) nebulizers. Prolonged nebulization may result in increasing concentrations of the acetylcysteine remaining in the nebulizer, and thus require dilution with sterile water. Open vials should be covered, refrigerated and used within 96 hours.

Carbocysteine

Carbocysteine (S-carboxymethyl cysteine) is another cysteine derivative available in Europe. This compound does not have a free thiol group but instead the hydrogen is replaced by a carboxymethyl group. Despite this "blocked" thiol group, carbocysteine has been reported to cleave disulfide bridges between mucoglycoproteins *in vitro*.[75] In addition, some authors claim that the drug has an effect on the synthesis of glycoproteins within the cell that may be beneficial in decreasing mucus viscosity.[75]

Carbocysteine is administered orally usually in doses of 750 mg t.i.d. as a respiratory mucolytic. Although most trials have demonstrated a decreased sputum viscosity in chronic bronchitis patients, the subjective and objective clinical benefit of the drug has been variable.[102,103] Improvement in pulmonary function parameters has been noted by some authors,[103,104] but not all.[105] In addition, Thomson et al[105] was unable to document a difference in respiratory clearance, as determined by radiolabeled tracer techniques, between carbocysteine and placebo trials in patients with chronic bronchitis.

Sodium 2-Mercaptoethane Sulphonate

Sodium 2-mercaptoethane sulphonate (mesna) is marketed in Europe as a mucolytic aerosol. It has a terminal thiol group and as such is capable of cleaving disulfide bonds. Mesna has been shown to liquefy sputum *in vitro* and *in vivo*.[91,106] Despite sputum changes, clinical trials have failed to show an improvement in pulmonary function or subjective clinical improvement in patients with chronic bronchitis.[91,107] In one limited study with cystic fibrosis patients, treatment with 2-mercaptoethane sulphonate produced no subjective improvement although selected pulmonary function tests were improved.[108] Again, further studies are needed to determine if this drug has any true benefit in patients with cystic fibrosis. Adverse side effects are few but include bronchospasm, nausea and vomiting, and a yellow staining of the teeth with prolonged use.

Enzymes

Proteases

The proteases trypsin and chymotrypsin can decrease the viscosity of sputum by digesting sputum proteins.[16,75] They are more effective on nonpurulent sputum probably, in part, because they are inhibited by the DNA of purulent sputum.[75] They are reported not to digest living tissue since both serum and viable cells contain specific inhibitors.[16] Anecdotal reports of using these proteases by inhalation or aerosol have claimed beneficial effects in tuberculosis, asthma, chronic bronchitis and alveolar proteinosis,[36,75] but there have been no controlled studies. The incidence of side effects associated with protease inhalation therapy is high and includes irritation of the throat and eyes, coughing, hoarseness, hemotypsis, bronchospasm, fever, generalized allergic reactions, and bronchial metaplasia. There is also a theoretical possibility of emphysematous changes with long term use, particularly in patients with α_1-antitrypsin deficiency. In view of these risks and the dubious benefits of therapy, inhalation treatment with trypsin or chymotrypsin is not generally recommended.

Deoxyribonuclease

Deoxyribonuclease has been used to liquefy purulent sputum where the DNA content is postulated to be elevated.[16,75] It has little effect on glycoprotein and is, therefore, without major effect on mucoid sputum.[75] When given as an aerosol, deoxyribonuclease can decrease sputum vicosity or increase its pourability.[75] Although some studies suggest that clinical improvement occurs in patients so treated, these trials are either subjective, poorly controlled or based on small numbers of patients.[75] Adverse reactions are similar to those described for proteases but in general are less frequent and severe. Since deoxyribonuclease offers no clear benefit over acetylcysteine, there seem to be few instances in which deoxyribonuclease would be preferred over acetylcysteine.

REFERENCES

1. Leith DE: Cough, in Brain JD, Procter DF, Reid LM (eds): Respiratory Defense Mechanisms, Vol 5. New York, Marcel Dekker, Inc, 1977, pp 545-592
2. Widdicombe JG: Respiratory reflexes and defense, in Brain JD, Proctor DF, Reid CM (eds): Respiratory Defense Mechanisms, Vol 5. New York, Marcel Dekker, Inc., 1977, pp 593-629
3. Irwin RS, Rosen MJ, Braman SS: Cough: A comprehensive review. Arch Intern Med 137:1186-1191, 1977
4. Salem H, Aviado DM: Physiology of the cough reflex, in Salem H, Aviado DM (eds): International Encyclopedia of Pharmacology and Therapeutics, Section 27, Vol I: Antitussive Agents. Oxford, Pergamon Press, 1970, pp 235-270
5. Godfrey RC: Diseases causing cough. Eur J Resp Dis 61 (Suppl 110):57-64, 1980
6. Clarke SW: The role of two-phase flow in bronchial clearance. Bull Physiopathol Resp 9:359-376, 1973
7. Irwin RS, Pratter: Treatment of cough. Chest 82:662-663, 1982
8. Irwin RS, Corrao WM, Pratter MR: Chronic persistent cough in the adult: The spectrum and frequency of causes and successful outcome of specific therapy. Am Rev Resp Dis 123:413-417, 1981
9. Poe RH, Israel RH, Utell MJ, et al: Chronic cough: Bronchoscopy or pulmonary function testing? Am Rev Resp Dis 126:160-162, 1982
10. Pharmaceutical Data Services: Business barometer: Share of total Rx's-6 leading therapeutic categories. Drug Topics, p 38, Oct. 15, 1984
11. Svedmyr N: General aspects on evaluation of drug effects on cough and expectoration. Eur J Respir Dis 61 (Suppl 110):81-92, 1980
12. American Pharmaceutical Association: Handbook of Nonprescription Drugs (ed 7). Washington, D.C., American Pharmaceutical Association, 1982
13. Howard P, Cayton RM, Brennan SR, et al: Lignocaine aerosol and persistent cough. Br J Dis Chest 71:19-24, 1977
14. Sanders RV, Kirkpatrick MB: Prolonged suppression of cough after inhalation of lidocaine in a patient with sarcoid. J Am Med Assoc 252(17):2456-2457, 1984
15. Stewart CJ, Coady TJ: Suppression of intractable cough. Br Med J 1:1660-1661, 1977
16. Salem H, Aviado DM: International Encyclopedia of Pharmacology and Therapeutics, Section 27, Vol III: Antitussive Agents. Oxford, Pergamon Press, 1970
17. Michelson AL, Schiller IW: The effect of a methoxy-poly(ethyleneoxy) ethyl p-butyl-aminobenzoate (Tessalon) on ventilation and lung volumes. J Allergy 28:514-518, 1957
18. American Medical Association Div of Drugs: Decongestant, cough and cold preparations, in AMA Drug Evaluations, United States, AMA, 1983, pp 563-567

19. McEvoy GK, McQuarrie GM: 48:00 Antitussives, expectorants and mucolytic agents, in McEvoy GK, McQuarrie GM (eds): American Hospital Formulary Service Drug Information 1985. Bethesda, American Society of Hosp Pharm, Inc, 1985, pp 1167-1178
20. Ziment I: Medications for cough and colds, in Ziment I (ed.): Respiratory Pharmacology and Therapeutics. Philadelphia, W.B. Saunders, Co., 1978, pp 282-339
21. Kuhn JJ, Hendlely SO, Adams KF, et al: Antitussive effect of guaifenesin in young adults with natural colds: Objective and subjective assessment. Chest 82(6):713-718, 1982
22. Packman EW, London SS: The utility of artificially induced cough as a clinical model for evaluating antitussive drug combinations. Part I: Liquid and solid formulations of systemic drugs. Current Therap Res 21:855-866, 1977
23. Bickerman HA: Clinical pharmacology of antitussive agents. Clinical Pharm and Ther 3(3):353-368, 1962
24. Jaffe JH, Martin WR: Opioid analgesics and antagonists, in Goodman LS, Gilman A (eds): The Pharmacological Basis of Therapeutics. New York, MacMillan Publ Co., 1980, pp 494-534
25. Salem H, Aviado DM: International Encyclopedia of Pharmacology and Therapeutics, Section 27, Vol II: Antitussive Agents. Oxford, Pergamon Press, 1970
26. Eckenhoff JE, Oech SR: The effects of narcotics and antagonists upon respiration and circulation in man. Clin Pharmac Ther 1:483-524, 1960
27. Eddy NB, Friebel H, Hahn KJ, et al: Codeine and Its Alternates for Pain and Cough Relief. Switzerland, World Health Organization, 1970
28. Sevelius H, McCoy JF, Colmone JB: Dose response to codeine in patients with chronic cough. Clin Pharmac and Ther 12(3):449-455, 1971
29. Aylward M, Maddock J, Davies DE, et al: Dextromethorphan and codeine: A comparison of plasma kinetics and antitussive effects. Eur J Resp Dis 65:283-291, 1984
30. Brown CT: The addiction liability of codeine. Milit Med 129:1077-1080, 1964
31. Committee on Drugs, American Academy of Pediatrics: Use of codeine and dextromethorphan containing cough syrups in pediatrics. Pediatrics 62(1):118-122, 1978
32. Cass LJ, Frederik WS, Andosca JB: Quantitative comparison of dextromethorphan hydrobromide and codeine. Amer J Med Sci 227:291-296, 1954
33. Levis S, Preat S, Moyersoons F: Evaluation of the antitussive activity of some esters of phenylcycloalkanecarboxylic acid and study of different pharmacologic properties of the most effective among them. Arch Internat Pharmacodyn 103:200-211, 1955
34. Lilienfield LS, Rose JC, Princiotto JV: Antitussive activity of diphenhydramine in chronic cough. Clin Pharmac and Ther 19(4):421-425, 1976
35. Wax J, Winder CV, Peters G: An antitussive property of diphenhydramine in dogs. Proc Soc Exp Biol 110:600-603, 1962
36. Ziment I: Mucokinetic agents, in Ziment I (ed): Respiratory Pharmacology and Therapeutics. Philadelphia, W.B. Saunders, Co., 1978, pp 60-104
37. Mossberg B: Drug effects on visco-elasticity—clinical importance? Eur J Resp Dis 61 (Suppl 110):193-194, 1980

38. Physicians' Desk Reference (ed. 39) Oradell, New Jersey, Medical Economics Co., Inc., 1985
39. Boyd EM: Respiratory Tract Fluid, Springfield, Illinois, Charles C Thomas, 1972
40. Ziment I: What to expect from expectorants. JAMA 236(2):193–194, 1976
41. Hirsch SR: In vitro evaluation of expectorant and mucolytic agents. Bull Physiopathol Resp 9:435–438, 1973
42. Hirsch SR, Kory RC: Expectorant effect of glyceryl guaiacolate. Chest 64:544–545, 1973
43. Chodosh S, Medici TC: Expectorant effect of glyceryl guaiacolate. Chest 64:543–544, 1973
44. Yeates DB, Cohen VR, Davis AL, et al: Effect of glyceryl guaiacolate on bronchial clearance in patients with chronic bronchitis. Am Rev Resp Dis 115 (Suppl 14):182, 1977
45. Chodosh S: Objective sputum changes associated with glyceryl guaiacolate in chronic bronchial diseases. Bull Physiopathol Respir 9:452–456, 1973
46. Thomson ML, Pava D, McNichol MW: A preliminary study of the effect of guaiphenesin on mucociliary clearance from the human lung. Thorax 28:742–747, 1973
47. Buchanan GR, Martin V, Levine PH, et al: The effects of 'anti-platelet' drugs on bleeding time and platelet aggregation in normal human subjects. Am J Clin Path 68:355–359, 1977
48. Boyd EM: Expectorants and respiratory tract fluid. Pharmacol Rev 6:521–524, 1954
49. Marriott C, Richards JH: The effects of storage and of potassium iodide, urea, N-acetylcysteine and Triton X-100 on the viscosity of bronchial mucus. Brit J Dis Chest 68:171–182, 1974
50. Liberman J, Kurnick NB: The induction of proteolysis in purulent sputum by iodides. J Clin Invest 43:1892–1904, 1964
51. Carson S, Goldhamer R, Carpenter R: Mucus transport in the respiratory tract. Am Rev Respir Dis 93 (Suppl):86–92, 1966
52. Bernecker C: Intermittent therapy with potassium iodide in chronic obstructive disease of the airways: A review of 10 years' experience. Acta Allerg 24:216–225, 1969
53. Pelz HH: Chronic obstructive pulmonary disease: A plea for simple therapy. Clin Med 80:18–19, 1973
54. Falliers CJ, McCann WP, Chai H, et al: Controlled study of iodotherapy for childhood asthma. J Allergy 38(3):183–192, 1966
55. Committee on Drugs, American Academy of Pediatrics: Adverse reactions to iodide therapy of asthma and other pulmonary diseases. Pediatrics 57(2):272–274, 1976
56. Takeda H, Abe Y, Misawa M, et al: The role of vagal reflex in mechanism of secretagogic action of bromhexine. Japan J Pharmacol 35:445–450, 1984
57. Irvani J, Melville GN: Wirking von Bromhexin-Metabolit VIII and einem neuer adrenergen staff auf die mukozilare. Funktion des Respirationstraktes, Arzneim Forsch, 24:849–853, 1974

58. Irvani J, Melville GN: Mucociliary function of the respiratory tract as influenced by drugs. Respiration 31:350-357, 1974
59. Bruce RA, Kumar V: The effect of a derivative of vascine on bronchial mucus. Br J Clin Pract 22:289-292, 1968
60. Lachmann B: The effect of ambroxol in newborn and adult animals with surfactant deficiency, in Cosini EV, Scarpelli EM (eds): Pulmonary Surfactant System, Symposia of the Giovanni Lorenzini Foundation, Vol 16. Amsterdam, Elsevier Science Publ., 1983, pp 237-248
61. Wauer RR: Medical treatment of neonatal hyaline membrane disease using bromhexine, ambroxol, and CDP-choline, in Cosini EV, Scarpelli EM (eds): Pulmonary Surfactant System, Symposia of the Giovanni Lorenzini Foundation, Vol 16. Amsterdam, Elsevier Science Publ., 1983, pp 173-188
62. Bertoli L, Rizzato G, Banfi F, et al: Action of ambroxol on mucociliary clearance, in Cosini RV, Scarpelli EM (eds.): Pulmonary Surfactant System, Symposia of the Giovanni Lorenzini Foundation, Vol 16. Amsterdam, Elsevier Science Publ., 1983, pp 349-360
63. Thomson ML, Pavia D, Gregg I, Starke JE: Bromhexene and mucociliary clearance in chronic bronchitis. Br J Dis Chest 68:21-27, 1974
64. Armstrong ML: Double-blind crossover trial of bromhexine in the treatment of chronic bronchitis. Med J Aust 1:612-617, 1976
65. Christensen SB, Kjer J, Ryskjaer S, et al: Mucolytic treatment of chronic bronchitis during two winter periods. Scand J Resp Dis 52:48-57, 1971
66. Stark JE: A controlled trial of the effects of bromhexine on the symptoms of out patients with chronic bronchitis. Brit J Dis Chest 67:49-60, 1973
67. Hamilton WFD, Palmer KNV, Gent M: Expectorant action of bromhexine in chronic obstructive bronchitis. Brit Med J 3:260-261, 1970
68. Gent M, Knowlson PA, Prime JF: Effect of bromhexine on ventilatory capacity in patients with a variety of chest diseases. Lancet 2:1094-1096, 1969
69. Langlands JHM: Double-blind clinical trial of bromhexine as a mucolytic drug in chronic bronchitis. Lancet 1:448-450, 1970
70. Wiesman KJ, Niemeyer K: Klinische ergebnisse bei der behandlung der chronisch obstruktiven bronchitis mit ambroxol im vergleich zu bromhexin. Arzneim Forsch 28(5a):918-921, 1978
71. Boyd EM, Boyd CE: Expectorant activity of water in acute asthma attacks. Am J Dis Child 116:397-399, 1968
72. Wanner A, Aswath R: Clinical indications for and effects of bland, mucolytic and antimicrobial aerosols. Am Rev Respir Dis 122 (Suppl):79-87, 1980
73. Gibson LE: Use of water vapor in the treatment of lower respiratory disease. Am Rev Respir Dis 110 (6, pt 2):100-103, 1974
74. Morrow PE: Aerosol characterization and deposition. Am Rev Resp Dis 110 (6, pt. 2):88-99, 1974
75. Richardson PS, Phipps RJ: The anatomy, physiology, pharmacology and pathology of tracheobronchial mucus secretion and the use of expectorant drugs in human disease. Pharmac Ther B 3:441-479, 1978
76. Parks CR, Alden ER, Standaert TA, et al: The effect of water nebulization on cough transport of pulmonary mucus in the mouth-breathing dog. Am Rev Resp Dis 108:513-519, 1973

77. Doershuk CF, Matthews LW, Gillespie CT, et al: Evaluation of jet type and ultrasonic nebulizers in mist therapy for cystic fibrosis. Pediatrics 41:723-732, 1968
78. Matthews LW, Doershuk CF, Spector S: Mist tent therapy of the obstructive pulmonary lesion of cystic fibrosis. Pediatrics 39:176-185, 1967
79. Taussig LM: Mists and aerosols: New studies, new thoughts. J Pedia 84:619-622, 1974
80. Eschenbacher WL, Boushey HA, Sheppard D: Alteration in osmolarity of inhaled aerosols cause bronchoconstriction and cough, but absence of a permanent anion cause cough alone. Am Rev Resp Dis 129:211-215, 1984
81. Barton AD, Aerosolized detergents and mucolytic agents in the treatment of stable chronic obstructive pulmonary disease. Am Rev Resp Dis 110 (6, pt. 2):104-110, 1974
82. Paez PN, Miller WF: Surface active agents in sputum evacuation: A blind comparison with normal saline solution and distilled water. Chest 60:312-317, 1971
83. Sturgess JM: Mucous secretions in the respiratory tract. Pediatric Clinics of N Am 26:481-501, 1979
84. King M: Mucus and mucociliary clearance. Basics of Resp Dis 11(1):1-8, 1982
85. King M: Viscoelastic properties of airway mucus. Fed Proc 39:3080-3085, 1980
86. Webb WR: New mucolytic agents for sputum liquification. Postgrad Med 36:449-455, 1964
87. Cato AE, Scott JA, Sisson AM: The clinical significance of the hypertonicity of acetylcysteine preparations. Respir Care 22:731-735, 1977
88. Perruchoud A, Ehrsam R, Heita M, et al: Atelectasis of the lung: Bronchoscopic lavage with acetylcysteine. Experience in 51 patients. Eur J Resp Dis 61 (Suppl 111):163-168, 1980
89. Millman M, Goodman AH, Goldstein IM, et al: Status asthmaticus: Use of acetylcysteine during bronchoscopy and lavage to remove mucous plugs. Ann of Allergy 50:85-93, 1983
90. Hirsch SR, Kory RC: An evaluation of the effect of nebulized N-acetyl-L-cysteine on sputum consistency. J Allergy 39:265-273, 1967
91. Hirsch SR, Viernes PF, Kory RC: Clinical and physiological evaluation of mucolytic agents nebulized with isoproterenol: 10% N-acetylcysteine versus 10% 2 mercaptoethane sulfonate. Thorax 25:737-743, 1970
92. Kory RC, Hirsch SR, Giraldo J: Nebulization of N-acetylcysteine combined with a bronchodilator in patients with chronic bronchitis. Dis Chest 54:504-509, 1968
93. Pulle DF, Glass P, Dulfano MJ: A controlled study of the safety and efficiency of acetylcysteine-isoproterenol combination. Curr Ther Res 12:485-492, 1970
94. Grater WC, Cato AC: Double-blind study of acetylcysteine-isoproterenol and saline-isoproterenol in non-hospitalized patients with asthma. Curr Ther Res 15:660-671, 1973
95. Denton R, Kwart H, Litt M: N-acetylcysteine in cystic fibrosis. Am Rev Respir Dis 95:643-51, 1967
96. Wood RE, Boat TF, Doershuk CF: Cystic fibrosis. Am Rev Resp Dis 113:833-878, 1976
97. Aylward M, Maddock J, Dewland P: Clinical evaluation of acetylcysteine in the

98. treatment of patients with chronic obstructive bronchitis: A balanced double-blind trial with placebo control. Eur J Respir Dis 61 (Suppl 111):81-89, 1980
98. Boman G, Bäcker U, Larsson S, et al: Oral acetylcysteine reduces exacerbation rate in chronic bronchitis: Report of a trial organized by the Swedish Society for Pulmonary Diseases. Eur J Respir Dis 64:405-415, 1983
99. Multicenter Study Group: Long-term oral acetylcysteine in chronic bronchitis. A double-blind controlled study. Eur J Resp Dis 61 (Suppl 111):93-108, 1980
100. Roomans GM, Tegner H, Toremalm NG: Acetylcysteine and its derivatives: Functional and morphological effects on tracheal mucosa *in vitro*. Eur J Respir Dis 64:416-425, 1983
101. Lawson D, Saggus BA: N.A.C. and antibiotics in cystic fibrosis. Br Med J 1:317, 1965
102. Aylward M: A between patient double-blind comparison of s-carboxymethylcysteine and bromhexine in chronic obstructive bronchitis. Curr Med Res Opin 1:219-227, 1973
103. Edwards GF, Steel AE, Scott JK, et al: S-carboxymethylcysteine in the fluidification of sputum and treatment of chronic airway obstruction. Chest 40:506-513, 1976
104. Aylward M: An assessment of s-carboxymethylcysteine in the treatment of chronic bronchitis. Curr Med Res Opin 2:387-394, 1974
105. Thomson ML, Pavia D, Jones CJ, et al: No demonstrable effect of S-carboxymethylcysteine on clearance of secretions from the human lung. Thorax 30:669-673, 1975
106. Hirsch SR, Zastrow JE, Kory RC: Sputum liquifying agents: Comparative *in vitro* evaluation. J Lab Clin Med 74:346-353, 1969
107. Steen SN, Ziment I, Freeman D, et al: Evaluation of a new mucolytic drug. Clin Pharmac Ther 16:58-62, 1974
108. Weller PH, Ingram D, Preece MA, et al: Controlled trial of intermittent aerosol therapy with sodium 2-mercaptoethane sulphonate in cystic fibrosis. Thorax 35:42-46, 1980

Richard J. Martin
Robert D. Ballard

8

Respiratory Stimulants

Respiratory stimulants will be defined as agents that increase the respiratory response to alterations in chemical control (hypoxia and hypercapnia) of breathing, augment ventilation without increasing the chemical control of breathing and/or improve ventilation during certain periods of the 24-hour cycle, (e.g., during sleep). These agents can be useful during both the awake and sleep cycles, but they are mostly used for respiratory disorders related to sleep. The first four drugs discussed—medroxyprogesterone acetate, the carbonic anhydrase inhibitors, protriptyline (antidepressants) and oxygen—are mainly, but not exclusively used for sleep related respiratory problems. The second four agents—almitrine, aminophylline, doxapram, and naloxone—are used over a broader day-night cycle.

PROGESTERONE

Mechanism of Action

Progesterone is a respiratory stimulant that increases minute ventilation. The increased progesterone blood levels in the last trimester of pregnancy,[1] and the last portion of the menstrual cycle[2] are associated with a reduced $PaCO_2$ as a result of an increased ventilation. Administration of progesterone to healthy male subjects stimulates ventilation and results in a significant fall in the $PaCO_2$ within 48 hours,[3] and the maximum effect seen within 7 days with the $PaCO_2$ decreasing by 5 mmHg. Progesterone does not necessarily increase the response to exogenous CO_2, but the ventilatory response to exercise is increased. Additionally, a medroxyprogesterone acetate related material has been found in the cerebrospinal fluid, and progesterone (hormonal) receptors have been found to be concentrated in the hyptholamus and hippocampus. These sites appear to work in a feedback system for hormonal control and probably directly or indirectly enhance ventilation.

Progesterone also produces a diuresis that may benefit respiration in certain disease states. In patients with cardiac decompensation, progesterone may lead to improvement in cardiac function, which reduces pulmonary congestion and improves oxygenation, and this in turn may help ventilation centrally (see below, effects of increased oxygen tension).

Indications

Lyons and Huan[4] and Sutton, et al[5] have demonstrated the efficacy of progesterone in a group of patients with probable respiratory abnormalities during sleep. Since polysomnographic studies were not done, it is not possible to determine the exact type of abnormality present in these subjects. In one study of patients with upper airway obstruction, a response to progesterone in four of nine subjects[6] was associated with a low PaO_2 and a tendency towards carbon dioxide retention, while in another,[7] there was no overall response to progesterone in seven patients. In the latter study the apnea time was reduced in five patients, but four still had between 259 and 456 apneic episodes per night. Daytime hypersomnolence did improve slightly, but it still interfered with normal routine functioning.

Clinical experience at our institution has shown that the administration of progesterone successfully treats patients with primary alveolar hypoventilation (i.e., individuals in whom ventilation is reduced, so that $PaCO_2$ is increased). It appears that a subgroup of patients with upper airway obstruction may also respond to this therapy, but this has not been fully elucidated, and further investigation is needed for better definition of the potential responders.

Progesterone has also been used to correct chronic carbon dioxide retention and improve hypoxemia while awake and asleep, in patients with chronic obstructive pulmonary disease (COPD) (8–10). When progesterone (20 mg) was taken orally three times a day for four weeks, there was a significant decrease in arterial carbon dioxide tension while awake (54 ± 2 to 47 ± 2 mmHg) and during nonrapid eye movement (non-REM) sleep (57 ± 2 to 49 ± 2 mmHg)[9]. The fall in carbon dioxide tension was primarily due to an increase in minute ventilation, the tidal volume and mean inspiratory flow (a reflection of neural output) being increased both while awake and during all sleep stages. Correspondingly there was an increase in PaO_2 from 46 ± 3 to 52 ± 4 mmHg during non-REM sleep. It is generally accepted that progesterone therapy will not result in improvement of a PaO_2 of 45 mmHg or less to an acceptable level, and other forms of therapy are required.

The use of progesterone in a healthy population is obviously limited to a specific set of conditions. An example is during sleep when climbing at high altitudes where progesterone has been shown to significantly reduce the number of central apneas. It is of interest in that oxygen desaturation and arousals from sleep were only minimally effected in this study.[11] These findings are in contradistinction to results seen with another respiratory stimulant, acetazolamide, which is discussed below.

Contraindications

The presence of thrombophlebitis and thromboembolic disorders are felt to be a contraindication to the use of progesterone, but there is no evidence to support this contention in the absence of a combination medication with estrogen. Other contraindications are liver abnormalities, breast or genital organ malignancy, and undiagnosed vaginal bleeding.

Dosage

For use as a respiratory stimulant, progesterone is generally given orally at a dose of 20–40 mg three times a day.

Side Effects and Management

Side effects are infrequent, but those which occur most commonly are impotency and alopecia in the male, and glucose intolerance. The impotency may be corrected by supplemental testosterone,[5] and new hair growth occurs following cessation of progesterone.[6] If there is a family history of diabetes mellitus, the blood sugar should be examined frequently in the first several months; otherwise, an occasional blood sugar can be obtained.

Drug Interactions

There are apparently no adverse drug interactions with progesterone.

CARBONIC ANHYDRASE INHIBITORS

The carbonic anhydrase inhibitor (CAI) used most commonly as a respiratory stimulant is acetazolamide (Diamox, Lederle Laboratories, Wayne, New Jersey 07470). Of equal, if not greater, potency and longer duration of action, is dichlorphenamide (Daranide Merck Sharp & Dohme, West Point, Pennsylvania, 19486). Both agents can be used in a wide variety of clinical settings.

Mechanism of Action

The increase in ventilation following administration of acetazolamide is felt to be due to impeding carbon dioxide transport, with resultant increase in cerebrospinal fluid and cerebral PCO_2 and hydrogen ion concentration. These alterations result in a sustained increase in alveolar ventilation. This agent augments the ventilatory response to hypoxia, and causes a parallel shift in the hypoxic ventilatory response curve but does not truly change the slope of the response (i.e., the sensitivity).[12]

Dichlorphenamide causes a similar parallel shift in the ventilatory response to CO_2.[13] The stimulation of ventilation parallels the development of metabolic acidosis, and tissues CO_2 accumulation does not appear to occur.[14] In fact, the cerebrospinal PCO_2 and mixed venous PCO_2 fall by the same amount as the arterial PCO_2. These results suggest that the primary site of action of this agent occurs in the kidney, where a metabolic acidosis is produced, which stimulates ventilation. Additionally, dichlorphenamide differs from acetazolamide in that it produces a chloruresis so that a severe metabolic acidosis is less likely to occur.

Indications

Both carbonic anhydrase inhibitors are particularly useful in those sleep disorders in which central apnea or primary alveolar hypoventilation occurs. Dichlorphenamide has also been shown to improve gas exchange. In patients with chronic obstructive pulmonary disease who have carbon dioxide retention, dichlorphenamide has resulted in clinical improvement associated with an increase in ventilation and improvement in arterial blood gas tensions both at rest and during exercise,[13,14] while acetazolamide has not been shown to lower the $PaCO_2$.

At altitude, acetazolamide raises the mean arterial oxygen saturation during sleep and significantly decreases arousals, while moderately reducing the amount of periodic central apneic type breathing in healthy subjects,[11,12] and in patients.[15] In the latter study there was an overall decrease in the apneas by 69 percent with better quality of sleep and less daytime somnolence. Although there have not been any studies reported, dichlorphenamide has been used successfully for central sleep apneas or primary alveolar hypoventilation in our laboratory, and is the drug of choice.

Contraindications

Carbonic anhydrase inhibitors are contraindicated in patients suffering from hyponatremia or hypokalemia, marked kidney and liver dysfunction or acidosis. In addition, long-term administration of these agents in patients with chronic noncongestive angle closure glaucoma may cause organic closure of the angle, which may not be apparent because of the lowered intraocular pressure. These agents can potentiate the development of calculi so they should not be used in patients with renal calculi.

Dosage

The dosage for acetazolamide is 250 mg orally four times a day and for dichlorphenamide, the dosage is 50–100 mg orally twice daily.

Side Effects

In addition to the long list of potential side effects, which are possible with many drugs, hypokalemia and significant acidosis can develop. The hypokalemia can be corrected by supplemental potassium. If a patient is also on corticosteroids, frequent assessment of serum potassium levels is necessary as the potential for hypokalemia is heightened in this situation.

Acidosis is more likely to occur with acetazolamide. Severe metabolic acidosis is uncommon unless the patient has an underlying process that predisposes him to acidosis. If the pH is less than 7.30, close follow-up is required. While on dichlorphenamide, the pH tends to return towards the predrug baseline.

Drug Interactions

Since carbonic anhydrase inhibitors alkalinize the urine, the excretion of amphetamine, procainamide, quinidine, and tricyclic antidepressants is reduced, so that concomitant administration with these drugs increases their blood levels. Conversely, administration of carbonic anhydrase inhibitors increases the excretion of weak acids, such as phenobarbitol and salicylates. Similarly, the excretion of lithium is also increased. The effectiveness of antibiotics that require an acidic urinary environment in order to be effective in urinary tract infections, (e.g., methenamine), is reduced. These agents are mild diuretics and thus can potentiate the effects of other diuretics.

PROTRIPTYLINE

Protriptyline (Vivactil, Merck Sharp & Dohme, West Point, Pennsylvania 19486) which is in the tricyclic antidepressant category of drugs, has been the most widely evaluated of these agents with regard to respiratory effects. The other tricyclics are likely efficacious to some degree, but they have not been fully evaluated probably because of their sedative effects. Therefore, we will only discuss protriptyline that has very little sedative effect.

Mechanism of Action

Protriptyline is used primarily in patients suffering from obstructive sleep apnea. It is not a respiratory stimulant, in that in most reports the $PaCO_2$ is not affected, but the respiratory pattern is altered. How the change in breathing pattern associated with upper airway obstruction is produced remains unclear, but there are several possible mechanisms. In general, protriptyline is thought to produce competitive blockade of presynaptic α-receptors.[16] Indeed, anecdotal reports have suggested that sleep apnea worsens in patients receiving antihypertensive agents, which may have presynaptic α-agonistic activity.

Another possible mechanism of action is direct or reflex alteration of airway tone by the anticholinergic effects of protriptyline. Many patients placed on this agent state that they are able to swallow food better and no longer have a "choking" sensation. In one study,[17] protriptyline reversed the inspiratory to expiratory flow characteristics suggestive of an upper airway problem in three of four patients.

Lastly, protriptyline decreases the REM stage of sleep, in which the most severe sleep apnea usually occurs. In addition, the apnea time in other stages of sleep is improved, so that the total apnea time during sleep is reduced.

Indications

Protriptyline should be reserved for patients suffering from obstructive sleep apnea, in whom several reports have shown benefits,[17-20] although the success is variable. Although improvement was reported in as much as 58 percent of patients, the overall benefit would appear to be about 15-20 percent. We do not recommend treating other types of apneas or respiratory disorders with this medication.

Contraindications

Protriptyline is contraindicated in patients receiving a monoamine oxidase inhibitor. In addition, it should not be administered during the recovery phase following myocardial infarction, because of the arrhythmias and hypotension that can occur.

Dosage

A wide dose range has been reported, but our suggested schedule is to begin with 10 mg orally one hour before sleep for one week. If the patient does not have significant complaints about a dry mouth or urinary hesitancy, then the dose is increased to 20 mg. It is important to recognize that the effect on the apneas may not be seen for 2-3 weeks after initiation of therapy.

Side Effects

The two most common side effects, dry mouth and urinary hesitancy or retention, which are related to its anticholinegic action, limit the use of this medication. The dry mouth can usually, but not always, be tolerated, but if urinary problems develop, the dosage should be cut back or the drug discontinued.

As indicated earlier, there is a potential for cardiac arrhythmias to develop, because of a direct effect on cardiac conduction and myocardial contractility.[21] However, arrhythmias may actually be less common if there is improvement of the sleep disorder. Protriptyline related arrhythmias have been more prevalent in our laboratory when the dose used was greater than 20 mg. Orthostatic hypotension is another common cardiovascular event that can occur.

Vague psychiatric, neurologic, allergic, hematologic, gastrointestinal, and endocrine effects have also been reported uncommonly.

Drug Interactions

Protriptyline has an additive effect when given with central nervous system depressants, antipsychotic agents, and sympathomimetic drugs. When used in combination with monoamine oxidase inhibitors hyperpyrexia, seizures and hypertensive crises can occur, and if α-adrenergic antihypertensive agents are being administered, hypertension can be worsened.

OXYGEN

Supplemental oxygen is not classically regarded as a respiratory stimulant. In fact, hypoxia increases ventilation as a result of stimulation of the peripheral chemoreceptors, while hyperoxia blunts the receptor output. There is, however, evidence that under certain conditions, "hyperoxia" is a respiratory stimulant.

Mechanism of Action

Since the exact mechanism underlying improvement in respiration during oxygen breathing in patients with sleep apnea is not known, several hypotheses have been entertained.[22] Each involves the relationship between the depressant effect of hyperoxia on peripheral chemoreceptor function and the stimulatory or beneficial effects of oxygen.

Hypoxia by itself stimulates the peripheral chemoreceptors, but depresses central chemoreceptors.[23] In healthy adult humans, there is a transient decrease in ventilation when 100 percent oxygen is breathed, but the long-term effect appears to be stimulatory.[24] The ventilatory stimulation has been attributed to a decrease in cerebral blood flow and an increased PCO_2 in the cerebral tissue by some[25] but others have suggested maintenance of cerebral blood flow if the decrease in arterial PCO_2 is prevented.[26] In premature infants, oxygen decreases or abolishes periodic breathing and stimulates regular respirations.[22-28] Also, ventilation is increased more with high oxygen concentrations containing 2 percent carbon dioxide than with 21 percent oxygen and carbon dioxide,[28] suggesting that the central drive to ventilation is impaired in preterm infants and that this is overcome by breathing oxygen. Our demonstration[22] of a decrease in the number of apneas occurring during sleep when supplemental oxygen was administered could also represent relief of hypoxic ventilatory depression. The time course of the response to the oxygen further suggested that the overall response was the result of two or more divergent effects of increased oxygenation, the benefit coming from the relief of hypoxic disruption of some central nervous system function. The increase in arterial saturation with oxygen was virtually complete after 7.5 minutes, but the decrease in percent apnea time progressed throughout a 30 minute period. This time lag might reflect an alteration in the concentration of some PO_2-sensitive metabolite. Oxygen decreased the percent apnea time and improved the ventilation of seven of the eight patients, but in the one patient, the percent apnea time increased because of prolongation of the apneas without a decrease in frequency, further supporting the likelihood of divergent effects.

Oxygen might also influence the respiratory pattern through an alteration of the interaction between hypoxic and hypercapnic stimuli. Generally, hypoxic and hypercapnic stimuli interact and produce a greater than additive effect. Under certain conditions, however, the combined effect of these two stimuli on ventilatory output may be less than additive and may even be inhibitory. Thus Ou and coworkers[28] showed a negative interaction between hypoxia and eucapnia or hypercapnia in cats.[29] This has also been demonstrated in premature infants,[29] as well as in adults during artificially induced sleep.[30] The severe hypoxemia that is commonly found during sleep in "apnea" patients, may also represent a negative interaction which is obviated by supplemental oxygen.

Finally, the effects of hyperoxia may be due to a diminished gain of the carbon dixoide sensor. For example, the periodic respiration that develops at high altitude or when breathing through a dead space is eliminated by oxygen administration, and this may be due to increased gain of the carbon dioxide sensor produced by hypoxemia.[31]

Indications

All types of apnea (i.e., upper airway obstruction, central apnea and mixed apnea), may be improved by supplemental oxygen.[22,32] It must be stressed, however, that not all patients respond favorably, and it is important to evaluate potential responders. This can be determined in the laboratory,[22] so that a prolonged home trial is not indicated.

Contraindications

At the present time, no true contraindication to oxygen is known, although hypercapnia and acidemia may be aggravated in some patients. Clearly there should be no smoking when oxygen is being administered. Although certain patients may not improve with oxygen and the duration of apneas during sleep may lengthen, cardiac arrhythmias do not become more prevalent.[22,32,33]

Dosage

Oxygen should be administered via nasal prongs at a flow rate between 2-6 liters/min depending on the degree of hypoxemia. If oxygen is not beneficial then alternate forms of therapy are required.

Side Effects

As for any group of patients the side effects of low-flow oxygen include drying of the mucous membrane of the upper airways, minimal epistaxis, ear discomfort, skin reactions from the tape and tubing, and sinusitis.

Drug Interactions

No interactions with other drugs are known.

DOXAPRAM

Doxapram, a respiratory stimulant that became available in 1962,[34] was used initially to treat patients suffering from hypoventilation secondary to general anesthesia.[35] More recently, doxapram has been shown to be effective in other settings, including acute respiratory failure in patients with COPD,[36] and patients with primary alveolar hypoventilation.[37] It has also been used successfully to stimulate ventilation in the newborn,[38] and to treat apnea associated with prematurity.[39]

Mechanism of Action

The mechanism of doxapram's respiratory activity has been studied in animals,[40] anesthetized[41] and awake humans,[42,43] and patients with primary alveolar hypoventilation.[37] The drug produces an increase in resting ventilation, which is manifested primarily by an increase in tidal volume as well as a slight increase in respiratory rate. Its initial effects are mediated through the peripheral carotid chemoreceptors, but as the dosage is increased, the central respiratory center is stimulated with a subsequent change in central timing components, and an increase in respiratory frequency.[43]

Indications

Use of doxapram should be considered in patients who are hypoventilating post-operatively because of general anesthesia, and in patients suffering mild depression of the central nervous system secondary to a drug overdose. It may also be used temporarily when acute respiratory failure develops in COPD. In this situation, concurrent therapy must be directed at reducing the work of breathing, and if necessary intubation and mechanical ventilation implemented to improve alveolar ventilation.

Another possible indication is in the treatment of hypoventilation and recurrent apnea in the newborn and premature infant.[38,39] Additional studies are necessary to evaluate the safety of doxapram in this age group.

Contraindications

Doxapram should not be used to treat patients suffering from respiratory insufficiency associated with other pulmonary conditions such as pulmonary embolism, pneumothorax, acute asthma, adult respiratory distress syndrome, chest wall trauma, restrictive diseases, or neuromuscular disorders. It should also not be used for prolonged periods of time (more than two hours) in any setting of acute respiratory failure in place of intubation and mechanical ventilation, nor should it be used to hasten weaning from mechanical ventilation.

Other contraindications include severe hypertension, coronary artery disease, severe congestive heart failure, and a history of a seizure disorder, hyperthyroidism, or pheochromocytoma. Its safety in pregnancy has not been evaluated.

Dosage

Doxapram is only available in an injectible form, and is best administered by continuous intravenous infusion. For post-anesthetic depression, infusion is begun at a rate of 5 mg/min and continued until there is an appropriate ventilatory response. At that time the infusion rate should be reduced to maintain ventilation with minimal side effects. The maintenance dose is usually in the range of 1–3 mg/min, which may be continued to a maximal total dose of 4 mg/kg, not to exceed 600 mg.

In a drug overdose, an initial dose of 2 mg/kg can be administered intravenously and repeated in 5 minutes. If the patient responds, a continuous infusion should be started at a rate of 1–3 mg/min. This should be continued until the patient awakens or two hours have elapsed, the total dose not to exceed 600 mg.

When acute respiratory failure develops in patients with COPD, a continuous infusion can be started at rate of 1–2 mg/min, and increased to a maximum of 3 mg/min if necessary. Administration should not be prolonged beyond two hours.

All patients undergoing therapy with doxapram should be monitored in an intensive care setting, with frequent arterial blood gases to detect progressive hypercapnia and acidosis, and to help determine appropriate infusion rates.

Side Effects

Patients receiving doxapram are often aware of a generalized sensation of warmth, most notable in the perineal region. They may suffer some central nervous system effects, including headache, dizziness, agitation, and disorientation. Rarely, seizures may occur. Other potential side effects include progressive dyspnea, bronchospasm, an elevated blood pressure, cardiac arrhythmias, various gastrointestinal complaints, and urinary retention. Severe side effects are uncommon at the recommended dosages, but should they occur, reduction of the infusion rate, or total discontinuation of the drug with symptomatic therapy is usually adequate to treat the complications.

Drug Interactions

Because of possible additive pressor effects, doxapram should be used very cautiously in patients receiving sympathomimetic or monoamine oxidase inhibiting drugs. Doxapram is known to increase epinephrine release, so that its administration should be delayed for at least 10 minutes after discontinuation of anesthetics such as halothane, cyclopropane, and enflurane, which are known to sensitize the myocardium to catecholamines.

NALOXONE

The respiratory depressant effects of exogenous opiates have been well described.[44] Endogenous opiates (endorphins) and opiate receptors have been found in high concentration in the medulla[45] so that a role for endorphins in the central control of respiration has been suspected.

In certain situations, endorphins may depress spontaneous ventilation in animals, and this is blocked by naloxone, an opiate antagonist. In humans, naloxone clearly blocks respiratory depression induced by exogenous opiates,[46] and is effective in reversing respiratory depression secondary to diazepam[47] and ethanol[48] overdose. There have also been reports of benefit in acute respiratory failure superimposed on COPD, as well as other acute illnesses.[49,50] However, conflicting data have been reported in normal subjects and stable patients with

COPD. In some studies, high doses of naloxone did not alter ventilatory and mouth occlusion pressure responses to hypercapnia and hypoxia in normal subjects[51] or change the breathing pattern significantly in patients with stable COPD.[52] Others reported that high doses of naloxone significantly increased ventilatory and mouth occlusion pressure responses to hypercapnia in both normal subjects and patients with stable COPD.[53] In addition, Santiago et al[54] showed that high dose naloxone could restore the load-compensating response in patients with COPD who previously lacked this response. It would appear that the respiratory effects of naloxone are small and variable, suggesting that this agent is of minimal use in the vast majority of respiratory disease patients.

Mechanism of Action

Although the mechanism of action of naloxone is not entirely understood, the majority of data suggest that it antagonizes the opioid effects of exogenous and endogenous opiates by competing for opiate receptor sites.

Indications

The use of naloxone is indicated to reverse CNS and respiratory depression due to opioids, including narcotics, propoxyphene, methadone, nalbuphine, pentazocine, and butorphanol, and respiratory depression secondary to diazepam or ethanol overdose. In addition, studies indicate that naloxone may be used effectively to treat acute respiratory failure in other settings, including that secondary to COPD where the goal is to increase ventilatory drive and thereby decrease CO_2 retention. However, results of such therapy in the latter situation have been extremely variable, and naloxone should not be considered an appropriate alternative to intubation and mechanical ventilation. Naloxone has been only briefly evaluated in the treatment of obstructive sleep apnea, with no apparent benefit.[55]

Contraindications

Naloxone should be used with caution in patients with preexisting cardiac disease. As there are no adequate studies in pregnant women, naloxone should be used in pregnancy only if it is clearly needed. Finally, naloxone therapy should never be considered as an appropriate alternative to intubation and mechanical ventilation when such therapy is clearly indicated.

Dosage

Naloxone is available for intravenous, intramuscular, and subcutaneous use. When a narcotic overdose is suspected, 0.4 mg to 2 mg of naloxone should be given intravenously, and may be repeated at 3 minute intervals to a maximal total dose of 10 mg. If there is no observed response, the diagnosis of narcotic toxicity should be questioned. Alternatively, continuous intravenous infusion may be instituted, in which case the infusion rate should be titrated according to each patient's response.

To reverse post-operative narcotic depression, smaller doses in the range of 0.1 to 0.2 mg should be administered. Alternatively, a continuous intravenous infusion at a rate of 0.066 microg/kg/min has been safely and effectively used.

Dosages ranging from 2–50 mg have been administered as intravenous boluses to healthy subjects, to patients with stable COPD, as well as to patients suffering from acute respiratory failure with variable results.

Side Effects

Little evidence of toxicity has been reported even at the highest doses. When reversing narcotic depression, however, the patient may experience nausea, emesis, diaphoresis, tachycardia, agitation, and elevated blood pressure. In addition, there are reports of hypotension, hypertension, and cardiac arrhythmias in the post-operative setting, but a causal relationship to naloxone has not been clearly established.

Drug Interactions

No interaction with other drugs is known.

ALMITRINE

Almitrine bimesylate is an interesting agent that is continuing to undergo extensive clinical evaluation in both the United States and Europe. It is a piperazine derivative that stimulates ventilation in animals, healthy individuals, and patients with COPD.[56-59] In addition, it would appear to improve ventilation-perfusion matching in patients with COPD.[60,61]

Mechanism of Action

Almitrine stimulates the peripheral chemoreceptors, and has very little effect on the medullary respiratory center.[56] It increases ventilation, and alters the pattern of breathing.[62] It also augments the hypoxic ventilatory response significantly, but increases the ventilatory response to hypercapnia minimally in normal subjects and COPD patients.[57,58] Others have found the ventilatory effects of almitrine to be variable, noting that improvement in oxygenation is often disproportionate to any observed increase in minute ventilation. It has subsequently been demonstrated that ventilation-perfusion inequality is reduced after almitrine in patients with COPD,[63] an effect that is felt to be secondary to enhanced hypoxic pulmonary vasoconstriction.[60,61,64]

Indications

Current data suggest that almitrine may be beneficial in the long term therapy of COPD patients. One large multicenter trial demonstrated that six months of daily therapy with oral almitrine was associated with a reduction in dyspnea and an increase in ventilation. The patients demonstrated persistent, significant improvements in PaO_2 and $PaCO_2$, with a reduction in the number of hospitalizations for acute exacerbations.[59] Because it apparently has the dual effects of stimulating ventilation and improving gas exchange, almitrine will no doubt prove to be very effective in the treatment of acute respiratory failure superimposed on COPD. It should be noted, however, that almitrine is still under investigation and ongoing clinical trials are necessary to determine its future role in the treatment of respiratory disease.

Finally, almitrine has been found to be useful in the treatment of nocturnal hypoxemia in patients with COPD,[65] and to decrease the mean duration of hypopneas, obstructive, and mixed apneas in non-REM sleep.[66] On the other hand, almitrine does not reduce the frequency or duration of central apneas.[65,66]

Contraindications

Almitrine has been well tolerated in multiple age groups with various coinciding illnesses. It has been suggested that liver insufficiency may alter the pharmacokinetics and absorption of the drug, so that it should be used with caution in patients with liver disease.[67]

Dosage

Doses of 50 and 100 mg given orally once or twice a day are effective and well tolerated in the long term therapy of patients with COPD,[59] and doses up to 400 mg/day have been well tolerated.[68] Because of the long half-life of almitrine (35-64 hours) it may take 10-15 days for the serum level to reach a plateau.

Almitrine has also been administered intravenously at a dose of 0.25-1.0 mg/kg/hr, which resulted in significant augmentation of the hypoxic ventilatory drive with only minimal side effects.[57]

Side Effects

Side effects of almitrine at doses previously used have been relatively minor, with only slight increases in heart rate and blood pressure reported. When administered in the fasting state, some subjects have complained of mild headache and nausea. At high doses, an increased sensation of dyspnea may be experienced during physical exertion.

Drug Interactions

Except for some evidence that calcium antagonists may block the vasoconstrictor effect of almitrine in an *in vitro* animal model,[69] no drug interactions have been reported at the present time.

THEOPHYLLINE

Theophylline is a dimethylated xanthine, and its bronchodilator effects in acute and chronic airway obstruction have been discussed in an earlier chapter. This agent also stimulates breathing, and was used as early as 1930 to restore normal ventilation in patients with Cheyne-Stokes respiration.[70] Subsequent investigators found that administration of aminophylline increases minute ventilation and hypoxic ventilatory drive, while decreasing arterial PCO_2[71,72] in healthy subjects.

In addition, aminophylline has been shown to improve diaphragmatic contractility and to render it less susceptible to fatigue in normal humans[73,74] and in a patient after high cervical cordotomy.[75] In view of the recent studies demonstrating less than expected bronchodilator activity of aminophylline in normal and asthmatic subjects,[76,77] it may be that the drug's effect on ventilatory drive and the diaphragm are more significant in the clinical setting than previously suspected.

Mechanism of Action

The mechanism by which theophylline augments ventilatory drive is unclear. It has been suggested that the drug may increase the ventilatory response to hypoxia by increasing the metabolic rate,[78] or by stimulating the central and peripheral chemoreceptors directly.[79]

The ability of theophylline to augment diaphragmatic contractility has also been offered as a partial explanation for the drug's apparent effect on hypoxic drive.[73] The mechanism by which the drug affects the diaphragm is poorly understood. The methyl xanthines' ability to inhibit cyclic nucleotide phosphodiesterases may alter cyclic AMP metabolism, facilitating neuromuscular transmission.[73] Alternatively, the drug may interact with the endoplasmic reticulum or plasma membrane of muscle cells to mobilize calcium ions, thereby affecting the contractile elements.[73]

Indications

As described in Chapter 2, theophylline is effective in the treatment of asthmatic patients during acute exacerbations, as well as the long-term therapy of the stable patient. The use of theophylline is also clearly indicated in the treatment of recurrent apnea of prematurity,[80] where it has been shown to decrease the frequency and duration of apneic episodes.

Theophylline is also indicated when acute respiratory failure develops in patients with COPD, where its beneficial effects include improvement of ventilatory drive and diaphragmatic contractility, as well as bronchodilation. For these reasons, we feel that theophylline is beneficial in the long-term therapy of the stable patient with COPD, even in the face of spirometric evidence suggesting irreversible airways obstruction.

Theophylline has been only briefly evaluated in the therapy of obstructive sleep apnea, with no apparent benefit.[55] In our experience, theophylline may be useful in patients suffering from progressive neuromuscular disorders, which often terminate in acute respiratory failure, but more studies are required.

Contraindications

The contraindications to the use of theophylline are well described in Chapter 2, and include medical illnesses (particularly severe congestive heart failure) which prolong the half-life of the drug, and thus may elevate serum theophylline to toxic levels. It is important to stress that intravenous aminophylline therapy is an important adjunct to therapy of acute respiratory failure but should not be utilized as a substitute for intubation and mechanical ventilation when they are clearly indicated.

Dosage

The dose of theophylline administered for the management of bronchoconstriction is well described in Chapter 2. As indicated there, individual doses and schedules should be adjusted to each patient to maintain a serum theophylline level that is associated with the maximum FEV_1 and no side effects, usually between 10 and 20 mcg/ml.

In management of the apnea of prematurity, a loading dose of 5 mg/kg followed by doses of 2–2.5 mg/kg two to three times a day is usually optimal. Serum concentrations in the range of 5 to 10 mg/ml appear adequate in this setting.

Side Effects

The side effects of theophylline have been described in Chapter 2. Briefly, they include nausea, emesis, abdominal pain, diarrhea, palpitations, cardiac arrhythmias, and multiple central nervous system symptoms, including headache, agitation, seizures, and even coma. Note that theophylline is dialyzable, and charcoal hemoperfusion should be considered in severe toxic reactions. Alternatively, oral charcoal has also been demonstrated to increase theophylline clearance.

Interactions

Again, these are discussed in detail in an earlier chapter. Theophylline is known to interact with many drugs. For example, tobacco smoking, phenytoin, phenobarbital, and carbamazepine are known to increase theophylline clearance. Propanolol, corticosteroids, troleandomycin, erythromycin, and cimetidine have been shown to decrease clearance. Theophylline has also been known to increase the metabolism of phenytoin, so that phenytoin serum levels are lowered. Finally, the concurrent use of aminophylline and halothane may provoke cardiac arrhythmias, probably secondary to release of catecholdmines and sensitization of the myocardium to catecholamines by halothane.

References

1. Goodland RL, Reynolds JG, Pommerenke WT: Alveolar carbon dioxide tension levels during pregnancy and early puerperium. J Clin Endocrinol 14:522–530, 1954
2. Doring GH, Loescheke HH: Atmung und saure-basengleichgewicht in der schwangerschast. Pfluegers Arch Gesumte Physiol Menschen Tiere 249:437–451, 1947
3. Skatrud JB, Dempsey JA, Kaiser DG: Ventilatory response to medroxyprogesterone acetate in normal subjects: Time course and mechanism. J Appl Physiol: Respir Environ Exercise Physiol 44:939–944, 1978
4. Lyons HA, Huang CT: Therapeutic use of progesterone in alveolar hypoventilation associated with obesity. Am J Med 44:881–888, 1968
5. Sutton FD, Zwillich CW, Creagh CE, et al: Progesterone for outpatient treatment of Pickwickian Syndrome. Ann Intern Med 83:476–479, 1975
6. Strohl KP, Hensley MJ, Saunders NA, et al: Progesterone administration and progressive sleep apnea. J Am Med Assoc 245:1230–1232, 1981
7. Orr WC, Imes NK, Martin RJ: Progesterone therapy in obese patients with sleep apnea. Arch Intern Med 139:109–111, 1979
8. Skatrud JB, Dempsey JA, Bhansuli P, et al: Determinants of chronic carbon dioxide retention and its correction in humans. J Clin Invest 65:813–821, 1980
9. Skatrud JB, Dempsey JA, Iber C: Correction of CO_2 retention during sleep in patients with chronic obstructive pulmonary disease. Am Rev Respir Dis 124:260–268, 1981
10. Skatrud JB, Dempsey JA: Relative effectiveness of acetazolamide versus medroxyprogesterone acetate in correction of chronic carbon dioxide retention. Am Rev Respir Dis 127:405–412, 1983
11. Weil JV, Kruger MH, Scoggin CH: Sleep and breathing at high altitude. In: Guil-

leminault C, Dement W, eds. Sleep apnea syndrome. New York: Alan R. Liss 119-136, 1978
12. Sutton JR, Houston CS, Mansell AL, etc: Effect of acetazolamide on hypoxemia during sleep at high altitude. N Engl J Med 301:1329-1331, 1979
13. Naimark A, Brodovsky DM, Cherniack RM: The effect of new carbonic anhydrase inhibitor (dichlorphenamide) in respiratory insufficiency. Am J Med 28:368-375, 1960
14. Naimark A, Cherniack RM: Effect of dichlorphenamide on gas exchange and CSF acid-base state in chronic respiratory failures. Canad Med Assoc J 94:164-170, 1966
15. White DP, Zwillich CW, Pickett CK, et al: Central sleep apnea: Improvement with acetazolamide therapy. Arch Intern Med 142:1816-1819, 1982
16. Van Zwieten PA, Paver M, Van Spenning HW, et al: Interaction between centrally acting hypotensive drugs and tricyclic antidepressants. Arch Int Pharmacodyn Ther 214:12-30, 1975
17. Smith PL, Haponik EF, Allen RP, et al: The effects of protriptyline in sleep-disordered breathing. Am Rev Respir Dis 127:8-13, 1983
18. Clark RW, Schmidt HS, Schaal SF, et al: Sleep apnea: Treatment with protriptyline. Neurol 29:1287-1292, 1979
19. Brownell LG, West P, Sweatman P, et al: Protriptyline in obstructive sleep apnea. N Engl J Med 307:1037-1042, 1982
20. Conway WA, Zorick F, Piccione P, et al: Protriptyline in the treatment of sleep apnea. Thorax 37:49-53, 1982
21. Jefferson JW: A review of the cardiovascular effects and toxicity of tricyclic antidepressants. Psychosom Med 37:160-179, 1975
22. Martin RJ, Sanders MH, Gray BA, et al: Acute and long-term ventilatory effects of hyperoxia in the adult sleep apnea syndrome. Am Rev Respir Dis 125:175-180, 1982
23. Watt JG, Dumke PR, Comroe JH Jr: Effects of inhalation of 100 percent and 14 percent oxygen upon respiration of unanesthetized dogs before and after chemoreceptor denervation. Am J Physiol 138:610-617, 1943
24. Shock NW, Soley MH: Effects of breathing pure oxygen on respiratory volume in humans. Proc Soc Exp Biol Med 44:418-419, 1940
25. Lassen NA: Cerebral blood flow and oxygen consumption in man. Physiol Rev 39:183-238, 1959
26. Turner JE, Lambertsen CJ, Owen SG, et al: Effect of .08 and .8 atmosphere of inspired PO_2 upon cerebral hemodynamics at a "constant" alveolar PCO_2 of 43 mm H_2 (abstract). Fed Proc 16:130, 1957
27. Wilson JL, Long SB, Howard PJ: Respiration in premature infants: Response to variations of oxygen and to increased carbon dioxide in inspired air. Am J Dis Child 63:1080-1085, 1942
28. Ou LC, Miller MJ, Tenney SM: Hypoxia and carbon dioxide as separate and interactive depressants of ventilation. Respir Physiol 28:347-358, 1976
29. Rigatto H, Varduzco RT, Cates DB: Effects of O_2 on the ventilatory response to CO_2 in premature infants. J Appl Physiol 39:896-899, 1975
30. Honda Y, Natsui T: Effects of sleep on ventilatory response to CO_2 in severe hypoxia. Respir Physiol 3:220-228, 1967

31. Reite M, Jackson D, Cahoon RL, et al: Sleep physiology at high altitude. Electroencephalogr Clin Neurophysiol 38:463-471, 1975
32. McNicholas WT, Carter JL, Rutherford R, et al: Beneficial effect of oxygen in primary alveolar hypoventilation with central sleep apnea. Am Rev Respir Dis 125:773-775, 1982
33. Zwillich C, Devlin T, White D, et al: Bradycardia during sleep apnea: Its chracteristics and mechanisms. J Clin Invest 69:1286-1292, 1982
34. Ward JW, Franko BV: A new centrally acting agent (AHR-619) with marked respiratory stimulating, pressor and "awakening" effects. (Abstract) Fed Proc 21:325, 1962
35. Mauro AL, Labartino L, Mojdehi E, et al: Use of doxapram hydrochloride to restore respiration in anesthetized man. Am J Med Sci 250:269-274, 1965
36. Moser KM, Luchsinger PC, Adamson JS, et al: Respiratory stimulation with intravenous doxapram in respiratory failure. N Engl J Med 288:427-431, 1973
37. Lugliani R, Whipp BJ, Wasserman K: Doxapram hydrochloride: A respiratory stimulant for patients with primary alveolar hypoventilation. Chest 76(4):414-419, 1979
38. Gupta PK, Moore J: The use of doxapram in the newborn. J Obst Gynec Brit Comm 80:1002-1006, 1973
39. Sagi E, Eyal F, Alpan G, et al: Idiopathic apnea of prematurity treated with doxapram and aminophylline. Arch Dis Child 59(3):281-283, 1984
40. Hirsch K, Wang SC: Selective respiratory stimulating action of doxapram compared to pentylnetetrazol. J Pharm Exp Ther 189:1-11, 1974
41. Scott RM, Whitwam JG, Chakrabati MK: Evidence of a role for the peripheral chemoreceptors in the ventilatory response to doxapram in man. Br J Anesth 49:227-231, 1977
42. Calverley PM, Robson RH, Wraith PK, et al: The ventilatory effects of doxapram in normal man. Clin Sci 65(1):65-69, 1983
43. Burki NK: Ventilatory effects of doxapram in conscious human subjects. Chest 85(5):600-605, 1984
44. Weil JV, McCullough RE, Kline JS, et al: Diminished ventilatory response to hypoxia and hypercapnia after morphine in normal man. N Engl J Med 292:1103-1106, 1975
45. Atweh SF, Kuharsence MJ: Autoradiographic localization of opiate receptors in rat brain II—the brainstem. Brain Res 129:1-12, 1977
46. Akil H, Mayer DJ, Leibeskind JC: Antagonism of stimulation-produced analgesia by naloxone, a narcotic antagonist. Science 191:961-962, 1976
47. Jordan C: Respiratory depression following diazepam; reversal with high dose naloxone. Anesthesiology 53:293-298, 1980
48. Michiels TM, Light RW, Mahutte CK: Naloxone reverses ethanol-induced depression of hypercapnic drive. Am Rev Respir Dis 128:823-826, 1983
49. Ayres J, Rees J, Lee T: Intravenous naloxone in acute respiratory failure. Br Med J 284:927-8, 1982
50. Williams AJ, Tarn AC, DeBelder MA, et al: Naloxone in acute respiratory failure. Lancet 2(8313):1470, 1982
51. Fleetham JA, Clarke H, Dhingra S, et al. Endogenous opiates and chemical control of breathing in humans. Am Rev Respir Dis 121:1045-1049, 1980

52. Tobin MJ, Jenouri G, Sackner MA: Effect of naloxone on breathing pattern in patients with chronic obstructive pulmonary disease with and without hypercapnia. Respiration 44:419–424, 1983
53. Tabona MV, Ambrosino N, Barnes PJ: Endogenous opiates and control of breathing in normal subjects and patients with chronic airflow obstruction. Thorax 38:834–839, 1982
54. Santiago TV, Remolina C, Scoles V, et al: Endorphins and the control of breathing. N Engl J Med 304(20):1190–1195, 1981
55. Guilleminault C, Hayes B: Naloxone, theophylline, bromocriptine and obstructive sleep apnea: Negative results. Bull Eur Physio Pathol Respir 19(6):632–634, 1983
56. Laubie M, Schmitt H: Long lasting hyperventilation induced by almitrine: Evidence for a specific effect on carotid and thoracic chemoreceptors. Eur J Pharm 61:125–136, 1980
57. Stanley NN, Galloway JM, Gordon B, et al: Increased respiratory chemosensitivity induced by infusing almitrine intravenously in healthy man. Thorax 38:200–204, 1983
58. Stanley NN, Pieczora JA, Pauly N: Effects of almitrine bimesylate on chemosensitivity in patients with chronic airways obstruction. Eur J Respir Dis (Suppl 126) 64:233–237, 1983
59. Arnaud F, Bertrand A, Charpin J, et al: Long term almitrine bimesylate treatment in patients with chronic bronchitis and emphysema: A multicenter double-blind placebo controlled study. Eur J Respir Dis (Suppl 126) 64:323–329, 1983
60. Melot C, Naeije R, Rothschild T, et al: Improvement of ventilation-perfusion matching by almitrine in COPD. Chest 83(3):528–533, 1983
61. Castaing Y, Manier G, Guenard H: VA/Q ratios distribution and oral almitrine bimesylate in COPD patients under mechanical ventilation: Preliminary results. Eur J Respir Dis (Suppl 126) 64:243–247, 1983
62. Stradling JB, Nicholl CG, Cover D, et al: The effects of oral almitrine on pattern of breathing and gas exchange in patients with chronic obstructive pulmonary disease. Clin Sci 66:435–442, 1984
63. Wagner PD, Saltzman HA, West JB: Measurement of continuous distributions of ventilation-perfusion ratios: Theory. J Appl Physiol 36:588–599, 1979
64. Thenot A: Alitrine bimesylate: Facts, deductions and therapeutic perspectives. Eur J Respir Dis (Suppl 126) 64:331–332, 1983
65. Douglas NJ, Connaughton JJ, Morgan AD, et al: Effect of almitrine on nocturnal hypoxemia in chronic bronchitis and emphysema, and in patients with central sleep apnea. Bull Eur Physiopath Resp 19:631, 1983
66. Krieger J, Mangin P, Kurtz D: Effects of almitrine in the treatment of sleep apnea syndromes. Bull Eur Physiopath Resp 19:630, 1983
67. Bromet N, Courte S, Aubert Y, et al: Pharmacokinetics of almitrine bimesylate: Studies in patients. Eur J Respir Dis (Suppl 126) 64:363–375, 1983
68. Maclcod CN, Thomas RW, Bartlcy EA, ct al: Effects and handling of almitrine bimesylate in healthy subjects. Eur J Respir Dis (Suppl 126) 64:275–289, 1983
69. Lockhart A: Pharmacologic properties of almitrine bimesylate. Eur J Respir Dis (Suppl 126) 64:225–231, 1983
70. Vogl A: Uber den mechanisms und die behandlung der zentralen dyspnoe. Klin Wochenschr 9:783–786, 1930

71. Lakshminarayan S, Sahn SA, Weil JV: Effect of aminophylline on ventilatory responses in normal man. Am Rev Respir Dis 117:33–38, 1978
72. Sanders JS, Berman TM, Bartlett MM, et al: Increased hypoxic ventilatory drive due to administration of aminophylline in normal men. Chest 78(2):279–282, 1980
73. Aubier M, Detroyer A, Sampson M, et al: Aminophylline improves diaphragmatic contractility. N Engl J Med 305:249–252, 1981
74. Sigrist S, Thomas D, Hovall S: The effect of aminophylline in inspiratory muscle activity. Am Rev Respir Dis 126:46–50, 1982
75. Chevrolet JC, Reverdin A, Suter PM: Ventilatory dysfunction resulting from bilateral anterolateral high cervical cordotomy. Chest 84:112–115, 1983
76. Estenne M, Yernault JC, Detroyer A: Effects of parenteral aminophylline on lung mechanics in normal humans. Am Rev Respir Dis 121:967–971, 1980
77. Rossing TH, Fanta CH, Goldstein DH, et al: Emergency therapy of asthma: Comparison of the acute effects of parenteral and inhaled sympathomimetics and infused aminophylline. Am Rev Respir Dis 122:365–371, 1980
78. Richmond GH: Action of caffeine and aminophylline as respiratory stimulants in man. J Appl Physiol 2:16–26, 1949
79. Stroud MW, Lambertsen CH, Ewing JH, et al: The effects of aminophylline and meperidine alone and in combination on the respiratory response to carbon dioxide inhalation. J Pharm Exp Ther 114:461–469, 1955
80. Aranda JV, Turmen T: Methylxanthines in apnea of prematurity. Clin Perinatol 6:87–93, 1979

G. S. Worthen

9

Pulmonary Vasodilators

Agents that dilate the pulmonary blood vessels have been employed largely in an attempt to treat pulmonary hypertension, and the use of these agents in this disorder forms the basis of this chapter. The material presented illustrates that vasodilator treatment of pulmonary hypertension is fraught with hazard, frequently unsuccessful, and must be accompanied by objective measurements of physiologic response.

PULMONARY HYPERTENSION

Pulmonary hypertension, defined as a mean pulmonary artery pressure greater than 25 mmHg can be a primary or secondary feature of several types of lung disease. The sequelae of long-standing pulmonary hypertension include right ventricular (RV) hypertrophy, dilation, and failure, with accompanying peripheral edema, and an inability to increase cardiac output (CO) leading to exercise intolerance and syncope.

Physiology

The pulmonary artery pressure (PAP) is modulated by a variety of factors, which include pulmonary vascular resistance (PVR), left atrial pressure, and cardiac output.[1] The cardiac output may be altered by RV preload and RV contractility. In the normal pulmonary vasculature, a significant increase in cardiac output is associated with a minimal rise in PAP because of the great

DRUGS FOR THE RESPIRATORY SYSTEM
ISBN 0-8089-1818-4

Copyright © 1986 by Grune & Stratton, Inc.
All rights of reproduction in any form reserved.

distensibility of the pulmonary vascular bed, and (most important) by recruitment of new capillary beds.[2] With mild to moderate limitation or restriction of the capillary bed, PAP may remain within normal limits while at rest, but will increase during exercise. Similarly, pulmonary vasoconstriction—for instance, as a result of hypoxia, may occur in local areas of the lung. As a result, blood flow may be redistributed to other lung zones without resulting in an increase in PAP. These two situations help explain why pulmonary hypertension is often recognized only when it is long-standing, and thus, less susceptible to therapy.

Therapy

There is, at this time, no specific treatment for pulmonary hypertension of any etiology. Hopefully, the pathogenesis of all forms of pulmonary hypertension will be elucidated in the future, but at the present time, treatment of the primary form is so unsatisfactory that a thorough search for secondary causes is in order. This being the case, it is important at the outset to determine whether pulmonary hypertension is primary (or idiopathic) (i.e., there is no evidence of other lung disease), or secondary to a pathologic process within the heart and lung (Table 9-1). Such studies may include radionuclide scintigraphy, venography, complete assessment of lung function, echocardiography, and polysomnography, in addition to more routine studies.

If an underlying cause is found, initial therapeutic efforts should be directed at the cardiac or pulmonary pathology. Improvement in airflow resistance and in gas exchange in patients with right ventricular failure will usually markedly improve the failure.[3-5] Similarly, anticoagulation in patients with pulmonary emboli may prevent further occurrences and perhaps allow for resolution.[6] Further, mitral valve replacement in patients with pulmonary hypertension due to mitral stenosis frequently results in improvement (although slowly).[7] Thus, if the underlying pathologic circumstances can be altered, pulmonary hypertension is potentially reversible. On the other hand, this is not true of primary pulmonary hypertension, where the underlying pathogenesis is unknown. Accordingly, therapy has generally been targeted directly at the pulmonary vasculature using

Table 9-1
Causes of Pulmonary Hypertension

Idiopathic	Secondary
Primary Pulmonary Hypertension	Chronic Obstructive Lung Disease (Cor Pulmonale)
Pulmonary veno-occlusive disease	Alveolar Hypoxia
	Pulmonary thrombo-embolic disease
Pulmonary capillary hemangiomatosis	Mitral Stenosis

vasodilator agents. Unfortunately, to date, treatment with vasodilators has not been shown to prolong survival, or to alter the pathologic process.

Current treatment of a high PAP with vasodilators is based on the assumption that the high pressures are due to pulmonary vasoconstriction. In a few situations, particularly alveolar hypoxia, this is largely the case. In other situations, however, high PAP may be due to a restricted pulmonary vascular bed, and thus might not be expected to respond well to vasodilator agents. There is, however, evidence that recruitment of new vascular channels may occur even in pulmonary hypertension,[8] perhaps allowing for an increased cardiac output and pulmonary blood flow with exercise. In addition, the obliterative type of pulmonary hypertension may also be associated with vasospastic events.[9] Thus, the two forms (vasoconstriction vs. limited vascular bed) may overlap to some degree.

Vasodilators

General principles. As stated in a recent review,[10] the goals of vasodilators in pulmonary hypertension therapy, are "the sustained restoration of hemodynamic variables towards normal values both at rest and during exercise; the alleviation of clinical symptoms and enhancement of exercise tolerance; and ultimately, reversal of the pulmonary vasoconstrictive process, regression of RV hypertrophy and prolongation of life." How can this best be accomplished? The desired hemodynamic response would be a fall in PAP towards normal and a sustained or increased cardiac output without a deleterious effect on systemic blood pressure, but as yet, no vasodilator fulfills these criteria in more than a few percent of cases. Inherent in these goals is the need to measure hemodynamic parameters in order to quantify the response and evaluate the effectiveness of a given agent.

Given the limitations of vasodilator therapy, it is important to keep in mind the criteria above. Decreasing the PAP *per se* is of itself not particularly valuable, if it is accompanied by a fall in cardiac output and further exercise limitation. Decreasing the PVR if due to systemic vasodilation, increasing the cardiac output and pulmonary vascular recruitment almost certainly improve exercise tolerance even if PAP is not decreased.[11] Since survival in patients with pulmonary hypertension is in general predicted by the cardiac output and PVR,[12] there are reasons to suspect that improved PVR and cardiac output may improve mortality. Thus, the goal should be to selectively diminish the PVR. Rich and colleagues have suggested that selective pulmonary vasodilation would be reflected in a greater fall in PVR than in systemic vascular resistance (SVR).[13]

From the above discussion, it is apparent that there may be several different types of response following administration of pulmonary vasodilators. Systemic vasodilation due to vasodilators may be greater than that of the pulmonary vasculature. If such a response is accompanied by an increase in cardiac output due either to the inotropic effects of certain vasodilators,[14] sympathetic activation,[15] or improved venous return,[16] then the PAP may actually increase. If, on the other hand, the cardiac output fails to increase, severe systemic hypotension may result. Such hypotension may lead to poor perfusion of the RV and worsen its performance.[17] Similarly, the negative inotropic effects of some vasodilators may impede RV function and further contribute to RV failure. Finally, pulmonary vasodilators may prevent normal ventilation-perfusion matching that contributes to maintenance of normal oxygen tension.[18] Thus, hypoxemia may occur as a consequence of perfusion of poorly ventilated regions.

Specific Vasodilators (Table 9-2)

β-Adrenergic Agonists

Isoproterenol. Isoproterenol is a sympathomimetic amine specific for β-adrenergic receptors. Its infusion produces peripheral vasodilation, an increased heart rate and enhanced cardiac contractility through its positive inotropic effect on the heart, all tending to increase cardiac output.[19] PVR often decreases, but PAP may increase by a significant amount if the cardiac output increases in a patient with a limited vascular bed,[16,20] and this can be accompanied by severe chest pain and dyspnea.[16] Hypoxemia has been reported,[20] presumably due to increased mismatching of ventilation and perfusion in the lungs. In patients who have had salutory responses to the acute administration of isoproterenol, a few have been observed to have sustained responses to chronic-sublingual administration,[21] but they are in the minority.[20] Whether lack of response is secondary to disease progression, down-regulation of β-receptors,[22] or some other mechanism remains unclear.

The dosage of isoproterenol utilized is 1 μg/min I.V. increasing by 1 μg/min every five minutes to a maximum of 5 μg/min or until the heart rate reaches 120/min and the systolic PAP increases by 10 mmHg. On a chronic basis, the sublingual preparation, 10 mgm is taken every four hours.

α-Adrenergic Antagonists

The role of the sympathetic nervous system in pulmonary hypertension remains unclear. For instance, attempts to inhibit α-adrenergic action on the pulmonary vasculature in Primary Pulmonary Hypertension (PPH) using stellate ganglion blockade or sympathectomy have been disappointing. According, although α-antagonists have been used as pulmonary vasodilators for over 30 years,[23] it remains unclear whether vasodilating effects are secondary to α-blockade.[24]

Phentolamine. Phentolamine is an imidazoline α-adrenergic antagonist that inhibits both the pre- and post-synaptic receptors, although it may have

Pulmonary Vasodilators

direct vasodilating actions as well.[25] In a few patients, phentolamine has been successful in attenuating the increase in PAP with exercise, and there was a beneficial response to prolonged therapy,[26] but most patients have had poor responses.[17,13]

Phentolamine is administered I.V. (0.5mg/min) up to a maximum of 10 mg. On a chronic basis it is given orally 25 mgm every six hours, up to a maximum of 50 mgm every eight hours.

Prazosin. Prazosin exerts its α-adrenergic blocking effects only on the post-synaptic receptors.[27] Although this agent has been effective in decreasing PVR in a few patients, the benefits have not been sustained.[28]

Prazosin is given orally at a dose of 2.5 mgm t.i.d.

Direct Vasodilators

Diazoxide. Diazoxide, a potent vasodilator, has been employed in the treatment of PPH in recent years. Although initial studies described both acute and long term benefit,[29] subsequent studies have demonstrated a significant incidence of complications including severe systemic hypotension, complete heart block and asystole, as well as death.[30] In other patients PAP increased dramatically[17] and long-term treatment has been associated with fluid retention, nausea, vomiting, hirsutism, hyperglycemia, and hypotension.[31] As a result, the use of this agent appears to have diminished in the past few years.

The drug is administered slowly I.V.; 50 mgm initially, then doubled every 15 minutes up to a maximum dose of 300 mg. On a chronic basis it is given orally—100 mgm b.i.d.

Hydralazine. Hydralazine is a direct-acting vasodilator that may exert its action by inducing the release of prostacyclin (PGI_2).[32] Its effects on the systemic circulation have been studied extensively, and it dilates arterioles and venules. The cardiac output is increased by its vasodilating actions as well as via a positive inotropic effect. Acute and long-term beneficial effects of hydralazine have been reported in patients with PPH[33] and in patients with pulmonary hypertension secondary to obstructive and restrictive lung disease,[34] as well as pulmonary hypertension secondary to multiple emboli.[35] Again, subsequent reports have indicated serious complications, including systemic hypotension, hypoxemia, azotemia, drug-induced lupus, increased PAP, and chest pain, as well as death.[36] One group[37] has suggested that those patients with lesser elevations of PVR are likely to have a better response.

Generally one administers hydralazine acutely intravenously (10 mgm) and this can be repeated once after 10 minutes. For chronic use 25–50 mgm every six hours is prescribed.

Table 9-2
Pulmonary Vasodilators

Drug	Hemodynamic Effects	Dose for Acute Administration	Dose Half-Life	Dose for Chronic Administration	Adverse Effects
BETA-ADRENERGIC AGONISTS					
Isoproterenol	Increase CO and HR, decrease SVR, PVR and SBP, no change or increase in PAP	1 ug/min I.V., inc. by 1 ug/min every 5 min until HR 120 or PA systolic increases 10 torr	15 min	10 mg SL q4hr	Hypoxemia, increased PAP, chest pain, dyspnea
ALPHA-ADRENERGIC ANTAGONISTS					
Phentolamine	Modest increase CO and HR, small decrease in PVR, SVR, SBP, PAP	0.5 mg/min I.V. max dose 10 mg	1–2 hr	25 mg p.o. q6h max 50 mg q3h	Increased PAP, systemic hypotension, atrial arrhythmias
Prazosin	Increase in CO and HR, small decrease in SVR, SBP, PAP, bigger decrease in PVR	2–5 mg p.o.	6 hr	5 mg p.o. q8h	Tachyphylaxis, hypotension
DIRECT VASODILATORS					
Diazoxide	Increase CO and HR, decrease SVR, PVR, SBP, No change PAP	50 mg slow I.V., double dose q15 min to max 300 mg	10 hrs	100 mg p.o. b.i.d. max 150 mg q6h	Hypotension (may be severe), ventricular tachycardia, asystole, complete heart block, hirsutism
Hydralazine	Increase CO, HR, decrease SVR, PVR, SBP, no change PAP	10 mg I.V., repeated once after 10 min	3–6 hrs	25 mg p.o. q6h max 50 mg q6h	Hypotension (may be severe) azotemia, increase in PAP, RV failure, tachycardia, GI intolerance

Nitroglycerine	No or small increase CO, decrease PAP, PVR, and SBP, no change HR	10 ug/min, increase by 0.5 ug/kg/min every 5 min	5–10 min	Isordil 10 mg p.o. q6h, max 50 mg q6h, or transdermal nitroglycerin 2.5/24 mg/24 hrs, increase gradually	Decreased cardiac output, hypoxemia
Nitroprusside	No or small increase CO, decrease PAP, PVR, and SBP, no change HR	0.5 ug/kg/min, increase by 0.5 ug/kg min every 5 min	5–10 min	Isordil 10 mg p.o. q6h, max 50 mg q6h or transdermal nitroglycerin 2.5 mg/24 hrs, increase gradually	Decreased cardiac output, hypoxemia
CALCIUM CHANNEL BLOCKERS					
Nifedipine	Small to no increase in CO, HR, decrease PAP, PVR, SBP, SVR	10 mg SL, repeat after 15 min	2 hrs	10 mg p.o. q8h max 30 mg q6h	Systemic hypotension RV failure, junctional arrhythmia flushing
Verapamil	No change in HR, small decrease in CO, PVR & SVR, decrease in PAP and SBP	1 mg/min I.V. to total dose of 0.15 mg/kg	2–5 hrs	80 mg p.o. q8h max 160 mg q6h	RV failure, junctional rhythm, bradycardia
ANTIOTENSIN-CONVERTING ENZYME INHIBITORS					
Captropril	Decrease in SBP, No change in SVR	6 mg I.V. slow		12.5 mg p.o. q8h max 50 mg q8hr	Systemic hypotension, increased PAP
PROSTAGLANDINS (INVESTIGATIONAL)					
PGI_2	Increase in CO, HR, decrease PAP, SBP, PVR, SVR	2 ng/kg/min q15 min max 12 ng/kg/min	3 min		Systemic hypotension, QRS widening, bradycardia, headache, flushing, nausea and vomiting
PGE_2	Increase in CO, HR, decrease PAP, SBP, PVR, SVR	20 ng/kg/min	20 min		

Nitroglycerine and nitroprusside. These direct-acting vasodilators may exert their effects by inducing the release of prostacyclin from the vascular endothelium.[38] The hemodynamic effects of these agents are different from that of the other agents described above since, in addition to a peripheral vasodilating effect, they also appear to decrease venous return.[39] Consequently, cardiac output may not increase as much as with other agents, and the PAP is more likely to fall. This effect may be an advantage in some patients, such as those evaluated by Pearl and colleagues,[40] in whom intravenous nitroglycerine led to a fall in PAP, central venous pressure, and PVR without tachycardia or systemic hypotension. In these patients cardiac output increased, and long-term benefit was obtained with nitropaste.[40] However, another group of patients studied by Hermiller and colleagues experienced a decrease in PAP and PVR, but the cardiac output did not increase.[17] Since most workers believe the functional limitations in pulmonary hypertension are largely due to a limited cardiac output, such treatment is unlikely to lead to functional improvement. In another study, hydralazine led to a decrease in PVR and an increase in cardiac output, while nitroglycerine decreased central venous pressure, PAP and cardiac output but not PVR in patients with pulmonary hypertension secondary to cor pulmonale.[41] Similar responses to nitrates were observed by Chick and colleagues,[42] but in their patients oxygen tension and oxygen delivery also fell. Taken together, these data suggest that agents that decrease preload may not be ideal for patients with an obliterated vascular bed, but the discrepant results highlight the importance of proper study of each individual patient.

When given intravenously, the dose of nitroglycerine is 10 µg/kg/min, increasing by 0.5 µg/kg/min every five minutes, and of nitroprusside 0.5 µg/kg/min, increasing by 0.5 µg/kg/min every five minutes. For chronic administration, Isordil 10–50 mg every six hours or transdermal nitroglycerin is prescribed.

Calcium blocking agents. Constriction of vascular smooth muscle probably requires translocation of calcium from extra-to-intra-cellular sites.[43] Accordingly, the class of agents known as calcium channel blockers have been used in an attempt to reverse vasoconstriction, and animal studies have suggested that hypoxic vasoconstriction is attenuated by these drugs.[44]

In PPH, verapamil has not been successful, while nifedipine has been shown to produce significant acute and long-term benefit, decreasing PVR and increasing cardiac output in some studies[45] but results have been more varied in other studies. Packer and co-workers[46] found no increase in cardiac output with varapamil or nifedipine, an effect that was apparently associated with a significant decrease in RV performance, several patients developing marked systemic hypotension. Similar results have been reported by other workers.[47] Differences between patient groups almost certainly exist, but no consistent theory yet explains these quite discrepant results.

In patients with pulmonary hypertension secondary to cor pulmonale, the data on use of calcium channel blockers are also confusing. Patients studied by Sturani had a salutary hemodynamic response persisting for eight weeks, but an unclear clinical response, with clinical worsening in two out of eight patients.[48] In addition, nifedipine has been shown to result in hypoxemia in patients with PPH,[46] and it is reasonable to suspect that a similar effect may occur in patients with cor pulmonale.

Nifedipine is administered sublinqually (10 mgm) or orally (10–30 mg every six hours). Verapamil can be given intravenously (1 mg/min to a total dose of .15 mg/kg) or orally (80–160 mg every eight hours).

Angiotensin-converting enzyme inhibitors. There is little evidence that the renin-angiotensin system is involved in pulmonary hypertension in humans. Nonetheless, since captopril has been of use in patients with left ventricular failure, there have been efforts to employ it in pulmonary hypertension. Except for a few case reports suggesting benefit, most studies suggest that captopril has no salutary effect on cardiac output or PAP.[49]

It is given slowly intravenously (6 mg) or orally (12.5–50 mg every eight hours).

Prostaglandins. Prostaglandins may modulate pulmonary blood flow,[50] and a deficiency or imbalance in the production of vasodilator prostaglandin has been proposed as a pathogenetic mechanism in PPH.[51] Indications for their use are unclear, however, since chronic therapy can only be undertaken currently with continuous ambulatory intravenous infusion.[52] It has been suggested that the hemodynamic response to prostacyclin (PGI$_2$) may predict responsiveness of the pulmonary vasculature to other oral agents.[53] Further testing is required to substantiate this notion. Little is known about the actions of prostaglandins in patients with cor pulmonale, and their use in pulmonary hypertension of any etiology should certainly be considered investigational.

They have been utilized intravenously at a dose of 2 ng/kg/min every 15 minutes up to 12 ng/kg/min (PGI$_2$) and 20 ng/kg/min (PGE$_2$).

Indications. Currently, the indications for the use of vasodilators in pulmonary hypertension remain unclear. They should not be used as a first-line therapy in patients who have pulmonary hypertension secondary to a pathologic process in the heart or lungs. Only when the accepted therapeutic modalities for the underlying condition have been exhausted and the patient manifests evidence of pulmonary hypertension, such as RV failure, exercise intolerance, syncope or radiographic evidence of persistent RV hypertrophy, and PA enlargement, should one proceed to evaluation of the efficacy of vasodilators. Once again, it is important to emphasize that such evaluation should be done only where appropriate hemodynamic monitoring facilities exist to study patients over a period of several days, while at rest and during exercise.

For patients who appear to have primary pulmonary hypertension, the situation may be different. Arguably, these patients should begin vasodilator treatment as soon as the disease is detected (which is, admittedly, usually late). Considerable controversy remains about the advisability of lung biopsy in primary pulmonary hypertension. Wagenvoort[54] has reported some morbidity, but no mortality in a series of patients with pulmonary hypertension who underwent open lung biopsy, and the lung biopsy may reveal the presence of thromboembolic disease that may be difficult to detect under other circumstances. Similarly, lung biopsy may reveal pulmonary vaso-occlusive disease and pulmonary capillary hemangiomatosis that may not be detected without microscopic evaluation, and it is unclear whether these two disorders respond to vasodilators at all.

Contraindications. Since every patient who receives vasodilators must be individually evaluated, there are few absolute contraindications, except for known hypersensitivity.

Side effects. The potential side effects of the vasodilators are shown in Table 9–2. As can be seen, the major adverse effects are in cardiac rhythm and output, systemic blood pressure, and gas exchange.

SUMMARY

The preceding sections are not meant specifically to discourage vasodilator treatment of pulmonary hypertension, but rather to emphasize the dangers and limitations inherent in such attempts. Foremost in the case of any patient with pulmonary hypertension must be a thorough search for antecedent causes that are treatable. Only when such causes have been either ruled out or found and treated should an attempt be made to use vasodilator therapy. In such circumstances, an array of different measurements should be used to evaluate the response. A practical approach to the use of these agents has recently been presented by Palevsky and Fishman.[55] In addition, follow-up studies are important to assure that vasodilating agents, which have significant side effects, continue to exert a favorable effect.

REFERENCES

1. Oakley C, Glick G, Luria MN, et al: Some regulatory mechanisms of the human pulmonary vascular bed. Circulation 26:917–930, 1962
2. Harris P, Heath D: The Human Circulation. Edinburgh, Churchill-Livingstone, 2nd Ed, 1977
3. Nocturnal oxygen therapy trial group. Continuous or nocturnal oxygen therapy in hypoxemic chronic obstructive lung disease. Ann Intern Med 93:391–398, 1980

4. Parker JO, Kelkor K, West RO: Hemodynamic effects of aminophylline in cor pulmonale. Circulation 33:17–25, 1966
5. Barer GR, Gunning AJ: Action of a sympathomimetic drug and theophylline on the pulmonary circulation. Circ Res 7:383–389, 1959
6. Dantzker DR, Bower JS: Partial reversibility of chronic pulmonary hypertension caused by pulmonary thromboembolic disease. Am Rev Respir Dis 124:129–131, 1981
7. Ferrer MI, Harvey RM, et al: Circulatory effects of mitral commissurotomy with particular reference to selection of patients for surgery. Circulation 12:7, 1955
8. Charms BL, Brofman BL, Kohn PM. Pulmonary resistance in acquired heart disease. Circulation 20:850–855, 1959
9. Hyman AL. Pulmonary vaso-constriction due to non-occlusive distension of large pulmonary arteries in the dog. Circ Res 23:401–413, 1968
10. Packer M: Vasodilator for primary pulmonary hypertension: Limitations and hazards. Ann Int Med 103:258–270, 1985
11. Rubin LJ, Peter RH: Oral hydralazine therapy for primary pulmonary hypertension. N Engl J Med 302:69–73, 1980
12. Rich R, Levy PS: Characteristics of surviving and non-surviving patients with primary pulmonary hypertension. Am J Med 76:573–578, 1984
13. Rich S, Martinez J, Lam W, et al: Reassessment of the effects of vasodilator drugs in primary pulmonary hypertension: Guidelines for determining a pulmonary vasodilator response. Am Heart J 105:119–127, 1983
14. Lee TD, Roveti GC, Ross RS: Hemodynamic effects of isoproterenol on pulmonary hypertension in man. Am Heart J 65:361–367, 1963
15. Kronzon I, Cohen M, Winer HE: Adverse effect of hydralazine in patients with primary pulmonary hypertension. JAMA 247:3112–3114, 1982
16. Elkayan U, Frishman WH, Yoram C, et al: Unfavorable hemodynamic and clinical effects of isoproterenol in primary pulmonary hypertension. Cardiovasc Med 3:1177–1180, 1978
17. Hermiller JB, Bambach D, Thompson MJ, et al: Vasodilators and prostaglandin inhibitors in primary pulmonary hypertension. Ann Int Med 97:480–489, 1982
18. Dantzker DR, Bower JS: Pulmonary vascular tone improving V/Q matching in obliterative pulmonary hypertension. J Appl Physiol 51:607–613, 1981
19. Silove ED, Inove T, Grover RF: Comparison of hypoxia, pH, and sympathomimetic drugs on bovine pulmonary vasculature. J Appl Physiol 24:355–365, 1968
20. Daoud FS, Reeves JT, Kelly DB: Isoproterenol as a potential pulmonary vasodilator in primary pulmonary hypertension. Am J Cardiol 42:817–822, 1978
21. Pietro DA, LaBresh KA, Shulman RM, et al: Sustained improvement in primary pulmonary hypertension during six years of treatment with sublingual isoproterenol. N Engl J Med 310:1032–1034, 1984
22. Shettigar UR, Hultgren HN, Specter M, et al: Primary pulmonary hypertension: Favorable effect of isoproterenol. N Engl J Med 295:1414–1415, 1976
23. Halmagyi DF: Role of the autonomic nervous system in the genesis of pulmonary hypertension in heart disease. J Chronic Dis 9:525–535, 1959
24. Dresdale DT, Schultz M, Michton RJ: Primary pulmonary hypertension: Clinical and hemodynamic study. Am J Med 11:686–705, 1951
25. Miller RR, Fennel WH, Young JB, et al: Differential systemic arterial and nervous

actions and consequent cardiac effects of vasodilator drugs. Prog Cardiovasc Dis 24:353–374, 1982
26. Ruskin JN, Hutter AM, Jr: Primary pulmonary hypertension treated with oral phentolamine. Ann Intern Med 90:772–774, 1979
27. Gilman AG, Goodman LS. The Pharmacologic Basis of Therapeutics, 8th Ed, New York, MacMillan Publishing Co, 1980, p. 806
28. Levine TB, Rose T, Kane M, et al: Treatment of primary pulmonary hypertension by alpha-adrenergic blockade. (Abstract). Circulation 62:SIII, 26, 1980
29. Klinke WP, Gilbert JA: Diazoxide in primary pulmonary hypertension. N Engl J Med 302:91–92, 1980
30. Buch J, Wennerold A: Hazards of diazoxide in pulmonary hypertension. Br Heart J 40:401–403, 1981
31. Honey M, Cotter L, Davies N, et al: Clinical and hemodynamic effects of diazoxide in primary pulmonary hypertension. Thorax 35:269–276, 1980
32. Rubin LJ, Lazar JD: Influence of protaglandin synthesis inhibitors on pulmonary vasodilatory effects of hydralazine in dogs with hypoxic pulmonary vasoconstriction. J Clin Invest 67:193, 1981
33. Rubin LJ, Peter RH: Oral hydralazine therapy for primary pulmonary hypertension. N Engl J Med 302:69–72, 1980
34. Rubin LJ, Peter RH: Hemodynamics at rest and during exercise after oral hydralazine in patients with cor pulmonale. Am J Cardiol 47:116–122, 1981
35. Rubin LJ, Handel F, Peter RH: The effects of oral hydralazine on right ventricular end-diastolic pressure in patients with right ventricular failure. Circulation 65:1369–1373, 1982
36. Packer M, Greenberg B, Massie B, et al: Deleterious effects of hydralazine in patients with pulmonary hypertension. N Engl J Med 306:1326–1331, 1982
37. Lupi-Herrera E, Sandoral J, Seoane M, et al: The role of hydralazine therapy for pulmonary arterial hypertension of unknown cause. Circulation 65:645–652, 1982
38. Levin RI, Weksler BB, Jaffe EA: Nitroglycerine induces production of prostacycline by human endothelial cells. Clin Res 28:471A, 1980
39. Mason DT, Braunwald E: The effects of nitroglycerine and amyl nitrate on arteriolar and venous tone in the human forearm. Circulation 32:755–766, 1965
40. Pearl RG, Rosenthal MA, Schroeder JS, et al: Acute hemodynamic effects of nitroglycerine in pulmonary hypertension. Ann Intern Med 99:9–13, 1983
41. Brent BN, Berger HJ, Matthay RA, et al: Contrasting acute effects of vasodilators (nitroglycerine, nitroprusside, and hydralazine) on right ventricular performance in patients with chronic obstructive pulmonary disease and pulmonary hypertension. A combined radiomilide-hemodynamic study. Am J Cardiol 51:1682–1689, 1983
42. Chick TW, Kochukoshy KN, Matsumoto S, et al: The effect of nitroglycerine on gas exchange, hemodynamics, and oxygen transport in patients with chronic obstructive pulmonary disease. Am J Med Sci 276:105–111, 1978
43. Bergofsky EH, Holtzman S: A study of the mechanisms involved in the pulmonary arterial pressor response to hypoxia. Circ Res 20:506–519, 1967
44. McMurtry IF, Davidson AB, Reeves JT, et al: Inhibition of hypoxic pulmonary vasoconstriction by calcium antagonists in isolated rat lungs. Circ Res 38:99–104, 1976
45. Rubin LJ, Nicod P, Hillis LD, et al: Treatment of primary pulmonary hypertension

with nifedipine: A hemodynamic and oscintigraphic evolution. Ann Intern Med 99:433–438, 1983
46. Packer M, Medina N, Medina M: Adverse hemodynamic and clinical effects of calcium channel blockage in pulmonary hypertension secondary to obliterative pulmonary vascular disease. J Am Coll Cardiol 4:890–901, 1984
47. Farber HW, Karlinsky JB, Fuliny LJ: Fatal outcome following nifedipine for primary pulmonary hypertension. Chest 83:708–709, 1983
48. Sturani C, Bassein L, Schivina M, et al: Oral nifedipine in chronic cor pulmonale secondary to severe chronic obstruction pulmonary disease (COPD). Chest 84:135–142, 1983
49. Leier CV, Bambach D, Nelson S, et al: Captopril in primary pulmonary hypertension. Circulation 67:155–161, 1983
50. Alpert JS, Haynes FW, Knutson PA, et al: Prostaglandins and the pulmonary circulation. Protaglandis 3:759–765, 1983
51. Hadhazy P, Visi ES, Megyar K, et al: Relaxation of human isolated pulmonary arteries by prostacyclin (PGI$_2$). Lung 161:123–130, 1983
52. Higgenbottam T, Wheeldon D, Wells F, et al: Long-term treatment of primary pulmonary hypertension with continuous intravenous epoprostenol (prostacyclin). Lancet 1:1046–1047, 1984
53. Rubin LJ, Graves BM, Reeves JT, et al: Prostacyclin-induced acute pulmonary vasodilation in primary pulmonary hypertension. Circulation 66:334–338, 1982
54. Wagenvoort CA: Lung biopsies and pulmonary vascular disease, in: Weir EK, Reeves JT (eds) Pulmonary Hypertension. Mt. Kisco: Future Publishing Co, 393, 1984
55. Palevsky HI, Fishman AP: Vasodilator therapy for primary pulmonary hypertension. Ann Rev Med 36:563–578, 1985

Robert A. Sandhaus

10

Newer Agents

Many pulmonary diseases are not treated effectively with current agents and several pulmonary processes have no therapy at this time. While it is impossible to predict which new agents will prove most effective, current research reveals several broad categories that are likely to provide us with new tools for the treatment of lung disease. Some of these agents are drugs already in use for treatment of nonpulmonary processes, while others are novel agents that will provide us with new classes of drugs and actions, as well as unforeseen side effects and interactions.

In view of the experimental nature of most of these therapies, it would be inappropriate to provide dosage information and specific indications. Instead the current rationale for the use of each group of agents in the treatment of lung disease will be discussed. Specific agents will be mentioned, where applicable. The selection of agents for inclusion is necessarily subjective, and those chosen are intended to represent a spectrum of current research.

CALCIUM CHANNEL BLOCKERS

Calcium channel blocking agents are widely used in the treatment of cardiovascular disorders. Agents such as nifedipine, verapamil, and diltiazem are already well integrated into our armamentarium against cardiac arrhythmias, congestive heart failure, hypertension, and coronary occlusive disease.[1] The influx of calcium ions into smooth muscle cells is associated with contraction of these cells. As indicated in previous chapters, this leads to the consideration of the use of calcium channel blockers in asthma[2,3] and in pulmonary hypertension.[4,5] Their use in asthma has gained further support through the demonstration that sodium cromoglycate and ketotifen, two agents currently in use in the treatment of reactive airway disease, possess calcium channel blocking activity.[6,7]

An additional role for intracellular influx of calcium has been suggested by studies of mediator release from effector cells such as the mast cell and basophil. The absence of calcium ions inhibits the release of mediators from these cells. Calcium channel blockers have been reported to reduce release of mediators such as slow reacting substance of anaphylaxis and histamine both *in vitro* and *in vivo*.[8,9]

The molecular mechanism of action of these agents is currently unknown. Since each appears to have a distinct spectrum of effects within the cardiovascular system and lung, and a distinct chemical structure, it seems likely that there are distinct molecular mechanisms for each as well.[10]

The use of calcium channel blockers in pulmonary hypertension is discussed in a previous chapter, therefore, the discussion here will only deal with their use in airway diseases in animals and humans. Most studies, both *in vitro* and *in vivo*, have examined the use of nifedipine or verapamil. Using tracheal and parenchymal strips of guinea pig lung tissue, some investigators report that nifedipine is effective at relaxing induced bronchoconstriction,[11] while other investigators, using a similar system, found that nifedipine had no effect.[12] Studies of human lung tissue, examined *in vitro*, have found nifedipine to be effective at reducing both antigen-induced bronchoconstriction[13] and that induced by histamine and acetylcholine.[14]

In vivo effects in humans have been quite variable and virtually never lead to complete reversal of induced bronchospasm.[15,16] The reasons for this variability are not known but may relate to the relative effectiveness of the currently available calcium channel blockers in lung cells, since these agents were developed primarily for their cardiovascular effects. One consistent relationship has emerged, however. Although the magnitude of the effect is extremely variable, calcium channel blockers show a consistent ability to reduce chemically-induced[17,18] and exercise-induced[19] airway reactivity, yet often fail to block antigen-induced bronchoconstriction.[20]

The future role of calcium channel blockers in lung disease will likely depend on the development of more specific pulmonary-acting agents. Until then these agents will be adjuncts to our current therapy. Individuals with both cardiovascular disease and reactive airways may well be candidates for a trial of calcium channel blocking agents, especially in lieu of β-blocking agents. The individual with an element of reactive airways disease, pulmonary hypertension, and cardiac problems (not an unusual combination) may be the ideal candidate for an effective calcium channel blocking agent.

SURFACTANT REPLACEMENTS

The surface active lining of the alveoli, functionally composed primarily of phospholipids, counterbalances the forces that would tend to collapse these respiratory units. In the neonatal respiratory distress syndrome, the lungs appear to lack the ability to produce adequate surfactant material; in the adult respiratory distress syndrome, and other processes that lead to alveolar disruption, this lining material is destroyed or no longer produced.

As a result, surfactant replacements have been used in these diseases, although the majority of experience has been gained in neonates. The surfactant replacements have been of two types: synthetic and natural. The synthetic surfactants are made in the laboratory by mixing phospholipids and other constituents, usually including a nonionic detergent, to produce a material of desired surface active properties. The detergent aids in delivery and spreading of the artificial surfactant over the internal surface of the lung. The natural surfactants are purified from pulmonary lavage material of animals (usually a bovine source) or of humans.

In addition to these source differences, there are differences in the physical state of the surfactant materials that may modulate their efficacy.[21] Some are dry powders, others aqueous suspensions (with or without detergent), still others represent alcohol extractions. Another variable is the surfactant-associated protein concentration.

Evaluation of these variables is still underway at this time. Studies in human and animal neonates at risk of respiratory distress syndrome have led to some preliminary conclusions. The first is that it is better to administer a surfactant replacement prior to development of the disease. Giving artificial surfactant to high risk neonates reduced the incidence of respiratory distress[22] while administration after the development of severe disease led to virtually no improvement in morbidity or mortality.[23,24] In most cases, lung mechanics improved after administration of artificial surfactant, even without improvement in the clinical course.[25]

The use of these agents in the adult respiratory distress syndrome has been proposed[26] and is highly controversial. In spite of the similar nomenclature, there are striking differences between the neonatal and adult respiratory distress syndromes. One of the most prominent differences is anatomic. There is massive destruction of the alveolar architecture in the adult respiratory distress syndrome, and this leads to the caution that the administration of artificial surfactant may have little beneficial effect in this condition.

ANTIOXIDANTS

Oxidant injury to lung tissue, caused by toxic oxygen metabolites and free radicals, has been implicated in the pathogenesis of virtually all pulmonary processes that involve the inflammatory response, as well as injury caused by exogenous oxidizing agents inhaled from the environment. Lung cells themselves may generate intracellular oxidants in response to changes in their extracellular milieu.[27] The most ubiquitous exogenous source of inhaled oxidants is the cigarette. The combusion of tobacco leads to the generation of a multitude of toxic agents, many of them oxidants.

In the inflammatory response, phagocytic cells (neutrophils and monocytes/macrophages) are stimulated to accumulate in the area of inflammation. These cells are capable of producing oxidizing chemicals in response to the stimuli present during the inflammatory response. Several of these oxidants live only a short time before decaying to harmless substances but, while active, are able to directly injure the cells in the local environment. In addition, several crucial lung proteins, such as α1-proteinase inhibitor and bronchial mucus inhibitor, are extremely susceptible to oxidative inactivation, thus disrupting the normal protective screen of the lung. Finally, these agents can indirectly produce distant effects including the generation of toxic arachidonic acid metabolites[28] and interaction with cells and humoral components that can act on phagocytic cells and cause the release of substances that, in turn, are injurious to lung connective tissue and cells.[29-31]

The reaction below represents the cellular pathway of oxygen reduction:

$$O_2 \rightarrow \overset{\cdot}{O_2}{}^- \rightarrow H_2O_2 \rightarrow {}^\cdot OH \rightarrow H_2O$$
$$(a)\phantom{{}^- \rightarrow }(b)(c)$$

This reaction leads to the generation of the most common toxic oxygen metabolites (a) superoxide anion, (b) hydrogen peroxide, and (c) hydroxyl radical. Endogenous defenses against the action of these injurious agents include superoxide dismutase that catalyzes the reduction of superoxide anion to hydrogen peroxide. Catalase and glutathione peroxidase are able to reduce hydrogen peroxide directly to water, without generation of the highly toxic hydroxyl radical. Additional antioxidant defenses are provided by circulating erythrocytes and ceruloplasmin[32,33]

In view of the mounting evidence suggesting a role for oxidant injury in many pulmonary processes, the use of antioxidant therapy and oxygen radical scavengers in these processes would seem reasonable.[34] There are endogenous antioxidant substances within the lung. Thus antioxidant therapy could take the form of stimulation of endogenous antioxidants or administration of exogenous agents. Many drugs currently in use have some antioxidant (reducing) potential. Among those used in early clinical trials are vitamin C[35] and vitamin E.[36] Preliminary evidence has shown little promise in the diseases that have been studied. Newer, more powerful, and more specific antioxidants may prove effective but, at the current time, these are agents with an excellent rationale, but little direct evidence for their effectiveness.

Other exogenous agents that have been studied include vitamin A,[37] minerals, and trace metals such as selenium,[38] lipids,[39] and proteins.[40] These latter two appear to act primarily as substrates for oxidation, thus allowing the toxic metabolites to oxidize an "irrelevant" substrate rather than one that might prove injurious to the cell under attack.

Experimental oxidant injury to lung has been caused by a variety of agents in the laboratory. Toxic oxygen metabolite-generating chemicals have been infused and inhaled, drugs known to induce oxidant injury have been administered, and lung tissue has been exposed to the oxidants directly.[41,42,43] In many such experimental models, antioxidant chemicals have been effective at reducing the injury caused by these toxic mediators. In some experiments the evidence is indirect. Dietary deficiencies of the vitamins mentioned above and/or selenium appear to exacerbate the lung injury induced by several oxidant injuries.[44,45] However, the administration of supplemental vitamins or selenium to normal animals often fails to protect against injury.[46]

The most encouraging experimental data has been obtained when delivering antioxidant enzymes in a physical state that prolongs the short half-lifes of these agents. Two delivery systems have been used: entrapment of these enzymes in liposomes (microscopic synthetic lipid vesicals) and conjugation with polyethylene glycol. Liposomes containing superoxide dismutase and/or catalase have been shown to protect cultured cells against hyperoxic and hydrogen peroxide-mediated injury[47,48] and to prolong survival of rats exposed to hyperoxia.[49] However, impairment of neutrophil mediated bacterial killing has been demonstrated following liposome-antioxidant administration. This is presumed to be due to the inhibition of oxidant-mediated bactericidal activities within the neutrophil.[50]

Polyethylene glycol conjugation of these same enzymes appears to have the same protective effects as liposome entrapment[51] but does not appear to hinder neutrophil bacterial killing mechanisms.[52]

The final group of agents that may prove effective in future studies are the direct radical scavengers. These include dimethyl thiourea, N-acetyl cysteine, and dimethylsulfoxide. Each has some effectiveness *in vitro* as a scavenger of toxic oxygen metabolites. In addition, they each appear to have little inherent *in vivo* toxicity.

PROTEINASE INHIBITORS

The possible role of proteinases, enzymes capable of degrading proteins, in the etiology of some pulmonary disease processes was first suggested in the mid 1960s by proteinase instillation into the lungs of laboratory animals. Proteinases with the ability to degrade elastin, a lung connective tissue protein, produced lesions identical to those of human pulmonary emphysema. It has since been found that the neutrophil and pulmonary alveolar macrophage synthesize and release potent proteinases including elastases, proteinases capable of degrading elastin.

In humans, the primary defense against the action of many of these proteinases, including neurophil elastase, is the circulating glycoprotein α1-proteinase inhibitor (known previously as α1-antitrypsin). A hereditary deficiency of α1-proteinase inhibitor leads to the development of precocious emphysema in affected individuals, even in the absence of risk factors such as cigarette smoking.

Additionally, proteinases have been implicated in the pathogenesis of pulmonary diseases other than emphysema. These include chronic bronchitis,[53] the adult respiratory distress syndrome,[54,55] the neonatal respiratory distress syndrome,[56] and the lung damage that occurs during certain bacterial pneumonias.[57,58] In individuals that do not have a genetic lack of α1-proteinase inhibitor, the inability to defend against endogenous proteinase attack is believed due to the oxidative inactivation of the inhibitor molecule (see discussion of oxidative injury, above) or the delivery of overwhelming concentrations of enzyme.

Thus it would seem rational to devise a method of improving the body's defenses against proteinase attack, and the administration of exogenous proteinase inhibitors has been under investigation through most of this decade. Three primary approaches have been used: pooled human serum α1-proteinase inhibitor or the cloned gene product; α1-proteinase inhibitor genetically modified to reduce its susceptibility to oxidation or prolong its circulatory half-life; and totally novel proteinase inhibitors. No doubt, the coming years will see a flood of proteinase inhibitors aimed at treating lung disease as well as other proteinase dependent processes such as coagulation, thrombolysis, and the complement system.

Animal models of pulmonary emphysema have been the first disease conditions to be clinically modified by the use of exogenous proteinase inhibitors. Investigators have used chloromethyl ketone oligopeptides specifically designed to block the activity of elastase.[59,60] They demonstrated that inhibitor, administered to rodents orally or intraperitoneally, just prior to the intratracheal instillation of an emphysema-producing dose of elastase, prevented the production of pathologic and physiologic changes. Vered et al[61] produced a product from the Streptococcus pneumoniae bacteria that is capable of blocking the evolution of elastase-induced lung injury in laboratory rodents.

The design of safe, elastase-inhibiting agents for human use has been proposed by Powers,[62] and the search for such agents is the continuing work of several investigators[63] and major pharmaceutical companies. The experimental use of α1-proteinase inhibitor infusions[64] to treat individuals with the genetic deficiency of this crucial serum protein has begun. It has been demonstrated that sufficient α1-proteinase inhibitor can be administered to reconstitute the normal proteinase inhibitor screen in the lung.[65]

The demonstration of free, active proteinases, primarily neutrophil elastase, in the lavage fluid of individuals with the adult respiratory distress syndrome[66] indicates that the next area in which we are likely to see the application of proteinase inhibitors is in this highly lethal process. Individuals at high risk of developing this syndrome would be pretreated with a proteinase inhibitor in order to prevent or modify the course of the disease.

It should be emphasized that the use of proteinase inhibitors, as currently envisioned, should be considered entirely prophylactic. Once proteinases have been able to reach their substrates, (i.e., the proteins of the lung) the damage has been done. Thus, along with the development of proteinase inhibitors for therapy, there is an increased need for early detection of the diseases to be treated and a clear means of identifying the populations at risk. Similar considerations apply to the use of antioxidants and surfactant replacements.

REFERENCES

1. Henry PD: Comparative pharmacology of calcium antagonists: Nifedipine, verapamil and diltiazem, Am J Cardiol 46:1047–1058 1980
2. Russi EW, Ahmed T: Calcium and calcium antagonists in airway disease, Chest 86:475–482 1984
3. Fanta CH: Calcium-channel blockers in prophylaxis and treatment of asthma, Am J Cardiol 55:202B–209B 1985
4. Pack M: Therapeutic application of calcium-channel antagonists for pulmonary hypertension, Am J Cardiol 55:196B–201B 1985
5. Kennedy TP, Michael JR, Summer W: Calcium channel blockers in hypoxic pulmonary hypertension, Am J Med 78:18–26 1985
6. Tinkelman DG: Calcium channel blocking agents in the prophylaxis of asthma, Am J Med 78:35–38 1985
7. Naspitz CK: Use of calcium channel blocking agents in the management of childhood asthma, J Asthma 21:451–460 1984
8. Lee VY, Hughes JM, Swale JP, et al: Verapamil inhibits mediator release from human lung *in vitro,* Thorax 38:386–387 1983
9. Barnes PJ, Wilson NM, Brown MJ: A calcium antagonist, nifedipine, modifies exercise-induced asthma, Thorax 36:726–730 1981
10. Solway J: Calcium channel blocking agents in bronchial hyperreactivity, J Asthma 21:419–426 1984
11. Fanta CH, Venugopalan CS, Lacouture PG, et al: Inhibition of bronchoconstriction in the guinea pig by a calcium channel blocker, nifedipine, Am Rev Respir Dis 125:61–66 1982
12. Henderson AF, Heaton RW, Dunlop LS, et al: Effects of nifedipine on antigen-induced bronchoconstriction, Am Rev Respir Dis 127:549–553 1983
13. Weiss EB, Markowicz J: Inhibition of anaphylaxis in airways smooth muscle by the

calcium channel drugs, Verapamil and Nifedipine, Am Rev Respir Dis 123:(A)42 1981
14. Drazen JM, Fanta CH, Lacouture PG: Effect of nifedipine on constriction of human tracheal strips *in vitro*, Br J Pharmacol 78:687-691 1983
15. Matthews JI, Richey HM 3d, Ewald FW Jr, et al: Nifedipine does not alter methacholine-induced bronchial reactivity, Ann Allergy 53:462-467 1984
16. Hartmann V, Magnussen H: Effect of diltiazem on histamine- and carbachol-induced bronchospasm in normal and asthmatic subjects, Chest 87:174-179 1985
17. Williams DO, Barnes PJ, Vickers HP, et al: Effect of nifedipine on bronchomotor tone and histamine reactivity in asthma, Br Med J 283:348 1981
18. Patel KR: The effect of verapamil on histamine and methacholine-induced bronchoconstriction, Clin Allergy 11:441-447 1981
19. Cerrina J, Denjean A, Alexandre G, et al: Inhibition of exercise-induced asthma by a calcium antagonist, nifedipine, Am Rev Respir Dis 123:156-160 1981
20. So SY, Lam WK, Yu DY: Effect of calcium antagonists on allergen-induced asthma, Clin allergy 12:595-600 1982
21. Notter RH, Egan EA, Kwong MS, et al: Lung surfactant replacement in premature lambs with extracted lipids from bovine lung lavage: Effects of dose, dispersion technique, and gestational age, Pediatr Res 19:569-577 1985
22. Fujiwara T, Maeta H, Chida S, et al: Artificial surfactant therapy in hyaline-membrane disease, Lancet 1:55-59 1980
23. Halliday HL, McClure G, Reid MM, et al: Controlled trial of artificial surfactant to prevent respiratory distress syndrome, Lancet 1:476-478 1984
24. Robertson B: Lung surfactant for replacement therapy, Clin Physiol 3:97-110 1983
25. Morley C, Robertson B, Lachmann B, et al: Artificial surfactant and natural surfactant. Comparative study of the effects on premature rabbit lungs, Arch Dis Child 55:758-765 1980
26. Merritt TA, Cochrane CG, Hallman M, et al: Reduction of lung injury by human surfactant treatment in respiratory distress syndrome, Chest 83:27S-31S 1983
27. Martin WJ 2d, Powis GW, Kachel DL: Nitrofurantoin-stimulated oxidant production in pulmonary endothelial cells, J Lab Clin Med 105:23-29 1985
28. Tate RM, Morris HG, Schroeder WR, et al: Oxygen metabolites stimulate thromboxane production and vasoconstriction in isolated saline-perfused rabbit lungs, J Clin Invest 74:608-613 1984
29. Petrone WF, English DK, Wong K, et al: Free radicals and inflammation: Superoxide-dependent activation of a neutrophil chemotactic factor in plasma, Proc Natl Acad Sci USA 77:1159-1163 1980
30. Harada RN, Vatter AE, Repine JE: Macrophage effector function in pulmonary oxygen toxicity: Hyperoxia damages and stimulates alveolar macrophages to make and release chemotaxins for polymorphonuclear leukocytes, J Leukocyte Biol 35:373-383 1984
31. Weiss SJ, Lampert MB, Test ST: Long-lived oxidants generated by human neutrophils: Characterization and bioactivity, Science 222:625-628 1983
32. Galdston M, Levytska V, Schwartz MS, et al: Ceruloplasmin. Increased serum concentration and impaired antioxidant activity in cigarette smokers, and ability to prevent suppression of elastase inhibitory capacity of alpha 1-proteinase inhibitor, Am Rev Respir Dis 129:258-263 1984

33. Taylor JC, Oey L: Ceruloplasmin: Plasma inhibitor of the oxidative inactivation of alpha 1-protease inhibitor, Am Rev Respir Dis 126:476-482 1982
34. White CW, Repine JE: Pulmonary antioxidant defense mechanisms, Exp Lung Research 8:81-96 1985
35. McGowan SE, Parenti CM, Hoidal JR, et al: Ascorbic acid content and accumulation by alveolar macrophages from cigarette smokers and nonsmokers, J Lab Clin Med 104:127-134 1984
36. Elsayed NM, Mustafa MG: Dietary antioxidants and the biochemical response to oxidant inhalation. I. Influence of dietary vitamin E on the biochemical effects of nitrogen dioxide exposure in rat lung, Toxicol Appl Pharmacol 66:319-328 1982
37. Davies AW, Moore T: Interaction of vitamin A and E, Nature 147:794-796 1941
38. Elsayed NM, Hacker AD, Kuehn K, et al: Dietary antioxidants and the biochemical response to oxidant inhalation. II. Influence of dietary selenium on the biochemical effects of ozone exposure in mouse lung, Toxicol Appl Pharmacol 71:398-406 1983
39. Boyd MR, Catignani GL, Sasame HA, et al: Acute pulmonary injury in rats by nitrofurantoin and modification by vitamin E, dietary fat and oxygen, Am Rev Respir Dis 120:93-99 1979
40. Deneke SM, Gershoff SN, Fanburg BL: Potentiation of oxygen toxicity in rats by dietary protein or amino acid deficiency, J Appl Physiol 54:147-151 1983
41. Evans MJ: Oxidant gases, Environ Health Perspect 55:85-95 1984
42. Jackson RM, Frank L: Ozone-induced tolerance to hyperoxia in rats, Am Rev Respir Dis 128:425-429 1984
43. Skillrud DM, Martin JW, 2d: Paraquat-induced injury of type II alveolar cells. An in vitro model of oxidant injury, Am Rev Respir Dis 129:995-999 1984
44. Sevanian A, Elsayed N, Hacker AD: Effects of vitamin E deficiency and nitrogen dioxide exposure on lung lipid peroxidation: Use of lipid epoxides and malonaldehyde as measures of peroxidation, J Toxical Environ Health 10:743-756 1982
45. Combs GF Jr: Influences of dietary vitamin E and selenium on the oxidant defence systems of the chick, Poult Sci 60:2098-2105 1981
46. Niewoehner DE, Peterson FJ, Hoidal JR: Selenium and vitamin E deficiencies do not enhance lung inflammation from cigarette smoke in the hamster, Am Rev Respir Dis 127:227-230 1983
47. Freeman BA, Mirza Z: Hydrogen peroxide injury to cultured endothelial cells: Modulation by liposome-mediated increase in intracellular catalase specific activity, Am Rev Respir Dis 129:A302 1984
48. Freeman BA, Young SL, Crapo JD: Liposome-mediated augmentation of superoxide dismutase in endothelial cells prevents oxygen injury, J Biol Chem 258:12534-12542 1983
49. Turrens JF, Crapo JD, Freeman BA: Protection against oxygen toxicity by intravenous injection of liposome-entrapped catalase and superoxide dismutase, J Clin Invest 73:87-95 1984
50. Martin WJ, 2d: Neutrophils kill pulmonary endothelial cells by a hydrogen-peroxide-dependent pathway. An in vitro model of neutrophil-mediated lung injury, Am Rev Respir Dis 130:209-213 1984
51. White CW, Jackson JH, Freeman BA, et al: Intravenous polyethylene glycol (PEG)-conjugated superoxide dismutase (SOD) and catalase (CAT) prolongs survival of rats exposed to hyperoxia, Am Rev Respir Dis 129:A311 1984

52. McDonald RJ, Berger EM, White CW, et al: Effect of liposome-encapsulated or polyethylene glycol conjugated superoxide dismutase on neutrophil bactericidal activity in vitro and bacterial clearance, Am Rev Respir Dis (in press)
53. Snider GL, Lucey EC, Christensen TG, et al: Emphysema and bronchial secretory cell metaplasia induced in hamsters by human neutrophil products, Am Rev Respir Dis 129:155-160 1984
54. Lungarella G, Gardi C, de Santi MM, et al: Pulmonary vascular injury in pancreatitis: Evidence for a major role played by pancreatic elastase, Exp Mol Pathol 42:44-59 1985
55. Garcia-Szabo RR, Malik AB: Pancreatitis-induced increase in lung vascular permeability. Protective effect of Trasylol, Am Rev Respir Dis 129:580-583 1984
56. Ogden BE, Murphy SA, Saunders GC, et al: Neonatal lung neutrophils and elastase/proteinase inhibitor imbalance, Am Rev Respir Dis 130:817-821 1984
57. Abrams WR, Fein AM, Kucich U, et al: Proteinase inhibitory function in inflammatory lung disease. I. Acute bacterial pneumonia, Am Rev Respir Dis 129:735-741 1984
58. Fritz H: Proteinase inhibitors in severe inflammatory processes (septic shock and experimental endotoxaemia): Biochemical, pathophysiological and therapeutic aspects, Ciba Found Symp (75) 351-379 1979
59. Stone PJ, Lucey EC, Calore JD, et al: The moderation of elastase-induced emphysema in the hamster by intratracheal pretreatment or post-treatment with succinyl alanyl prolyl valine choromethyl ketone, Am Rev Respir Dis 124:56-59 1981
60. Janoff A, Dearing, R.: Prevention of elastase-induced experimental emphysema by a synthetic elastase inhibitor administered orally, Bull Eur Physiopath Respir 16s:399-405 1980
61. Vered M, Dearing R, Janoff A: A new elastase inhibitor from Streptococcus pneumoniae protects against acute lung injury induced by neutrophil granules, Am Rev Respir Dis 131:131-133 1985
62. Powers JC: Synthetic elastase inhibitors: Prospects for use in the treatment of emphysema, Am Rev Respir Dis 127:54-58 1983
63. Hassall CH, Johnson WH, Kennedy AJ, et al: A new class of inhibitors of human leucocyte elastase, FEBS-Lett 183:201-205 1985
64. Glaser C: Can alpha-1-protease inhibitor be used in replacement therapy?, Am Rev Respir Dis 127:47-53 1983
65. Gadek JE, Fells GA, Zimmerman RL, et al: Antielastases of the human alveolar structures. Implications for the protease-antiprotease theory of emphysema, J Clin Invest 68:889-898 1981
66. Lee CT, Fein AM, Lippman M, et al: Elastolytic activity in pulmonary lavage fluid from patients with adult respiratory distress syndrome, N Eng J Med 304:192-196 1981

Index

Page numbers in *italics* indicate illustrations.
Page numbers followed by *t* indicate tables.

Acetylcholine, mechanism of action of, 64–66
Acetylcysteine as mucolytic, 181–183
Adult respiratory distress syndrome (ARDS), corticosteroids for, 108–109
Adrenaline, development of, 1
α-Adrenergic antagonists as pulmonary vasodilators, 216–217, 218*t*
Adrenergic receptors, glucocorticoid effects on, 83
Adrenoceptors in bronchial smooth muscle, 2–4
Adrenoreceptor agonist(s), 5–11
  adverse effects of, 14–17
  carbuterol as, 7*t*, 11
  ephedrine as, 5, 6*t*, 8
  epinephrine as, 6*t*, 8
  fenoterol as, 7*t*, 10
  hexoprenaline as, 7*t*, 9
  isoetharine as, 7*t*, 9
  isoproterenol as, 6–7*t*, 8–9
  metaproterenol as, 7*t*, 9–10
  pulmonary vasodilators as, 216, 218*t*
  rimeterol as, 7*t*, 9
  salbutamol as, 7*t*, 10–11
  terbutaline as, 7*t*, 10
Aerosol, corticosteroid, 87–88
  side effects of, 124
Aerosol administration of β_2 agonists, 12–14
Aerosolized water therapy in cough management, 180
Airways, hyperreactive
  anticholinergic, antimuscarinic agents, 66–68
  β agonists for, 5–11
  corticosteroids for, 90–91
  cromolyn sodium for, 50
Allergic angiitis and granulomatosis, cytotoxic drugs for, 145
Allergic bronchopulmonary aspergillosis (ABPA), corticosteroids for, 91
Allergic rhinitis
  chronic corticosteroids for, 93–94
  cromolyn sodium for, 51
Almitrine as respiratory stimulant, 203–205
Alopecia from cyclophosphamide, 154
Alveolar hemorrhage, cytotoxic drugs for, 149–150
Ambroxol as expectorant, 179

Ammonium chloride as expectorant, 177
Anesthetics, local, as antitussives, 169–170
Angiitis and granulomatosis, cytotoxic drugs for, 145
Angio-immunoblastic lymphadenopathy, cytotoxic drugs for, 150
Angiotensin-converting enzyme inhibitors as pulmonary vasodilators, 219t, 221
Anticholinergic, antimuscarinic drugs
　adverse effects of, 71–72
　agents used concomitantly with, 72–73
　for bronchoconstriction, 66–68
　for bronchorrhea, 68–69
　contraindications to, 69
　dosage of, 70–71
　indications for, 66–69
　interactions of, with other drugs, 72–73
　mechanism of action of, 62–66
Anticonvulsants, corticosteroid action and, 128–129
Antigens, exposure to, cromolyn sodium for, 52
Antimuscarinic drugs; see also Anticholinergic, antimuscarinic drugs
　for bronchoconstriction, 66–68
　mechanism of action of, 66
Antioxidants, 229–231
Antitussive(s), 168–175
　caramiphen as, 174
　carbetapentane as, 174
　centrally acting, 171–175
　codeine as, 172
　demulcents as, 170
　dextromethorphan as, 173
　diphenhydramine as, 174–175
　expectorants as, 171
　hydrocodone as, 173
　local anesthetics as, 169–170
　narcotics of 171–172
　nonnarcotic, 173–175
　noscapine as, 174
　peripherally acting, 169–171
Apnea, recurrent, theophylline for, 25–26

Arachidonic acid, glucocorticoid effects on, immunosuppressive/anti-inflammatory, 82–83
Arrhythmias, cardiac, from adrenoreceptor agonists, 15
Arterial oxygen tension (PaO$_2$), effects of adrenoreceptor agonists on, 15
Arthritis, rheumatoid
　cytotoxic drugs for, 147–148
　corticosteroids for, 96
Aspergillosis, allergic bronchopulmonary, corticosteroids for, 91
Aspiration, gastric, ARDS following, corticosteroids for, 109
Asthma
　anticholinergic, antimuscarinic agents for, 66–68
　β agonists for, 5–11
　chronic, theophylline for, 24–25
　corticosteroids for, 90–91
　cytotoxic drugs for, 151
　occupational, cromolyn sodium for, 50–51
　perennial, cromolyn sodium for, 50
　reflex-induced, cromolyn sodium as modulator of, 47–48
　seasonal, cromolyn sodium for, 52–53
Atropine sulfate, 61–73; see also Anticholinergic, antimuscarinic drugs
　for bronchorrhea, 68–69
　as prophylaxis against vaso-vagal reactions, 69
Avascular osteonoecrosis from corticosteroids, 116–117
Azathioprine; see also Cytotoxic drugs
　drug interactions with, 157
　mechanism of action of, 141–142
　side effects of, 155–156
　special considerations for, 152

β_2 agonists, 1–17
　routes of administration of, 11–14
　　aerosol, 12–14
　　oral, 12
　　parenteral, 12

Bacterial infections, susceptibility to, increased, from corticosteroids, 119
Behcet's syndrome, cytotoxic drugs for, 146
Benign lymphocytic angiitis and granulomatosis, cytotoxic drugs for, 145
Benzonatate as antitussive, 170
Blood vessels, glucocorticoid effects on, immunosuppressive/anti-inflammatory, 82
Bone marrow depression
 from azathioprine, 155
 from chlorambucil, 156
 from cyclophosphamide, 152-153
Bronhexine as expectorant, 179
Bronchial smooth muscle, pharmacology of, 2-5
Bronchiolitis obliterans, corticosteroids for, 107-108
Bronchocentric granulomatosis, corticosteroids for, 101
Bronchoconstriction
 aminophylline for, 24-25
 anticholinergic, antimuscarinic drugs for, 66-68
 β agonists for, 5-13
 corticosteroids for, 90-91
Bronchodilator(s)
 anticholinergic, antimuscarinic drugs as, 61-73; see also Anticholinergic, antimuscarinic drugs
 catecholamine, biochemical characteristics of, 3-5
 sympathomimetic, 1-17
 theophylline as, 21-38
Bronchopulmonary aspergillosis, allergic, corticosteroids for, 91
Bronchorrhea, anticholinergic, antimuscarinic drugs for, 68-69
Bronchospasm, exercise-induced
 β agonists for, 1, 14
 cromolyn sodium for, 50, 52

Caffeine for recurrent apnea, 25-26
Calcium blocking agents as pulmonary vasodilators, 219t, 220-221
Calcium channel blockers in lung disease, 227-228
Calcium metabolism disturbances of, from corticosteroids, 121
Captopril as pulmonary vasodilator, 219t, 221
Caramiphen as antitussive, 174
Carbetapentane as antitussive, 174
Carbocysteine as mucolytic, 183
Carbonic anhydrase inhibitors as respiratory stimulants, 193-195
Carbuterol as bronchodilator, 7t, 11
Cardiac arrhythmias from adrenoreceptor agonists, 15
Cardiovascular effects of adrenoreceptor agonists, 15
Cataracts, subcapsular, posterior, from corticosteroids, 117
Catecholamine bronchodilators, biochemical characteristics of 3-5
Cellular elements, glucocorticoid effects on, immunosuppressive and anti-inflammatory, 80-82
Cellular metabolism, effects of corticosteroids on, 79-80
Charcoal, activated, for theophylline toxicity, 35-36
Chlorambucil; see also Cytotoxic drugs
 mechanism of action of, 142
 side effects of, 156-157
 special considerations for, 152
Chronic eosinophilic pneumonia, corticosteroids for, 103
Chronic obstructive pulmonary disease (COPD)
 β agonists for, 5-13
 corticosteroids for, 92-93
 theophylline for, 26-27
Churg-Strauss syndrome, cytotoxic drugs for, 145
Codeine as antitussive, 172
Connective tissue disorders, cytotoxic drugs for, 147-149

Corticosteroid(s), 77-129; see also
    Glucocorticoids;
    Mineralocorticoids
  for adult respiratory distress syndrome,
    108-109
  for allergic bronchopulmonary
    aspergillosis, 91
  alternate day therapy with, 86-97
  anti-inflammatory effects of, 80-83
  for asthma, 90-91
  avascular osteonecrosis from, 116-117
  for bronchiolitis obliterans, 107-108
  for bronchocentric granulomatosis,
    101
  for chronic allergic rhinitis, 93-94
  for chronic eosinophilic pneumonia,
    103
  for chronic obstructive pulmonary
    disease, 92-93
  clinical pharmacology of, 83-86
  clinical properties of, 85t
  for connective tissue diseases, 94-98
  contraindications to, 112-113
  Cushing's syndrome from, 113
  for dermatomyositis, 97-98
  for drug-induced hypersensitivity
    pneumonitis, 102
  drug interactions of, 126-129
  effects of, on adrenergic receptors, 83
  effects of, on cellular metabolism,
    79-80
  for eosinophilic granuloma of lung,
    107
  for fat embolism syndrome, 109
  gastrointestinal disorders from,
    113-114
  for Goodpasture's syndrome, 102
  for hypersensitivity pneumonitis,
    101-102
  for hypersensitivity vasculitides,
    100-101
  for idiopathic pulmonary fibrosis,
    105-107
  immunosuppressive effects of, 80-83
  indications for, 90-112
  for inhalation injury, 111
  for interstitial lung diseases, 103-108
  for Loeffler's syndrome, 102-103
  for lymphomatoid granulomatosis, 100
  mechanisms of action of, 78-83
  method of administration of, 86
  for mixed connective tissue disease, 98
  myopathy from, 114-115
  ocular side effects of, 117-118
  osteoporosis from, 115-116
  physiologic half of, 84
  plasma half-life of, 84, 85t
  for polymyositis, 97-98
  preparations of, 85t, 86
  for progressive systemic sclerosis,
    96-97
  for radiation pneumonitis, 111-112
  for rheumatoid arthritis, 96
  for sarcoidosis, 103-105
  side effects of, 113-126
    from aerosols, 124
    from excessive and prolonged
      therapy, 113-124
    gastrointestinal, 113-114
    growth-related, 122
    from inappropriately rapid
      withdrawal, 125-126
    infectious, 119-120
    metabolic, 120-121
    musculoskeletal, 114-117
    ocular, 117-118
    psychiatric, 118
    renal, 120-121
    reproductive, 123-124
  for Sjogren's syndrome, 97
  for smoke inhalation, 111
  for systemic lupus erythematosus,
    94-96
  for thermal injury of lungs, 111
  for tuberculosis, 110
  for tuberculous meningitis, 110
  for tuberculous pericarditis, 110
  for tuberculous peritonitis, 110-111
  for vasculitic syndromes, 99-101
  for Wegener's granulomatosis, 99-100
  withdrawal from, 88-90
Corticosteroid aerosol, 87-88
  side effects of, 124
Cough
  chronic, cromolyn sodium for, 50
  complications of, 168t

Index

disorders causing, 166t, 167t
management of
 antitussives in, 168–175; see also Antitussive(s)
 detergents in, 180
 drug therapy in, 165–185
 expectorants in, 175–179; see also Expectorant(s)
 fluids in, 179–180
 indications for, 167–168
 wetting agents in, 180
mechanisms of, 165–167
mucolytic therapy for, 180–185; see also Mucolytic therapy for cough
Cromolyn sodium, 44–54
 agents used concomitantly with, 54
 contraindications to, 53
 dosage of
  for long-term therapy, 51–52
  for short-term therapy, 53
 forms of, 49t
 indications for, 48–53
  for long-term therapy, 50–51
  for short-term therapy, 52–53
 interactions of, with other drugs, 54
 as mast cell stabilizer mode of action of, 46–47
 mode of action of, 46–48
 as modulator of reflex-induced asthma, 47–48
 side effects of, 53
Cushing's syndrome, iatrogenic, from corticosteroids, 113
Cutaneous disturbances from corticosteroids, 120
Cyclophosphamide; see also Cytotoxic drugs
 drug interactions with, 157
 mechanism of action of, 140–141
 for rheumatoid arthritis, 147–148
 side effects of, 152–154
 special considerations for, 151
 for Wegener's granulomatosis, 142–144
Cytotoxic drugs
 for alveolar hemorrhage, 149–150
 for angio-immunoblastic lymphadenopathy, 150

 for asthma, 151
 for Behcet's syndrome, 146
 for benign lymphocytic angiitis and granulomatosis, 145
 for Churg-Strauss syndrome, 145
 for connective tissue disorders, 147–149
 drug interactions with, 157
 indications for, 142–151
 for interstitial lung disease, 146–147
 for lymphomatoid granulomatosis, 144–145
 mechanism of action of, 140–142
 for mixed connective tissue disease, 149
 for neurological disease, 150
 for nonneoplastic disorders of respiratory system, 139–157
 for polyarteritis nodosa, 146
 for polymyositis/dermatomyositis, 148
 for progressive systemic sclerosis, 148
 for relapsing polychondritis, 151
 rheumatoid pulmonary vasculitis, 146
 for sarcoidosis, 149
 side effects of, 152–157
 for systemic lupus erythematosis, 148
 for vasculitides, 142–146
 for Wegener's granulomatosis, 142–144

Demulcents as antitussives, 170
Deoxyribonuclease as mucolytic, 184–185
Dermatomyositis
 corticosteroids for, 97–98
 cytotoxic drugs for, 148
Detergents in cough management, 180
Dextromethorphan as antitussive, 173
Diabetes mellitus from corticosteroids, 122–123
Dialysis, gastrointestinal, for theophylline toxicity, 35–36
Diazoxide as pulmonary vasodilator, 217, 218t
Diphenylhydantoin, corticosteroid action and, 128–129
Diphenhydramine ad antitussive, 174–175

Doxapram as respiratory stimulant, 199–201
Drugs, hypersensitivity pneumonitis induced by, corticosteroids for, 102

Edema from corticosteroids, 121
Enzymes as mucolytics, 184–185
Eosinophilic granuloma of lung, corticosteroids for, 107
Ephedrine
 as bronchodilator, 5, 6t, 8
 corticosteroid action and, 129
Epinephrine
 as bronchodilator, 6t, 8
 isolation of, 1
Exercise-induced bronchospasm, cromolyn sodium for, 50, 52
Expectorant(s), 175–179
 ambroxol as, 179
 as antitussives, 171
 bromhexine as, 179
 iodides as, 177–178
 vagally mediated, 176–177

Fat embolism syndrome, corticosteroids for, 109
Fenoterol as bronchodilator, 7t, 10
Fertility, corticosteroids and, 123
Fibrosis, pulmonary
 idiopathic
  corticosteroids for, 105–107
  cytotoxic drugs for, 146–147
 interstitial, from chlorambucil, 156
Fluids in cough management, 179–180
Food, theophylline absorption and, 37
Freon propellants in bronchodilator inhalers, adverse effects of, 16–17
Fungal infections, susceptibility to, increased, from corticosteroids, 119–120

Gas exchange, effects of adrenoreceptor agonists on, 15
Gastric aspiration, ARDS following, corticosteroids for, 109

Gastrointestinal dialysis for theophylline toxicity, 35–36
Gastrointestinal disorders
 from azathioprine, 155
 from chlorambucil, 156
 from corticosteroids, 113–114
Gastrointestinal hemorrhage from corticosteroids, 113–114
Glucocorticoids, 78; see also Corticosteroids
 anti-inflammatory effects of
  on blood vessels, 82
  on cellular elements, 80–82
  on lipid mediators, 82–83
 effects of, on adrenergic receptors, 83
 immunosuppressive effects of
  on blood vessels, 82
  on cellular elements, 80–82
  on lipid mediators, 82–83
Gonadal dysfunction from cyclophosphamide, 154
Goodpasture's syndrome
 corticosteroids for, 102
 cytotoxic drugs for, 149
Granuloma of lung eosinophilic, corticosteroids for, 107
Granulomatosis
 bronchocentric, corticosteroids for, 101
 lymphomatoid
  corticosteroids for, 100
  cytotoxic drugs for, 144–145
 Wegener's
  corticosteroids for, 99–100
  cytotoxic drugs for, 142–144
Growth retardation from corticosteroids, 122
Guaifenesin as expectorant, 176–177

Hair, loss of, from cyclophosphamide, 154
Hemorrhage
 alveolar, cytotoxic drugs for, 149–150
 gastrointestinal, from corticosteroids, 113–114

Index

Hemosiderosis, pulmonary, idiopathic, cytotoxic drugs for, 149–150
Hexoprenaline as bronchodilator, 7t, 9
Hydralazine as pulmonary vasodilator, 217, 218t
Hydrocodone as antitussive, 173
Hyperreactive airways, cromolyn sodium for, 50
Hypersensitivity pneumonitis, corticosteroids for, 101–102
Hypersensitivity vasculitides, corticosteroids for, 100–101
Hypertension
  intracranial, from corticosteroids, 118–119
  pulmonary, 213–222; see also Pulmonary hypertension
Hypokalemia from corticosteroids, 121
Hypothalamo-pituitary-adrenal (HPA) suppression from rapid corticosteroid withdrawal, 125–126

Idiopathic pulmonary fibrosis (IPF)
  corticosteroids for, 105–107
  cytotoxic drugs for, 146–147
Idiopathic pulmonary hemosiderosis (IPA), cytotoxic drugs for, 149–150
Immunosuppression from cyclophosphamide, 152–153
Immunotherapy, cromolyn sodium during, 51
Infection(s)
  from azathioprine, 155
  from chlorambucil, 156
  susceptibility to, increased, from corticosteroids, 119–120
Inhalation injury, corticosteroids for, 111
Interstitial lung diseases
  corticosteroids for, 103–108
  cytotoxic drugs for, 146–147
Interstitial pneumonitis
  lymphocytic, cytotoxic drugs for, 147
  plasma cell, cytotoxic drugs for, 147
Interstitial pulmonary fibrosis from chlorambucil, 156

Intracranial hypertension from corticosteroids, 118–119
Intraocular pressure, increased, from corticosteroids, 117–118
Iodides as expectorants, 177–178
Ipratropium bromide, 61–73; see also Anticholinergic, antimuscarinic drugs
Irritant(s), exposure to, cromolyn sodium for, 52
Isoetharine as bronchodilator, 7t, 9
Isoproterenol
  as bronchodilator, 6–7t, 8–9
  as pulmonary vasodilator, 216, 218t

Junctional transmission of neural impulse, atropine action and, 62–64

Ketotifen as mast cell stabilizer, 54–55
Kidneys, disorders of, from corticosteroids, 120–121

Lidocaine as antitussive, 169–170
Lipid mediators, glucocorticoid effects on, immunosuppressive/anti-inflammatory, 82–83
Lithium, concentrations of, theophylline therapy and, 36
Liver metabolism, corticosteroids and, 83–84
Lodoxamide as mast cell stabilizer, 55
Loeffler's syndrome, corticosteroids for, 102–103
Lung(s)
  disease of
    from azathioprine, 155–156
    chronic obstructive
      corticosteroids for, 92–93
      theophylline for, 26–27
    interstitial
      corticosteroids for, 103–108
      cytotoxic drugs for, 146–147
    eosinophilic granuloma of, corticosteroids for, 107

Lupus erythematosus, systemic
  corticosteroids for, 94–96
  cytotoxic drugs for, 148
Lymphadenopathy,
    angio-immunoblastic,
    cytotoxic drugs for, 150
Lymphocytes, glucocorticoid effects on,
    immunosuppressive/anti-
    inflammatory, 80–81
Lyphocytic interstitial pneumonitis,
    cytotoxic drugs for, 147
Lymphomatoid granulomatosis
  corticosteroids for, 100
  cytotoxic drugs for, 144–145

Macrolide antibodies, corticosteroid
    action and, 127–128
Malignancy
  from chlorambucil, 156
  from cyclophosphamide, 153–154
Marrow depression
  from azathioprine, 155
  from chlorambucil, 156
  from cyclophosphamide, 152–153
Mast cell(s)
  definition of, 43
  degranulation of, mediators released
    by, 43–44
  function of, 43
  stabilizers of, 43–56
    cromolyn sodium as, 43–56; see
      also Cromolyn sodium
    ketotifen as, 54–55
    lodoxamide as, 55
    nedocromil sodium as, 55
    sudexanox as, 56
    WY-41195 as, 56
    zaprinast as, 56
Meningitis, tuberculous, corticosteroids
    for, 110
Metabolism
  cellular, effects of corticosteroids on,
    79–80
  disturbances of, from corticosteroids,
    120–121
  liver, corticosteroids and, 83–84

Metabolites, effects of adrenoreceptor
    agonists on, 15–16
Metaproterenol as bronchodilator, 7*t*,
    9–10
Miliary tuberculosis, corticosteroids for,
    110
Mineralocorticoids, 78; *see also*
    Corticosteroids
Mixed connective tissue disease
    (MCTD)
  corticosteroids for, 98
  cytotoxic drugs for, 149
Monocyte-macrophage system,
    glucocorticoid effects on,
    immunosuppressive/anti-
    inflammatory, 81
Mucolytic therapy for cough, 180–185
  acetylcysteine in, 181–183
  carbocysteine in, 183
  enzymes in, 184–185
  sodium 2-mercaptoethane sulphonate
    in, 184
Muscles, smooth, bronchial,
    pharmacology of, 2–5
Myopathy from corticosteroids, 114–115

Naloxone as respiratory stimulant,
    201–203
Narcotics as antitussives, 171–172
Nebulizer in β_2 agonist administration,
    13
Necrosis, avascular, from
    corticosteroids, 116–117
Nedocromil sodium as mast cell
    stabilizer, 55
Nervous system, parasympathetic,
    anticholinergic drug action
    and, 62, *63*
Neural impulse, junctional transmission
    of, atropine action and, 62–64
Neurological disease, cytotoxic drugs
    for, 150
Neutrophils, glucocorticoid effects on,
    immunosuppressive/anti-
    inflammatory, 81

Index

Nifedipine as pulmonary vasodilator, 219*t*, 220–221
Nitroglycerine as pulmonary vasodilator, 219*t*, 220
Nitroprusside as pulmonary vasodilator, 219*t*, 220
Noscapine as antitussive, 174

Occupational asthma, cromolyn sodium for, 50–51
Oral administration of β_2 agonists, 12
Osteonecrosis, avascular, from corticosteroids, 116–117
Osteoporosis from corticosteroids, 115–116
Oxidant injury to lungs, 229–231
Oxygen as respiratory stimulant, 197–199

Pancreatitis, acute, from corticosteroids, 114
Parasitic infections, susceptibility to, increased, from corticosteroids, 120
Parasympathetic nervous system, anticholinergic drug action and, 62, *63*
Parenteral administration of β_2 agonists, 12
Peptic ulcer from corticosteroids, 113–114
Pericarditis, tuberculous, corticosteroids for, 110
Peritonitis, tuberculous, corticosteroids for, 110–111
Pharmacology
  of bronchial smooth muscle, 2–5
  clinical, of corticosteroids, 83–86
Phenobarbital, corticosteroid action and, 128–129
Phentolamine as pulmonary vasodilator, 216–217, 218*t*
Plasma cell interstitial pneumonitis, cytotoxic drugs for, 147

Pneumonia, eosinophilic, chronic, corticosteroids for, 103
Pneumonitis
  from cyclophosphamide, 154
  hypersensitivity, corticosteroids for, 101–102
  interstitial
    lymphocytic, cytotoxic drugs for, 147
    plasma cell, cytotoxic drugs for, 147
  radiation, corticosteroids for, 111–112
Polyarteritis nodosa, cytotoxic drugs for, 146
Polychondritis, relapsing, cytotoxic drugs for, 151
Polymyositis
  corticosteroids for, 97–98
  cytotoxic drugs for, 148
Potassium, loss of, from corticosteroids, 121
Prazosin as pulmonary vasodilator, 217, 218*t*
Pregnancy, corticosteroids in, 123–124
Progesterone as respiratory stimulant, 191–193
Progressive systemic sclerosis (PSS)
  corticosteroids for, 96–97
  cytotoxic drugs for, 148
Prostaglandins as pulmonary vasodilators, 219*t*, 221
Proteases as mucolytics, 184
Proteinase inhibitors for lung disease, 231–233
Protriptyline as respiratory stimulant, 195–197
Pseudotumor cerebri from corticosteroids, 118–119
Psychiatric disturbances from corticosteroids, 118
Pulmonary disease
  from azathioprine, 155–156
  chronic obstructive
    corticosteroids for, 92–93
    theophylline for, 26–27
  interstitial
    corticosteroids for, 103–108
    cytotoxic drugs for, 146–147

Pulmonary fibrosis
  idiopathic
    corticosteroids for, 105–107
    cytotoxic drugs for, 146–147
  interstitial, from chlorambucil, 156
Pulmonary hemosiderosis, idiopathic,
    cytotoxic drugs for, 149–150
Pulmonary hypertension, 213–222
  causes of, 214t
  physiology of, 213–214
  therapy for, 214–216; see also
    Vasodilator(s), pulmonary
Pulmonary vasodilators, 213–222; see
    also Vasodilator(s),
    pulmonary

Radiation pneumonitis, corticosteroids
    for, 111–112
Relapsing polychondritis, cytotoxic
    drugs for, 151
Renal disturbances from corticosteroids,
    120–121
Reproductive system, corticosteroid side
    effects involving, 123–124
Respiratory distress, acute, theophylline
    for, 23–24
Respiratory stimulant(s), 191–207
  almitrine as, 203–205
  carbonic anhydrase inhibitor as,
    193–195
  doxapram as, 199–201
  naloxone as, 201–203
  oxygen as, 197–199
  progesterone as, 191–193
  protriptyline as, 195–197
  theophylline as, 205–207
Rheumatoid arthritis, corticosteroids for,
    96
Rheumatoid disease, cytotoxic drugs for,
    147–148
Rheumatoid pulmonary vasculitis,
    cytotoxic drugs for, 146
Rhinitis, allergic
  chronic, corticosteroids for, 93–94
  cromolyn sodium for, 51
Rifampin, corticosteroid action and, 128
Rimeterol as bronchodilator, 7t, 9

Salbutamol as bronchodilator, 7t, 10–11
Sarcoidosis
  corticosteroids for, 103–105
  cytotoxic drugs for, 149
Scleroderma
  corticosteroids for, 96–97
  cytotoxic drugs for, 148
Sclerosis, systemic, progressive
  corticosteroids for, 96–97
  cytotoxic drugs for, 148
Seasonal asthma, cromolyn sodium for,
    52–53
Seizures from theophylline therapy,
    34–35
Sepsis, ARDS following, corticosteroids
    for, 108–109
Sjogren's syndrome, corticosteroids for,
    97
Skin disorders from corticosteroids, 120
Smoke inhalation, lung injury from,
    corticosteroids from, 111
Smooth muscle, bronchial,
    pharmacology of, 2–5
Sodium 2-mercaptoethane sulphonate as
    mucolytic, 184
Status asthmaticus
  β agonists for, 13
  corticosteroids for, 90
  Theophylline for, 23–24
Stimulant(s), respiratory, 191–207; see
    also Respiratory stimulant(s)
Sudexanox as mast cell stabilizer, 56
Surfactant replacements, 229
Sympathomimetic agents corticosteroid
    action and, 129
Sympathomimetic bronchodilators, 1–17
Systemic lupus erythematosus (SLE)
  corticosteroids for, 94–96
  cytotoxic drugs for, 148

Terbutaline as bronchodilator, 7t, 10
Terpin hydrate as expectorant, 177
Theophylline, 21–38
  for acute respiratory distress, 23–24
  adverse effects of, 34–36
  for chronic asthma, 24–25

Index

for chronic obstructive pulmonary
disease, 26–27
concentrations of, dosage adjustments
based on, 32–34
concomitant agents for, choice of,
36–37
dosage regimen for, 27–28
indications for, 23
interactions of, with other drugs,
36–37
mechanisms of action of, 22–23
product formulation for, 28–30
for recurrent apnea, 25–26
as respiratory stimulant, 205–207
sustained-release formulations of, 30
therapeutic drug monitoring for, 31–34
Thermal injury to lungs, corticosteroids
for, 111
Tolerance to adrenoreceptor agonists,
development of, 16
Troleandomycin (TAO), corticosteroid
action and, 127–128
Tuberculosis
corticosteroids for, 110
reactivation of, by corticosteroids, 119
Tuberculous meningitis, corticosteroids
for, 110
Tuberculous pericarditis, corticosteroids
for, 110
Tuberculous peritonitis, corticosteroids
for, 110–111

Ulcer, peptic, drom corticosteroids,
113–114
Urinary tract abnormalities from
cyclophosphamide, 153

Vasculitic syndromes, corticosteroids
for, 99–101

Vasculitides
cytotoxic drugs for, 142–146
hypersensitivity, corticosteroids for,
100-101
Vasculitis, pulmonary, rheumatoid,
cytotoxic drugs for, 146
Vaso-vagal reactions, prophylaxis
against, atropine sulfate as,
69
Vasodilator(s), pulmonary, 213–222
α-adrenergic antagonists as, 216–217,
218t
β-adrenergic agonists as, 216, 218t
angiotensin-converting enzyme
inhibitors as, 219t, 221
calcium blocking agents as, 219t,
220–221
contraindications to, 222
direct, 217, 218–219t, 220–222
general principles of, 215–216
indications for, 221–222
prostaglandins as, 219t, 221
side effects of, 218–219t, 222
Verapamil as pulmonary vasodilator,
219t, 220–221
Viral infections, susceptibility to,
increased, from
corticosteroids, 120

Wegener's granulomatosis
corticosteroids for, 99–100
cytotoxic drugs for, 142–144
Wetting agents in cough management,
180
Withdrawal, corticosteroid, 88–90
rapid, side effects of, 125–126
WY-41195 as mast cell stabilizer, 56

Zaprinast as mast cell stabilizer, 56